T0375201

Rights Come to Mind

Through the sobering story of Maggie Worthen and her mother Nancy, this book tells of one family's struggle with severe brain injury and how developments in neuroscience call for a reconsideration of what society owes patients at the edge of consciousness. Drawing on more than fifty in-depth family interviews, the history of severe brain injury from Quinlan to Schiavo, and his participation in landmark clinical trials such as the first use of deep brain stimulation in the minimally conscious state, Joseph J. Fins captures the paradox of medical and societal neglect even as advances in neuroscience suggest new ways to mend the broken brain. Responding to the dire care provided to these marginalized patients, after heroically being saved, Fins places society's obligations to patients with severe injury within the historical legacy of the civil and disability rights movements, offering a stirring synthesis of public policy and physician advocacy.

JOSEPH J. FINS, M.D., M.A.C.P., is the E. William Davis Jr., M.D., Professor of Medical Ethics and Chief of the Division of Medical Ethics at Weill Cornell Medical College where he also serves as Professor of Medicine, Professor of Health Care Policy and Research, and Professor of Medicine in Psychiatry. He is the founding chair of the Ethics Committee of New York–Presbyterian Weill Cornell Medical Center where he is an attending physician and Director of Medical Ethics. Dr. Fins co-directs the Consortium for the Advanced Study of Brain Injury and is an adjunct faculty member and senior attending physician at Rockefeller University and Rockefeller University Hospital. The author of more than 250 publications, Fins is a co-author of the landmark 2007 *Nature* paper describing the first use of deep brain stimulation in the minimally conscious state. He is an elected Member of the Institute of Medicine of the National Academy of Sciences, a Fellow of the American Academy of Arts and Sciences, and an *Academico de Honor* of the Royal National Academy of Medicine of Spain.

Rights Come to Mind

Brain Injury, Ethics, and the Struggle for Consciousness

JOSEPH J. FINS
Weill Cornell Medical College
Cornell University

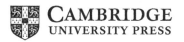

CAMBRIDGE
UNIVERSITY PRESS

CAMBRIDGE
UNIVERSITY PRESS

University Printing House, Cambridge CB2 8BS, United Kingdom

One Liberty Plaza, 20th Floor, New York, NY 10006, USA

477 Williamstown Road, Port Melbourne, VIC 3207, Australia

4843/24, 2nd Floor, Ansari Road, Daryaganj, Delhi - 110002, India

79 Anson Road, #06-04/06, Singapore 079906

Cambridge University Press is part of the University of Cambridge.

It furthers the University's mission by disseminating knowledge in the pursuit of
education, learning and research at the highest international levels of excellence.

www.cambridge.org
Information on this title: www.cambridge.org/9780521887502

© Joseph J. Fins 2015

First published 2015
Reprinted 2016

A catalogue record for this publication is available from the British Library

Library of Congress Cataloging in Publication data
Fins, Joseph, author.
Rights come to mind : brain injury, ethics, and the struggle for
consciousness / Joseph J. Fins.
      p. ; cm.
Brain injury, ethics, and the struggle for consciousness
Includes bibliographical references and index.
ISBN 978-0-521-88750-2 (hardback) – ISBN 978-0-521-71537-9 (pbk.)
I. Title. II. Title: Brain injury, ethics, and the struggle for consciousness.
[DNLM: 1. Brain Injury, Chronic–psychology. 2. Brain Injury, Chronic–rehabilitation.
3. Patient Rights–ethics. 4. Unconsciousness–psychology. WL 354]
RC451.4.B73
617.4′81044–dc23   2015003339

ISBN 978-0-521-88750-2 Hardback
ISBN 978-0-521-71537-9 Paperback

To the Memory of Drs. John L. Battenfeld, Martin Gardy, and Fred Plum,
who left legacies;
and Robin Heller Moss and Jerold B. Katz, who sustain our scholarship.
For Ruth and Hank Fins, who made everything possible,
and
Amy Ehrlich and Harrison Ehrlich Fins, who make it all worthwhile.

"But it's not about pity, it's about courage.... Here's a real person and here's what happened to her."

Nancy Worthen

Contents

Unless otherwise noted with an asterisk*, permission to use family names and other identifiable information has been given through a formal consent process for narrative interviews approved by the Weill Cornell Medical College Institutional Review Board.

* Names in this book, first identified by an asterisk, are not the individual's real name but pseudonyms.

Acknowledgments

A book like this could not have been written without the families that so generously shared their stories. I hope their confidence in me has resulted in a book that is worthy of their courage and commitment.

I am also indebted to my colleagues who have taught me so much about brain injury and disorders of consciousness. No one could ask for a better teacher or colleague than Niko Schiff who graciously agreed to be interviewed about his research and also generously read and critiqued multiple versions of the manuscript. I also owe a big debt to Joe Giacino, now at Spaulding Harvard Rehabilitation Hospital, for our many years of collaboration and for his willingness to talk with me about the origins of the minimally conscious state and to share documentary evidence about what emerged as the Aspen Criteria.

I am especially grateful to the Robert Wood Johnson Foundation for an Investigator Award in Health Policy Research and the leadership of David Mechanic who has inspired generations of scholars. I am also incredibly indebted to Robin Moss and the Buster Foundation for their early and ongoing support of my scholarship. I am also deeply appreciative of Jerrold B. Katz, the Katz Foundation, and the entire Katz family for their generous support of both Dr. Schiff and myself.

Guy McKhann and Carolyn Asbury of the Charles A. Dana Foundation deserve special mention for underwriting this line of research dating back to the pioneering work of Fred Plum. I am honored to be part of this legacy. I am also most appreciative of the generosity of my friends, Eva and John Usdan.

Institutionally we are indebted to Weill Cornell Medical College and Rockefeller University for their willingness to host the Consortium for the Advanced Study of Brain Injury that Dr. Schiff and I co-direct. We are grateful to the staff of both institutions who make it possible for us to do our research and are especially grateful for the Weill Cornell leadership of Tony Gotto and Laurie Glimcher and Barry Coller at Rockefeller. We have benefited from their strategic advice and support.

A special word of thanks goes to Jennifer Hersh who did a spectacular job as a research coordinator conducting interviews and always ensuring that our families were treated with kindness and compassion when they came to New York. Jen transcribed and organized the interviews and quickly became an essential source of knowledge and insight into the families' experiences. Barbara Pohl joined Jennifer and brought a keen editorial eye to the project.

I am personally grateful to my three chairmen: Andy Schafer, Al Mushlin, and Jack Barchas, each of whom has steadfastly defended the importance of scholarship in academic medicine and been incredibly supportive. In the Division of Medical Ethics, I have relied on the skill and professionalism of Cathy Acres, Ellen Meltzer, Inma de Melo Martin, Kim Overby, and Pablo Rodriguez del Pozo who have made it possible for me to focus on this volume with the confidence that our divisional activities would continue to thrive without interruption.

The dedication of my (present and past) neuroscience and neuroethics colleagues at Weill Cornell is inspiring and I am honored to have worked with and learned much from them. My thanks go out to Jon Victor, Mary Conte, Keith Purpura, Andy Goldfine, Peter Forgacs, Henning Voss, Shawniqua Williams, Lexi Suppes, Maria Master, Diana Rodriguez Moreno, Sudin Shah, Erik Kobylarz, Peter Forgacs, Esteban Fridman, and Jon Bardin. Their deep regard for our patients and their generosity to each other is their secret ingredient to individual and collective success.

Beyond Cornell the many others who have shared their work and insights with me constitute a *Who's Who of Neuroscience*. They include Jerry Posner, Kathy Foley, Donald Pfaff, Jim Bernat, Steven Laureys, Doug Katz, Jaimie Henderson, Andre Machado, Jerry Vitek, Ken Baker, John Whyte, Ross Zafonte, Kathy Kalmar, C. Rees Cosgrove, Bart Nuttin, Alim Benabid, Luis Sanjuanbenito, Cindy Kubu, Carolyn McCagg, Emery Brown, David Menon, Richard Payne, Joseph Pancrazio, Kristi Kirschner, Joy Hirsch, Warren Grill, John Pickard, Jack Gallant, Adrian Owen, Martin Monti, Nathan Zasler, Caroline Schnakers, and the late Martin Coleman, Ron Cranford, Bryan Jennett, and Fred Plum.

In the sphere of medical ethics and neuroethics, I have benefited from countless colleagues who have graciously invited me to speak at their institutions or to collaborate on issues related to disorders of consciousness, deep brain stimulation, or neuroimaging. I am especially grateful to Judy Illes (now at the University of British Columbia) for co-convening a key meeting on neuroimaging and disorders of consciousness at Stanford in 2007 with support from the Greenwall Foundation. Judy has also provided countless opportunities for dialogue about this work, most notably in Vancouver with John Harris of the University of Manchester.

I am also appreciative of Thomas Schlaepfer of the *Europaische Akademie* and the University of Bonn Medical Faculty for his invitation to collaborate on a longitudinal project on the ethics of deep brain stimulation that included the opportunity to collaborate with Helen Mayberg and Reinhard Merkel and meet Matthis Synofzyk; Bill Winslade for his many valuable insights along the way and his generous invitation to present *The John P. McGovern Award Lecture in the Medical Humanities* at The Institute for the Medical Humanities, University of Texas Medical Branch, Galveston in 2010; Alan Weintraub of Denver's Craig Hospital for the invitation to speak at its 2012 Brain Injury Summit; Adela Cortina of the Universidad de Valencia for the chance to gain a cross-cultural perspective on brain injury during its 2012 meeting at the Facultad de Filosophia; and Walter Sinott-Armstrong and Ross McKinney of Duke University for the opportunity to present the 2013 Nancy Weaver Emerson Lecture through the Trent Center for Bioethics.

I am also grateful to Kip Ludwig of the National Institute of Neurological Diseases and Stroke for an opportunity to present at the 2012 Neural Interface Meeting in Salt Lake, the Brocher Foundation for the chance to attend a valuable conference on deep brain stimulation in Geneva, and Marianne Lovstad of the Sunnas Rehabilitation Hospital and the University of Oslo for allowing me to present my work at a meeting on disorders of consciousness.

I have also benefited from the wisdom of Dan Callahan, Al Jonsen, Frank Miller, Martha Farah, Diego Gracia Guillén, John Banja, Mark Siegler, Art Caplan, Paul Wolpe, Hilde Lindemann, Debjani Mukherjee, Marilyn Martone, Eric Racine, David Magnus, Beatrix Hoffman, Rachel Grob, Chuck Bosk, Jean Berube, George Zitany, Johnathan Moreno, John Paris, Jim Nelson, Myra Christopher, Walter Glannon, Paul Ford, Cindy Kubu, Bob Klitzman, Steve Hyman, Susan Wolf, Emily Bell, Jason Karlawish, Lainie Ross, Ben Rich, Franscoise Baylis, Jeffrey Baker, Carla Keirns, Jane Polin, Debra Matthews, Ruth Fischbach, Linda Gerber, Hunter Peckham, Larry Casalino, Art Derse, Jorge Ferrer, Mark Schlesinger, Rosemary Stevens, Rod Nichols, Arleen Salles, Bill Andereck, Ruth Faden, Jeremy Sugarman, Stuart G. Finder, Bob Woodruff, Stephen Xenakis, and Ken Goodman. And, of course, Amy Ehrlich, Hank Fins, and Robin Fins. Each has been a source of inspiration and astute analysis.

I owe a special debt to several legal colleagues who helped me develop the disability and civil rights arguments. I am grateful to Michael Freeman for the chance to present an early version of this part of the work at Bentham House, University College London Faculty of Laws in 2009; Hank Greely of Stanford for his ever-wise legal counsel; and Hal Edgar and Abbe Gluck for invitations to present at Columbia Law School as well as Steve Latham, Madeleine Schachter, Nancy Dubler, Beth Roxland, Mary Beth Morrissey, Stephen Morse, and Kathleen Burke. Professor Gluck and Harriet Raab at Rockefeller University gave me pivotal advice when they suggested that I meet with Chai Feldblum at the U.S. Equal Opportunity Commission to discuss the Americans with Disabilities Act. The insights of Professor Feldblum and her superb colleagues was a key turning point in my thinking.

I also want to thank George Makari and Diane Richardson of the Oskar Diethelm History of Psychiatry Library at Weill Cornell Medical College for access to their collection on psychosurgery; Valerie Gillispie and Suzy Taraba of the Wesleyan University Archives for files on C. P. Snow's visit to campus; and Lisa Mix, archivist at the New York–Presbyterian Weill Cornell Medical Center Archives, and Susan Plum for access to the Fred Plum papers.

I have a special debt of gratitude to Professor Anne Greene, the director of the Wesleyan Writer's Conference. Her invitation to speak at the conference was kind and her ongoing and sustained interest in the writing of this book was more than generous. I stand in a long line of authors who deeply respect her opinion and ever will be grateful for her sound counsel and encouragement.

Madeliene Schachter has been a true friend and fine colleague, always generous and wise. Joel Kurtzberg of Cahill Gordon has provided indispensable legal advice and been a true advocate for this book and its content.

I am especially appreciative of Tomi Kushner, editor of the *Cambridge Quarterly of Healthcare Ethics*, for suggesting that I speak with Beatrice Rehl of Cambridge University Press when I was contemplating this book. It was good advice and ever since I have been the beneficiary of Beatrice's uncanny editorial skills and direction and her fine colleagues at Cambridge, Isabella Vitti, Elisabeth Traugott, and Christine Dunn. I hope Beatrice's insistence on excellence has been borne out here.

Fundamentally, this is a book about families and I want to thank mine for allowing me to write this book. Witnessing what other families have experienced makes me appreciate how precious even the most ordinary moments can be.

Introduction

I

By now the scene is familiar and the story predictable. An expectant family is in my office at Weill Cornell Medical College sharing the story about how a son or daughter, husband or wife, mother or father sustained a brain injury. They have come to Cornell to participate in scientific studies designed to understand how the brain recovers from disorders of consciousness, serious conditions like the vegetative and minimally conscious states. Their goals are modest. They want to know if their loved one is aware and if they will get better, be able to understand, speak, and love again.

When they arrive, most are worn out. They are like refugees, having been cast aside by an indifferent health care system that provided brilliant emergent care only to abandon them thereafter. Irrespective of differences in race, ethnicity, class, or state of origin, a stereotypic pattern of neglect emerges.

Although each case is unique, the overall story becomes rather predictable. Families face a pervasive nihilism with practitioners assuming a static notion of brain injury. Despite stunning scientific evidence to the contrary, the prevailing view in the clinic is that all brain injuries are immutable. From this perspective, it is preordained that the injured brain cannot recover and that the humane course is to pursue palliative care, to let nature take its course.

At the bedside, this translates into early – some might say premature – decisions to withhold or withdraw life-sustaining therapies, writing do-not-resuscitate orders or removing of ventilators, even before patients have had a chance to declare themselves. More worrisome have been reports of families urged to turn their loved ones into organ donors before their prognosis is clear.

Most families do choose a palliative course, knowing that even under the most optimistic of scenarios their loved ones will need ongoing medical care and years of rehabilitation. Theirs is a reasonable choice, and perhaps a logical one, appreciating the considerable challenges, when early optimism and the promise of recovery do not get translated into desired outcomes. For these families, death is preferable to survival and what some would describe as an even worse outcome, a diminished or extinguished ability to interact with others.

But the families we interviewed are put together differently. Although the advent of palliative care has its origins in patients' rights, the families we spoke to did not view such recommendations as enfranchising. To them, the palliative care option, often promoted forcefully, is a choice that they cannot sanction. Instead, the recommendation was often seen as overly prescriptive and an affront to their exercise of choice. These families can't seem to let go. It is not about religiosity but a different kind of devotion, a depth of obligation to their family member and a sense that the world would be intolerably incomplete without their loved one.

From afar, their choices may seem selfish, compelling others to endure a life that no one would choose for themselves. But that's the point. These families *didn't* choose the outcomes with which they must now contend. Like all families suddenly summoned to an emergency room or the waiting room outside an operative suite, they hoped and prayed that their family member would survive only to have their appeals answered – in part. But unlike the more fortunate, they have learned a cruel lesson. They have come to appreciate that choice in those circumstances is a charade.

Families might think they are directing care when they authorize a treatment or sign a consent, but outcomes are determined by the nature of the injury, when and where the injury occurred, the skill of the surgeon, and just plain luck.

No, the families we interviewed did not wish lives of cognitive and physical impairment for their loved ones, but once it became apparent that would be the outcome, they felt compelled to sustain the life that their loved one's had been dealt. That too was a choice out of their hands and really the only thing to do. Unless their loved one was in intractable pain, they were not going to acquiesce to those who urged that care be withheld or withdrawn. They would continue to care and to hope.

Given their desire for ongoing treatment, families find their goals completely out of sync with the chronic care system to which patients will be discharged. If patients survive their acute injuries, and their families withstand pressures to remove life support contrary to their wishes, a pattern of neglect emerges. Patients are often discharged prematurely while still unstable and then they find themselves in facilities that are unequipped to provide necessary care. Once in chronic care, families must wage war with bureaucrats and utilization reviewers to qualify for ongoing rehabilitation. Many simply struggle to obtain a credible diagnosis, importantly trying to determine if their loved one is conscious.

This book seeks to give voice to their struggles and to explain why the scientific study of brain injury, whose mysteries constitute a holy grail of science, has had so little impact on the lived experiences of patients who have a tenuous grip on consciousness. Brilliant science and rather indifferent care. It is a paradox worthy of a book, and one ripe for denial.

And therein lies the challenge of writing such a volume. This is difficult terrain: healthy people, generally in their prime, struck down by an injury that will threaten their lives and forever alter them and their relationships. The prospect of a brain injury is a scenario our conscious selves would prefer not to imagine. It is a problem space that can be disavowed when considered in the aggregate, a distant probability that can be avoided. It is much harder to ignore when it becomes personal.

So this book is a story about an individual, Margaret Worthen. Maggie was a senior at Smith College when she sustained a brain injury in 2006. Her story, as told by her mother Nancy, is one that can neither be denied nor forgotten. Like all the many narratives that comprise this book, Maggie's story, as Nancy reminds us, is about "... a real person and ... what happened to her."

Maggie's young life, full of promise, was interrupted and nearly severed, only to resume at the edge of known neuroscience. And here she is joined by nearly forty others whose families agreed to be interviewed. Their family narratives, comprising nearly ninety hours of interviews and 2,750 pages of transcripts, fill out a broader canvas that depicts a landscape of clinical neglect now challenged by scientific discovery.

That pioneering work, not yet influencing clinical practice, but increasingly gaining attention in the media and the wider scientific community, is also the subject of this book, which will consider its emergence and ultimate relevance to clinical practice. Although the history of medicine is lamentably marginalized, the intellectual history of disorders of consciousness is a tale that must be told, lest we misunderstand how so much scientific promise has been discounted in the clinic.

To tell this story, I return to Maggie's and draw upon the confluence of the scientific and historical: the progression a patient makes from acute injury to recovery tracks precisely with the historical advent of each of these brain states. So as Maggie makes the progression from coma into the vegetative state (VS) and on to the minimally conscious state (MCS), we will consider how these states were first described and how modern science is refining what we think we know.

Although the structure of the book follows the arc of Maggie's life after her injury, we will digress from her story to share other narratives as rich and textured as hers. Each is worthy of their own book, but in this effort they are cast in a supporting role. They are here to provide an additional detail or share a variation on a theme. In some cases these digressions can encompass a chapter or two, as in the case of pivotal cases or my discussion of the first effort to use deep brain stimulation (DBS) in the MCS. I hope that the reader finds these excursions useful and that they help to place Maggie's experience within the context of a broader canvass. By doing so, her tale becomes less an anecdotal account of one patient and more the representative trajectory of many other patients and families.

Maggie's medical history continues with a discussion of the origins of the vegetative state. Here I draw upon historic accounts of my late teacher, and later colleague, Dr. Fred Plum, co-originator of the persistent vegetative state (PVS) and the court-appointed neurologist in the Quinlan right-to-die case in 1976. Plum's seminal work, with the Scottish neurosurgeon Bryan Jennett on the vegetative state, first published in *The Lancet* in 1972, will be complemented by recounting the remarkable story of Terry Wallis and how the MCS emerged as a diagnostic category thirty years later.

Along the way, I will consider the role that neuroimaging has had on our growing understanding of the injured brain, most notably the disturbing, yet fascinating, finding that neuroimaging can reveal a discordance between what is observed on clinical examination with what is inferred from brain scans. Such discrepancies, when a scan seemingly refutes a diagnosis of unconsciousness, portend a reconfiguration of diagnostic categories and ethical norms for patient care.

My consideration of the neuroscience of disorders of consciousness will coalesce around my Cornell colleague, neurologist and neuroscientist Dr. Nicholas Schiff. Schiff has studied the capability of minimally conscious patients to process language and led the first studies using DBS in the MCS. That work culminated in a landmark 2007 *Nature* publication.

I was privileged to serve as a co-investigator on the DBS in MCS study, designing the ethical framework enabling that effort to continue. That study, its origins, ethical justification, and surgery, is told through first-person accounts from many of the investigators, and most notably, the subject's mother, Corinth Pecco. Up until now, Ms. Pecco had preferred to remain anonymous. This is the first and only account of her recollections of and response to the historic surgery performed on her son Greg.

DBS, along with new drug therapies and the use of neuroimaging, are discussed collectively as constituting a new era of neuroprosthetic communication through which patients will be enabled to communicate with the assistance of device, drug, or machine. This potential, and the science that is revealing the potential of the seemingly silent brain to speak when given help, is a story that is just being written. These developments will have profound implications for how we think about the utility (versus the futility) of intervening in the injured brain and consequently how we structure and finance ongoing rehabilitation and chronic care for patients, many of whom now only know neglect.

II

The potential is astounding, but so too are the barriers, notwithstanding progress made in the past decade. These threats transcend the real challenges posed by neuroscience. They speak to the place of science in society and the forces that can promote or retard the translation of new insights into clinical practice. One key barrier is health care financing and how we pay for rehabilitation. The paradox is striking: the promise of neuroscience and the challenge of reimbursement schema that truncates the potential for recovery.

Brains recover by biological standards, not reimbursement criteria. To impose the latter on the former is to fail to take account of time frames needed for recovery by the injured brain, which as a nonlinear system resists simple predictive models. Yet that is precisely what *medical necessity* presupposes. It dictates the length of rehabilitation, access to brain-injury treatment programs, and other benefits. A reimbursement construct, written into federal law, medical necessity is seen by families as scripting dire outcomes. It is an affront to patients and families because it denies care notwithstanding our evolving understanding of biomarkers of the recovering brain.

Although medical necessity is currently the object of a class action lawsuit that might temper its effects, how these reforms – if they come to pass – will affect patients with severe brain injury remains unclear. As we shall see, this population of patients is a deeply marginalized class who conceivably may not benefit from revisions to medical necessity provisions.

And whatever happens to medical necessity, it will take place against the larger backdrop of what might come to pass under the Affordable Care Act, President Obama's health care plan, which laudably seeks to broaden access and provide efficient and evidence-based care. But what of access for those whose injuries are so biologically complex so as to defy simple notions of efficiency? Put another way, if we do not yet understand how brains recover from the MCS, and the time it might take, how could anyone say progress is delayed? Or that a patient is an inefficient outlier whose benefits should be curtailed?

And as the family narratives amply show, this is what happens. Rehabilitation is curtailed and stopped. Patients not "showing progress" are discharged from rehabilitation programs to nursing homes where they linger without rehabilitation or diagnostic oversight. The impact of a medical necessity determination is high, potentially depriving a patient of the opportunity to recover or, as critically, be placed in a medical context in which an emerging recovery might be identified.

This is not a trivial problem. Recent data reveals that the diagnostic error rate of patients with traumatic brain injury in nursing homes diagnosed as vegetative may in fact be as high as 40 percent, with those patients actually being in the MCS. This is troubling data and a significant error rate with profound implications. It means that a large number of patients are taken to be permanently unconscious when in fact they may be conscious, albeit in the MCS. Although there is a risk to the following speculation, I am haunted by it: imagine lying in a nursing home bed, cognitively impaired and wondering why the staff and even your family are treating you as if you are not there. What could possibly be the reason? Don't they care? Don't they know I am here?

These are questions we can only imagine being asked. That is, until we can probe the brains of patients whose partial or absent motor output suggests a lack of consciousness but whose neuroimages show activations potentially consistent with the ability to sustain thought, language, and emotion. So, absent proper support for rehabilitation and diagnostic assessment, the conscious can easily be mistaken for the unconscious.

As a first step toward reform, I suggest that we reconsider the place of *medical necessity*, a reimbursement category used to assess progress in conditions whose pace of recovery is well understood. In such conditions, physicians and policy makers can predict additional recovery based on the achievement of certain milestones and make fiscal (and ethical) judgments about the utility of additional therapies or rehabilitation. Because that is still not possible with patients in the MCS, we will need to develop new constructs that incorporate elements of the patient's history, clinical exam, and imaging and EEG studies to better predict outcomes. These constructs will need to broaden the definitions of progress currently embedded in medical necessity, which require the demonstration of *physical* improvement versus better indicators of brain-based changes that might portend additional recovery.

In tandem with these efforts, families should have a better opportunity to appeal discharge decisions and determinations about a patient's rehabilitative status and have access to expert, if not simply better, assessment to remediate the unacceptably poor state of evaluation to which this population is subjected. This will require cross-training of internists and geriatricians who primarily staff chronic care facilities. These physicians are not typically trained to provide neurological or physiatry assessments, and they will need to learn more about the assessment and management of patients with disorders of consciousness, if more expert evaluators are not available.

But it will take more than cross-trained physicians to better assess and rehabilitate these patients. In addition to the reform of professional education, I would also suggest that we reframe our conception of rehabilitation and view this process through the prism of an educational reform. I make this argument because, as we will see, there is early scientific evidence that the brain recovers from severe injury utilizing processes, like axonal regeneration, seen in normal development. Although this remains speculative, it appears that the brain makes reparative connections much the way it originally made connections in the naturally maturing and developing brain. It seems that developmental processes, honed over millennia of evolution, are being recast to serve a regenerative function.

If the brain regenerates by recapitulating a process normally reserved for development, might it not make good sense to recast therapeutic efforts geared toward the injured brain like a kind of reeducation, in which the object is not the developing youth, but the developmental processes that may undergird recovery? That means that rehabilitation centers will need to transform into schools. They will need to meet patients along their new developmental continuum and help them achieve their maximal potential.

Practically, this would require a theoretical reconsideration of the methods and the quantity of rehabilitative efforts. It would seem prudent to have rehabilitation experts work collaboratively with early age educators who shepherd early learners in motor tasks, the acquisition of language and linguistic skills, and behavioral norms for communal living.

Reframing rehabilitation as education would also necessitate us asking how much intervention is appropriate. Educators speak of more, not less early childhood education and the critical importance of pre-K education on the developing brain's long-term prospects. And preschools incrementally increase the amount of time their little learners go to school, starting slow but eventually extending the school day until they approximate older children.

Given the constraints of fatigue and injury, should not the same strategy be invoked for patients undergoing recovery or, might we say, the redevelopmental process from brain injury? The amount of rehabilitation given to brain-injured patients is paltry if compared to educational interventions. As educational experts speak of extending the school day and the school year, rehabilitation specialists might consider increasing the amount and frequency of their ministrations.

Of course, rehabilitation efforts will be severely limited if next-generation assistive devices are not available to patients, as therapist-teachers instruct their patient-students in how to use these prosthetic tools in the service of their reeducation and recovery. But absent support for the development of neuroprosthetics, patients identified as conscious will remain forever unable to translate their thoughts into words. They will remain condemned to a life of isolation and cognitive imprisonment that might find some degree of liberation through the machinations of modern neuroscience.

So it is essential that the National Institutes of Health (NIH) and the private sector work together to develop these tools for this population. Their development will redound to benefit others less severely afflicted. They will serve a dual purpose as probative devices of discovery helping to elucidate the circuitry that underlines brain injury and neurological and psychiatric disorders, like Parkinson's disease and depression, which are now understood as diseases that result from disordered brain wiring.

Therefore, any agenda for reform must contend with barriers to the development of these devices. A central challenge is one of classification when it comes to funding streams. For better or worse, tools like DBS and neuroimaging can both serve as platforms for therapeutic/restorative and diagnostic/investigative purposes. Because of their current and potential diagnostic or therapeutic capabilities, they are cast as clinical whose primary support is not the basic science purview of the NIH, but the commercial realm of the private sector. Truth be told, these prostheses can operate at both the basic science and therapeutic levels. But this dual purpose leaves them stuck in a funding gulf, starving from levels of funding and investigative freedom only available from the NIH or prone to the market pressures of industry, which seeks more immediate product development.

We are at a pivotal time in the development of the neurosciences and the confluence of technologies from engineering, imaging, and informatics that make accelerated and substantive process possible in ways not previously envisioned. It is a golden moment that could represent a renaissance in the neurosciences all in the service of patients whose very existence has been demonstrated by this same technology. Without neuroimaging we would not now be contending with the ethical challenge of what we owe those who are behaviorally inactive but demonstrate awareness on brain scans. Here, technology has revealed the discordance between brain and body and the dependency of these patients upon others for access to communication and community. We need to see such developments as an ethical obligation that confers responsibilities on society. A failure to restore functional communication is much more than a denied entitlement or a failed investment in a scientific curiosity. It is the perpetuation of the segregation that has placed conscious individuals outside the medical mainstream and sequestered them in chronic care far from the neuroscience that might make their integration back into civil society possible.

A failure to attend to the present needs of these patients, and to support the forward-looking science that will serve them decades hence, will silence the untapped capability of these conscious individuals to engage with others. It will deprive those who are conscious, but unable to speak, the solidarity of human community, something only made possible by the restoration of functional communication.

Some might cast the provision of medical care toward such goals as a discretionary benefit or an entitlement that can be funded or not, depending upon the prevailing political and fiscal winds. But I see such care – and the scientific advances that will make it possible – efforts geared toward the restoration of functional communication, as an intervention that is far more fundamental. I view it as reconstituting a basic human right, in which the restoration of voice is now made possible by neuroprosthetics. And through the restoration of functional communication, patients segregated from their families and from society can be more maximally integrated into the community.

This possibility has now been demonstrated – at least at the level of a proof of principle – through DBS and functional neuroimaging. And though the techniques remain preliminary, almost crude, they foreshadow a certain future in which restorative neuroprosthetic technologies will have the power of giving voice to those silenced by severe brain injury. Realizing this scientific potential and affirming the civil rights of those who will benefit from these innovations is the normative objective of this book.

Make no mistake. This challenge is not simply invoking an appeal to legislation like the Americans with Disabilities Act (ADA) to these individuals. Although the ADA's intent to maximally integrate people with disabilities into community, a goal achieved in part by the restoration of functional communication, is laudable, invoking the enforcement power of the ADA will not be possible without a change in societal attitudes.

It would be far easier if the ADA could address the needs of these patients and remediate their marginalization. But it has not, as yet. Patients with disorders of consciousness linger on the fringes of society. Sadly, before society views these patients as properly covered by disability rights legislation, they first need to been seen as a class that might benefit from such protections.

But to date, these patients have been seen as invariably hopeless or worse, outside the human scope of such legislation as the status quo attests. They remain sociologically – if not legally – outside the regulatory protection of the ADA. The neglect and disregard continues, making the sad point that before this population is deemed worthy of disability rights, society needs to acknowledge even more fundamental rights of citizenship.

This is not the first time in the long march of civil rights that individuals were seen as somehow exempted from the rights enjoyed by a dominant class. It is a recurring theme. From Seneca Falls to Stonewall and Selma, our nation's history has borne witness to marginalized groups that had to appeal for rights enjoyed in full by other citizens. And so it is with those with severe brain injury.

But unlike predecessor groups that have achieved some measure of success, it is still early in the struggle for those with severe brain injury. Perhaps the argument is premature. The science that will restore voice is still new and the technical challenges profound. But I have little doubt that the science will outpace society's ability to fully vest those with severe brain injury with the rights enjoyed by other citizens.

If we take the American civil rights movement as the prototype, we recall that norms, values, and laws can evolve. It was only a little more than half a century ago when our African American brethren were still segregated and excluded from the rights and privileges, even as other Americans enjoyed the fruits of citizenship, the right to vote, access to schools and public accommodations. As the neglect of those with severe brain injury is tolerated, so too have been the practices of discrimination and segregation directed to black America. Those exclusionary practices were accepted and considered normative, until social norms and conventions evolved – and continue to evolve – beyond the tragic legacy of slavery and entrenched discrimination.

The analogy to the American civil rights movement is particularly instructive because it demonstrates how conventional thinking can evolve over time, revealing logical and ethical inconsistencies that make long-accepted practices untenable. When segregation was finally viewed as contrary to American norms and values in *Brown v. Board* in 1954, the Supreme Court recognized the illogic inherent in its 1896 *Plessy v. Ferguson* "separate but equal" decision, appreciating that equality was completely and fully incompatible with segregation.

With all due respect to the heroic legacy of the civil rights movement, a similar transformation needs to occur with respect to patients with severe brain injury. They need to be seen as individuals deserving of the same civil protections owed the rest of us, notwithstanding significant disabilities that paradoxically have placed them beyond society's protective gaze. Their basic rights of citizenry need to be secured so that they can enjoy the benefits of existing protections like the ADA and the inevitable fruits of a generative period of neuroscience.

III

These are serious arguments and that brings me to its messenger. To focus our gaze on the plight of these patients, the story has to be grounded and made personal. It has to have a basis in lived experience and accurately reflect the sociology of severe brain injury in America. To do this one needs testimony and first-person accounts. For this reason this first attempt at an ethnography of this population owes a tremendous debt to my interlocutors and respondents. Their stories lend authenticity to this volume and constitute a data source of tremendous value, and I am deeply indebted to the families who entrusted their stories with me. I hope that I have shared them with the authenticity and deep respect they deserve.

As the custodian of these narratives, I have edited the narratives for ease of reading seeking to be ever-faithful to what was communicated and context. In the cases of Angilee Wallis and Corinth Pecco, excess redaction would remove primary source material about two cases that will be important in the history of the neurosciences: the recovery of Terry Wallis; and the first use of DBS in MCS in Greg Pearson, Ms. Pecco's son. Although I will seek to interpret their accounts and testimony, I feel it is important to maintain the voice of these families to help the reader appreciate fully the emotional angst and, yes, sadness that is part of their stories. Their words resonate deeply and express the daunting task of navigating uncertainty without clear guidance and support.

Collectively, these narratives call out for a change in practice, a call that would be weakened if the occasional inelegance of these articulations were edited out of the volume merely for literary reasons. When the stakes are high, and they are, the first-person authenticity of the narratives lends credibility to observation and urgency to reform. Theirs is an expertise borne of experience few have had and even fewer would want to endure.

And while some of this may appear the stuff of fiction, or perhaps science fiction, these are real stories. I neither created the characters in this work of narrative nonfiction nor the broader population they represent. The existence of patients in a liminal state of consciousness does not owe itself to my imagination, but to heroic medical measures that did not bring individuals back to full health. The patients described here are ones left in the middle: medicine saved their lives but left them only partially restored, leaving families with ethical questions for which they are unprepared.

Despite my advocacy, my intent is neither to glorify their circumstances nor romanticize these brain states. No one would wish this on themselves or others. But when these outcomes do occur it is wholly insufficient to avoid our collective responsibility because we are convinced that our good judgment would protect us from such a dire scenario for ourselves or for our loved ones.

1 Decisions

THE CALL

Maggie didn't make her trip to Weill Cornell Medical College to participate in studies of patients with severe brain injury. Left partially paralyzed and perhaps even permanently unconscious more than a year after a brainstem stroke during her senior year at Smith College, she was now fighting her third bout of pneumonia in succession. Her mother Nancy called to tell us she had to cancel the visit. Maggie was just too sick and the doctors at Good Samaritan Medical Center in Brockton, Massachusetts, wanted to reinsert a tracheostomy tube to help her breathe.

The procedure is relatively simple and safe. A small incision is placed into the neck just below the Adam's apple and a plastic tube is inserted to create a new airway to the trachea and lungs. Just twenty minutes in the operating room, but Nancy agonized over the decision. As she saw it, it was a step backward. Maggie had a trach placed weeks after her stroke in May 2006. That tube served its purpose and had been removed. Unfortunately, Maggie had not regained a level of consciousness that would help her manage her secretions. Instead of safely swallowing them, they would pool in her mouth and eventually lodge in her lungs, setting up infections.

Nancy worried that by agreeing to the tube she was destining her child to a return to a breathing machine, which could be the next step in a series of medical escalations that were seemingly excessive in light of Maggie's utter lack of responsiveness. But the doctors were pushing hard for the trach tube and a bronchoscopy to take a look at the lungs. Harmless enough, but they would have to put her on a breathing machine to do the bronchoscopy. The pressure was intense. The doctors told her, "she's going to die, not for sure, but this is going to happen if you don't do something."

Nancy was close to saying no and letting this end peacefully. She had watched her beautiful daughter, the child who had dreamt of becoming a veterinarian, traveled to Spain, and had amazing friends, struck down before her prime. In a photo taken before the stroke her eyes shone brightly full of hope and promise. She was now bald and swollen with eyes that were barely open.

This had gone on for a long time and there was no visible improvement. Perhaps this pneumonia would be the one that went untreated. Letting nature take its course was a real option, but Nancy's ex-husband, wavered.

He had been less close to the daily drama of caring for Maggie and needed time to adjust. He too loved his daughter and was quite clear that treatment should continue.

Nancy was bighearted and sympathetic. "Then her father and I," she paused, "well I can't say we had a total disagreement, but I invited him to be part of the discussion, and he was adamant that she should have the trach ... there was no question in his mind. That if she can live with a trach, she should have a trach."

Nancy worried that the trach would be permanent and an acknowledgment that this was as good as it would ever be. A permanent trach for a persistent pneumonia that would accompany Maggie's state of diminished consciousness. All "because it's so convenient for suctioning and she needed suctioning so badly."

A PERFECT TOOL

Nancy and Paul, accompanied by their best friends and Maggie's boyfriend huddled for a "crisis meeting" with the doctor. It was a "scene of angst" with Nancy thinking, "... maybe this is a natural process of, she's dying of pneumonia, but she's sick, and maybe this is the right thing. ..." She thought of the accumulated burden of care to that point. "I felt that she, that it's hard to go through what she's going through, and that she was being treated for pneumonia, I mean she had all kinds of medications." And more to the point, none of it was working, so she questioned the utility of yet "another intervention." She was at something of a crossroad. Maggie was helpless, already on a feeding tube and unable to do anything on her own. Nancy was perplexed by the choices, seemingly at a dead end, she "just didn't know."

Although the tube would make Maggie more comfortable – if she could perceive pain – placing the trach would somehow turn her daughter into a port for a ventilator and nothing more. "I was feeling like, and it's true, you have a trach then you just hook it up to a ventilator, it's what it was made for, being hooked up to a ventilator, it's like a perfect tool."

Her use of phrase, "a perfect tool," suggests an inversion of goals. The tracheostomy tube had become a receptacle for the ventilator, not an intervention to help Maggie, who was seemingly beyond help. Although Nancy understood the medical rationale for the tube's insertion, she needed to figure out why it was the right thing to do, beyond mere instrumentality and medical convenience of more efficient ventilation and what is described as "pulmonary toilet." The question was larger. It wasn't just about managing secretions, but thinking about her daughter's life. Did it seem proportionate given her prospects for recovery?

Mired in the medical facts, she was approached cautiously by a physician's assistant who asked to talk. A translator between Nancy's reality and the clinical context, and sympathetic soul, he told her, "I really want to talk with you about this because I think maybe you just need to hear it in a different language." He reminded Nancy of the questions that had consumed her: What exactly did Maggie know? Was she in there? Did she know her mother was at her side? That she loved her?

There was no way of reliably knowing by looking at her. Sometimes she turned her head to Nancy when she was talking to her. Other times she cried and struggled to make a sound in response to something. But these moments were rare and unpredictable. Her responses had nothing to do with instructions, which caused problems when the doctors tried to assess her. It was inconsistent. Simply put, "She doesn't do anything with a command."

Most of the doctors back at the nursing home where Maggie lived thought she was in the persistent vegetative state (PVS) like Terri Schiavo. "That's what the people where she's living every day, that's how they describe her, as being PVS." But Nancy had her doubts because of her rare responses. She didn't care too much about medical jargon but did want "... to know what the possibilities are, what the next steps are. . . ."

Until she could get an answer to her question, she insisted that the doctors avoid the harm of treating Maggie as if she were unconscious and not there. Although she acknowledged that the "behavior that they see does not show them that she's not in PVS," she did not want Maggie to be harmed if she was aware. It was a mother's plea for a most vulnerable daughter, until they knew otherwise that there was no possibility that she could understand. She told the nursing home doctors, "You have to treat Margaret as if she's conscious. I believe she is. You have to treat her as though she's conscious."

DR. KATZ WAS INTERESTED

But Nancy wondered if she was in denial about her daughter's brain state. Was she suffering from false optimism? She decided that she needed to get a more definitive answer from a specialist who she felt could provide a credible answer. Fortunately, she tracked down Dr. Douglas Katz, a highly skilled neurologist at Braintree Hospital in Boston whose practice is dedicated to patients with severe brain injury and disorders of consciousness. Unlike doctors who had become affixed to the vegetative label, Katz was *interested.*

He was also concerned. He wondered if Maggie might be demonstrating the "beginning of communication." And if this was the case, he thought she might be minimally conscious, a state of limited consciousness just above the vegetative state, but one in which the patient is conscious. This was a new category introduced into the literature in 2002.[1] Dr. Katz suggested to Nancy that she and her daughter travel to Weill Cornell in

New York to participate in neuroimaging and electroencephalogram studies aimed at understanding mechanisms of recovery from severe brain injury. Nancy hoped that bringing Maggie to Cornell might give her more insight into Maggie's condition, although we were careful to remind her that our work was still research and there could be no promises of useful, much less reliable information.

But she was not overly optimistic. Her daughter had promise, was poised to make a contribution. Now that she couldn't do so in the way that all had expected, perhaps she could contribute to science, a genuine expression of altruism and purpose from a still grieving mother. Indeed, participation was something of a memorial, "It would give her life meaning because she had things she wanted to do and she probably won't do some of those things. ..." Continuing, Nancy recounted all the usual experiences that her daughter will never have. Taking an inventory of these losses, she noted that, "... it would be unlikely that she'll have children, that she'll hike the Appalachian Trail, that she'll become a veterinarian." And even in the event that she had some recovery, it is unlikely that her functional level would ever get her to do those things.

So in a quest for meaning amidst the tragedy with which she was struggling, Nancy thought that participation in scientific studies would help her cope and might make a difference for others. She also invoked what bioethicists call substituted judgment, deciding as Maggie would if she could communicate, sharing that "I know that she would want to be part of this if she had a choice." And then invoking her daughter's voice, which had been silenced, she said that Maggie would say, " 'let's do the research part for me, but also for other people' ... it was a way to have her contribute."

The physician's assistant reminded her of all of that. He told her, "you wanted to do this research, maybe she should be alive. She can't be dead and have this research done, you know, so you should think about that, and that's important to you, and this is important to Margaret."

And so it was. Nancy had the doctors replace the tracheostomy tube. Studies in New York would have to wait, but she would get there soon enough.

2 The Injury

COMMENCEMENT

It was May 10, 2006 and the end of the semester of her senior year at Smith College. Graduation was approaching, but that morning things were not right. Maggie did not feel well. She called her father and told him, "I have a really bad headache. It's behind my ear, kind of different than any headache I've ever had." He told her to go to the infirmary, but she didn't. She stayed in her single room.

That afternoon one of her friends heard an "odd sound" coming from Maggie's room. She tried to break into the room and asked friends for help. They couldn't open the door because Maggie was on the floor pressed up against it. Security couldn't get in either, so one of her enterprising girlfriends climbed out through the dorm window into the adjoining room. She found Maggie unconscious.

No one knew what had happened and why she was unconscious. But once she was in the ambulance en route to the local community hospital near Smith, she began to have seizures. Perhaps that explained the noises coming from her room. In retrospect Nancy thinks it "was her banging around a bit."

It was a truly disturbing picture that was outside anyone's control. The doctors at the local community hospital did a computerized axial tomography or CAT scan and found serious abnormalities whose treatment was beyond their abilities. They realized that they were over their heads and Maggie would need to go to a bigger hospital that had a full complement of neurologists and neurosurgeons. It was not the sort of problem that a small hospital could handle. They were going to airlift her to Worcester Hospital but fog set in, and so a ninety-minute trip was made by ambulance.

At Worcester Hospital, specialists determined that Maggie had a blockage in a major artery in her brainstem, in the lower part of the brain just above the spinal cord. This blockage resulted in a stroke and her state of unconsciousness. After midnight she was taken to surgery to extricate a blood clot in the basilar artery, a thin little vessel responsible for supplying the brainstem with blood flow. Among the most important vascular territories in the body, good flow in the basilar is of critical importance because there is scant collateral circulation to step in should something go wrong, as it did with Maggie. Her basilar was occluded, blocked, by a blood clot. The point of the surgery was to put a catheter into the vessel and remove the clot or shunt it with a bypass.

As Nancy tells it, "They took a catheter and they pulled or pushed the clot that was in her basilar artery and removed it or whatever they do, broke it up, and then they put in a ... I think it's called a shunt into that artery. And that's basically" her story. Told with a bit of an understatement, Nancy's comments belie the life-altering drama of that first night, a temporal divide that would forever mark a before and after, a time when the challenges of everyday life would seem quaint compared with the burdens and responsibilities for which neither Nancy nor Maggie were prepared.

IN AN INSTANT

Maggie's arrival at the second hospital set in motion a frantic search for her parents. From the hospital's perspective it was prompted by a need for a family member to provide consent for surgery. But for the recipients, the notification is so much more. It immediately calls for decisions about medical care and signed consents about conditions and procedures that are unfamiliar and frightening.[1] Becoming a surrogate decision maker for a loved one with brain injury occurs "in an instant," as the title of Lee and Bob Woodruff's memoir of the ABC News anchor's near fatal brain injury from an improvised explosive device in Iraq attests.[2,3] In that time, the world is changed forever for the patient and upon those whom she must depend.

Although brain injury is the leading cause of death and disability among young people in the United States,[4] most of us are ill-prepared for the sudden call that alters the status quo and dramatically changes everything. One moment your family is secure and safe. Then, an urgent call from an emergency room or notification by the police that there has been an accident, and that security and sense of well-being is disrupted, forever. The news is unanticipated, unlike the deterioration of a long-suffering patient with cancer or heart failure. In that case, the news, though not welcome, is certainly not unanticipated. With brain injury, it is different. Abruptly, lives that had been thought to be shatterproof become broken, often irrevocably, without warning or preparation.

Nancy was on vacation in Paris and recounts the anxious hours when she was unable to be there for her daughter. With a twinge of (unjustified) remorse and concern that her absence might have compromised the timing and outcome of the surgery, she told me that hospital officials reached her ex-husband Paul and actually sent a limousine to quickly bring him to the hospital, "... so that he could sign papers for the surgery that needed to be done." But her report of the circumstances was infused with doubt, "I don't think his arrival delayed the surgery ... I mean, I think that they ...

got there in time. ...." It was the uncertain recollection of a mother who was thousands of miles away from her only child, stranded in a foreign airport, awaiting news.

LAMENTS

Nancy's reaction is one I have seen in other families. They look back at the event and wonder if they had done something differently they might have cheated fate and avoided the outcome that they were dealt. Delays are second guessed, decisions questioned, and scenarios repeated endlessly trying to figure out their bad luck. Time freezes and is rehashed and relationships, whatever their state at that time, become a legacy that must be endured into the future.

Betty and Immanuel Wexler, older parents of a woman who had developed meningitis and a subsequent disorder of consciousness told us of warning signs that had been neglected. Recounting how their pregnant daughter Sarah had taken ill, they lament her unwillingness to seek timely medical care and admit their frustration. "Well, you know that one Sunday evening we received a phone call that told us that she had been found unconscious and moved to the hospital, and we knew that she was seven months pregnant at the time. We didn't know how serious the situation was. But we discovered very shortly, a day and a half [later], how serious it was."

And then the guilt and remorse: "... to put it quite succinctly, we were both totally devastated by what had happened, especially since we knew that the week before it happened she was complaining about flulike symptoms and we, from Connecticut through the phone, tried to persuade her to seek doctor's care and advice and even go to the ER. But Sarah, being very stubborn and very strong minded did not want to do that." But there is something else too, that complicates all further reflection. That is the unresolved emotions that get frozen in time, never to be resolved because the object of the ambivalence or even anger can no longer be engaged. Immanuel Wexler was candid in his report that he remained angry that Sarah did not take her parents' advice and seek medical care that might have prevented a severe infection. He told us, "... I must confess, and I don't know about Betty, but I must confess, that after the fact I was a bit angry with her for not actually following the advice and the urging of Betty."

It is a father's lament of a sequence of events that might have been avoided, if only Sarah had heeded some maternal advice. It is a regret couched in the past tense because it no longer makes sense to cast blame on a daughter who no longer understands her father's disappointment. Strangely, with her injury, his daughter has become an innocent. She is blameless now because she is no longer able to communicate or defend her actions. That guilt, that

remorse will always be in the background and part of the story. And no matter the extent of the recovery, blame seems unjustified because the consequences for Sarah were so disproportionate to her choice not to seek medical
attention more rapidly.

Pat Flores, mother of aspiring baseball player George Melendez, returned
to the scene of her son's car accident to try to visualize what had happened.
George's car went out of control and ended up partially submerged in a road-
side creek. Afterward, he was left with both traumatic brain injury and oxygen deprivation. Pat had to know, to understand what happened. She went
back to drive the road where catastrophe struck, testing the police report's
account of the spin out on a particular curve, "I know George's driving and
I tested that seventy mph thing on a curve many a times, and I didn't lose
control."

Like so many parents and spouses, Pat Flores just had to know what had
happened, much like those Gold Star mothers of World War II who wanted
to know how their boy had died. Knowledge of that fateful moment helped
take the ache away of not being there with a mother's protective balm when
it was needed most. The test drive around the curve was her way of making
peace by returning to a different sort of battlefield. So comforted, she could
even bring a bit of levity to her narrative. With a sense of resignation, indeed
irony, she told us that George, the baseball hopeful, had landed his car on the
property of the owner of the Cincinnati Reds. Later, one of the Reds officials
would kid George while he was in a coma, "Hey buddy we know you wanted
to make the big leagues but that was not the way to go about it."

Most poignantly, these events have the ability to freeze time and relationships. As a father, I often return to the haunting story of a father and teenage son whose relationship was abruptly interrupted by a severe brain injury.
Scott* was a high school senior. Each day he and his friends would get into
his car and rush off to get food during the thirty-minute lunch period. One
day on the way back the car slammed into a pole. The weather was good, the
car in good repair, and there was no evidence of intoxication. There was no
high speed damage but "... everything went wrong, the pole hit the car like a
razor blade" cutting through the front end of the vehicle, striking Scott while
leaving his two friends completely unharmed. A volunteer fireman who was
driving just behind Scott "thought it was going to be a fender bender." But as
he reported, "... it was insane, I've seen a million accidents; I've never seen
anything like this."

It was simply a horrible accident that also cut deeply into Scott's relationship with his dad, Phil*. Father and son had been "very close" when
Scott was growing up. That is until recently, when adolescence put a wedge
between them. His mother recalls, Scott "... was a character at that age; they
definitely fought." For most fathers and sons there is nothing unusual in that

development. It is part of maturation and individuation and fortunately for most it is a temporary estrangement, with loving reconciliation occurring when the young man reaches his twenties. There a new, deeper relationship of mutual respect and regard awaits. But not for Scott and his dad. The accident stranded father and son in a perpetual adolescence. That reconciliation "didn't happen."

Phil, for his part, tries to make things right by doing everything for Scott, even at the expense of his other kids. Helen* notes that, "... my husband felt very badly for [Scott], he does. That's why a neighbor said to him your other son needs you maybe more. But [Phil] can't think like that." He misses his old relationship with his son and is haunted by memories of the accident and how it changed everything.

Phil "thinks with his heart." But Helen sees the need to set reasonable limits. "My husband ... wants the best for [Scott] and he'll spend anything, do anything." But Helen notes that she has a responsibility for her retirement and two other children. She cannot rely on an extended family to help out and worries about her husband's health and the stress that he's under. "He's more emotional than I am ... I don't want him to have a heart attack, we're 10 years later, we're older, and I can't have [Phil's] back break. So I try to think of the whole family and I don't think [Phil] does that, I think he'd just say yes to anything when it comes to [Scott]."

Although the medical consequences can be quite subtle, they are far more overt than the psychological burdens that family members carry from the moment that they get the call that a loved one has been injured or taken ill. And the trauma can be recurrent, like a variant posttraumatic stress disorder, inflicting additional harm with even the most pedestrian of tasks. When Phil drops his daughter off at the high school that Scott attended, he has to drive by where their family's life took a tragic turn. Even as he lovingly takes his youngest child to school, he suffers again. As Helen tells it, he "... flips out, every time he goes, he gets so sad ... you still see the dent in the pole."

SHE COLLAPSED IN MY ARMS

For loved ones who witness the event the pain is perhaps greater. They too may reproach themselves for failing to act more forcefully and having sound counsel ignored. Burt Brody*, a lawyer whose wife Jean* had a brainstem stroke also lives with the legacy of not pushing hard enough for a trip to the hospital when she first took ill. He worries that had he gotten Jean medical care after a first warning headache, perhaps he could have averted the second more serious event.

In a script too reminiscent of Maggie's own exchange with her father the morning before her stroke, we see the power of self-denial, even in the face of the worst headache she had ever experienced. Although Jean had suffered from migraines, the one she experienced one summer morning in 2005 was far worse. She woke Burt up, and he suggested that she take "some Midrin, which was what her doctor had prescribed her." The first time she wakened Burt was three in the morning. He told her "... if we need to go to the hospital let's do it now." Jean responded, "Let's see what happens with the Midrin, if it helps." After fifteen or twenty minutes, "she said it was helping a lot and then we both went back to sleep."

But then it got far worse, "... at about five o'clock she woke up again almost in tears saying that the pain was back and that it was just the worst pain she had ever felt in her head." She was feeling nauseous and asked Burt to help get her to the bathroom. Then in tears, he tells us when he realized that everything changed, "I went to her side of the bed and helped her stand" – and he tears up and pauses – "she collapsed in my arms and lost total control of her bladder." Any sense of denial that this was one of Jean's typical headaches that had lingered from earlier that morning had vanished; now he knew "that something was really wrong."

When Jean collapsed in his arms, he fully appreciated that this headache was out of the ordinary. That fear was confirmed when he realized that Jean had become unconscious. He put her back onto the bed and called 911, worried that her "breathing was really quite shallow." But he was still hopeful and not fully appreciating the gravity of Jean's condition recalling that, "it took the EMS people over a half hour to get there so if it had been *something really serious* she would have died right then, or could have died right then."

It was very serious and the paramedics took Jean to the local hospital.

NIGHT FLIGHT

Everyone back in Massachusetts tried to spare Nancy the worst of the news so she would not worry while crossing the Atlantic from Europe, powerless to do anything. But during a layover in London she decided to call the hospital to see how Maggie was doing. It was then that Nancy discovered the truth about her daughter's condition and that selectively withholding medical information from one entitled to know almost certainly does not work. It usually leads to an innocent and often cruel disclosure by someone who is unaware that the bad news had been censored.

When Nancy left Paris she knew she had to come home but did not know exactly why, "And I didn't know until I was in London on my way home that she had had a stroke because they hadn't told me what was the matter. I guess they made the decision not to, I don't know why, but, but then I happened to call the hospital to check on her." She was shocked by the casualness of what she heard, "They said 'oh she's in surgery because they're trying to get the clot from her stroke' and I was like 'Stroke? What are you talking about?'"

Putting it mildly, Nancy notes, "... that was a bit awkward, because the social worker and my friends decided that it might be better for me to travel without [knowing]" but then evaluates their judgment, "I don't know what, I don't know what they were thinking."

During that conversation she also learned that Maggie was in a coma and this led to even more confusion, typical of all the families we have encountered who struggle with the range of terms used to describe severe brain injury. Nancy immediately equated a coma with a car accident, illustrating the need for medical personnel to be exceedingly careful with terms that can be misconstrued by laypeople. With the hindsight of wisdom that comes with being a surrogate for a patient with severe brain injury, she told us that was the start of her education in medical nomenclature.

"Yeah, they said that she was in a coma. So I thought that from that information, I had just assumed she had been in a car accident. Because I thought, why would someone be in a coma? Well, they'd be in a coma because they were in a car accident. Because she was supposed to be driving home that day, I knew she had a car, that was just my assumption." It was the logical thing to assume that "at three in the morning, when you get a phone call, it's sort of the first thing you think of."

But that was not the only false assumption. She also did not appreciate that her daughter was critically ill. As she put it, when she was flying back from London to Boston, "I didn't really know anything until I got back to the States." Nancy had "three pieces of information": that Maggie "had a stroke, was in a coma, and that she was having surgery." But she didn't piece it all together and appreciate how serious it was initially. This is not uncommon even when families are closer to home. This is new terrain for most and a type of injury with which few have experience.

FIRST NEWS

Diane Davidson, the mother of Chris Hammett, a West Point cadet, recalls how she learned that her son was in a car accident. He had been on an interim assignment at Fort Meade in Maryland when he and another cadet had their Honda Accord rear-ended by a Chevy Suburban going sixty miles an hour. The young cadet had been sleeping in a reclined passenger seat when the accident occurred. When they were hit his head had no support and his brain was prone to both shearing and rotational injury.

It was a bad accident but Diane's initial reaction was one of relief mixed with confusion and denial, "The biggest thing is you don't really, you hear but you don't really hear ... the medical doctors, the nurses, they come ...

they give you the medical, I mean they try to talk in English but you really don't understand the full extent of it." Gratitude that life was not lost also obscures the seriousness of the injury that remains, "I mean, that first night we were just grateful he was still alive. We were happy that he survived both the brain injury and the other operations. And that he was stable. So the first day we were just, we were just celebrating that Chris was still with us … but we had no idea that the extent of what his brain injury was."

The power of denial coupled with the *lingua franca* of brain injury is a combination ripe for misconstrual and miscommunication. Even with a "very kind and solicitous" family doctor who had been treating their family for years, Eve Baer, whose son Ian Berg has a severe brain injury, told us she remained hopeful despite a challenging reality that she would only later fully appreciate. Early in her son's course, their family doctor tried to paint an accurate picture, "… he also was factual. Like he didn't want us to think that this was something that Ian was just going to get better. He did not give us that impression. So he definitely let us know that it was a significant, serious injury. And even that he still might die."

Under optimal circumstances with a physician who knew and cared for her family for years, Eve admits that, "Although, although at that moment, I have no idea what the injury or recovery looked like, I had no idea…I don't think that I fully understood that the severity, although it was severe, I didn't know what severe even meant. I didn't know that it would mean that he wouldn't be talking for over 20 years." With decades of reflection, she adds, "I didn't know that, like I said, I'm just such an optimistic person, I thought it's serious, it might take him two or three months to get better, maybe six months. But, I thought that he would recover."

DON'T KNOW MUCH ABOUT THE BRAIN

Stephen Carrier, the husband of Mary Beth, who sustained a ruptured brain aneurysm, told us of his difficulty in appreciating the seriousness of her injury. A successful bond trader, he started his comments with a self-deprecating preface that, "this probably sounds stupid …" but he only "… knew something was really wrong when I got a sort of private conference room to sit in at the Mass General ER. … The fact that I got something solitary I thought was a little strange." That tipped him off to some extent. But even after a one-on-one meeting with a neurologist who told him that Mary Beth "had a very severe injury" and another clinician who "came in around the same time" to tell him "… there's nothing we could do for her…" Carrier still did not appreciate the full extent of his wife's brain injury.

In the sort of disbelief that only comes with the passage of time, he recalled that despite all the conversations with the doctors, he was unprepared to hear what was being said, "... it still wasn't dawning on me that it was that life threatening. I still thought, terrible headache or some strange thing." It was only later, "... when they finally came in again and said that she had hydrocephalus" did he appreciate the seriousness of the situation. And even then, he needed the facts and the medical discourse to be translated. He did not appreciate what was meant by hydrocephalus, "... I didn't know what that was at the time, but they explained the bleeding in the brain, the pressure, and they had to put a drain in to relieve the pressure." Only with some passage of time and a fuller explication did he know it "was thoroughly serious."

But thoroughly serious wasn't quite equated with consequential. Remarkably, he told us, "... even after she had undergone the brain aneurysm clipping procedure and had been in the Neuro-ICU for a couple of days we had a meeting with the neurologist and at one point he talked about ... 'she's going to have significant damage.'"

Still not understanding, Mr. Carrier recalled, "... and my question was, 'what kind of damage, you mean *brain damage*?' Like I still didn't get it, and that's when he said, 'yeah brain damage.'"

And when the diagnosis of the brain bleed was translated into a future-looking prognostic statement about outcomes, rehabilitation, and recovery, the weight of the injury really sunk in. He recalls medical staff, "... saying if she makes it through this we could be in a rehab for a year or more, and that's when it really kind of hit home, that it was that serious."

He did not think that his inability to grasp the severity of his wife's condition was just a function of new terminology but rather the charitable instincts of the doctors and nurses who were providing care. "Well I clearly didn't understand the terminology. But I think the not understanding was more a function of ... the kindness of the doctors and nurses." He pauses, as if to regroup, "I think they were trying to be as nice about it as possible."

It was a bit of countertransference. The medical staff identified with the Carriers – like them, young and successful – and saw in them a fate they would not wish for themselves. As Stephen put it, "You know, we were reasonably young, we were both forty, my wife was very attractive, and I think it was, it was as much as everyone was saying, seeing her come in there like that kind of *unnerved everybody*." And more charitably, the medical and nursing staff felt true sorrow for the familial consequences for the Carriers' children and how their lives would be affected. "They knew that I had two little kids at the time, and I think they were trying to be extra nice." The pathos is clear: they were a handsome couple whose lives had irretrievably been altered. Even success does not protect you from brain injury.

Stephen also reflected back on how unprepared he was for the enormity of the change taking place in his family's life and the hesitancy of medical staff to broach the tougher questions about quality of life that now weigh upon him years later. At that early meeting, when Mary Beth was in the intensive care unit or ICU, the question about a withdrawal of life-sustaining therapy never came up. He reflected back to those discussions, "... did I ever have, was there ever an option given to us that we should continue to try to save her or not?" His conclusion: "And nothing was ever overtly said like that."

It was far less explicitly stated. There was an implicit message, from that session, that this was the occasion to broach that delicate issue. It was, perhaps in retrospect an opportunity lost, "... I think that meeting was my chance to have said, *if I'd had the wherewithal*, I would have said, you know, 'what are we talking about in terms of damage? What will her life be like?' So I think that was the chance they were giving me to say, 'you know what, just pull back.'"

In retrospect while he continues to appreciate the kindness and competence of his wife's doctors, Stephen is also judgmental, "I think they could have done a better job letting us know that we had potential decisions to make." And hence the paradox. These early discussions between surrogates and physicians are marked by errors of omission and commission. In Stephen and Mary Beth's case, it was the failure to ensure that Stephen understood that there were choices available about the level of care to provide, including decisions to withhold or withdraw life-sustaining therapy.

In most others, that we have encountered, the discourse has been overly directed toward decisions to do less, not more. More guidance was necessary about where Mary Beth's care and case was headed and a failure to explicitly state the options was problematic. In all of these cases, the superior knowledge of the physician speaking with surrogates imposes an ethical obligation to provide guidance, without dictating or omitting a plausible outcome, a task made all the more difficult by the complete unfamiliarity of families with brain injury and its prognosis.

The doctor-surrogate relationship at this juncture in the evolution of a brain injury is highly asymmetrical. Families are wholly unprepared, unaware of the terminology and still in a state of disbelief, unwilling and unable to accept the new reality that has been thrust upon them. In contrast, medical professionals are experienced and not personally connected to those who have sustained injury. We should expect something better in terms of the quality of the explications given and the framing of the issues, explicit questions that prompt true reflection and do not obscure choices that may cease to be available later in the process of recovery. The obligation is squarely on the shoulders of the medical professionals who counsel surrogates during these pivotal early moments. As Mr. Carrier reminded us, "... let's face it, this is a complicated area and I know a lot about the bond market, but I don't know much about the brain."

3   Coming to Terms with Brain Injury

THE FEVERS

Stephen Carrier's point is very well taken. Unlike other areas in medicine where terms are more accessible, brain injury remains shrouded in mystery and is obscure to most. One mother of a child who sustained brain injury, herself a physician, confessed that neither she nor the child's father, who was also a doctor, had experience with brain injury. Even they were befuddled by the diagnostic categories. Indeed they were at a disadvantage because the treating physicians "assumed a lot more than we knew, and we didn't."

Terms like *coma, brain death,* and *persistent vegetative state* are used with families with the assumption that they are understood. But in our experience, surrogate decision makers are unprepared for this technical language. The nomenclature is foreign and sometime oxymoronic. How can someone be brain dead and still alive? How is a coma different than the vegetative state? Why is a vegetative state patient unaware when their eyes are open and darting about? Such questions confound daily reality and our usual operating assumptions when dealing with each other.

Surrogates of patients with brain injury have no reason to have become familiar with the complex language that describes their loved one's condition after severe injury. It is not part of routine experience. Yet, clinical terms like *coma* are used by clinicians with the expectation that they are understood, a potential error in the wake of the Schiavo case in which familiarity with these terms could be mistaken for actual understanding.

Consider Lucy Busby*, whose child, Sharon*, was in the vegetative state. Asked about their understanding of the vegetative state, she responded, "... it was in our minds quite a bit probably because I think it was 2005, that whole incident with Terri Schiavo." They "followed" that case when Schiavo had been described in the press as being in a variety of conditions, "... in either quote 'vegetative state' or 'minimally conscious state,' or 'coma,' – all those terms were being thrown around back then ... so we were pretty familiar with what that was all about."

Or so they thought. The Schiavo case was a source of a great deal of misinformation with politicians and others deliberately misusing medical terms for ideological purposes. This has left a residue of confusion in the public sphere that is amplified by physicians who either do not adequately distinguish between brain states or conflate diagnostic categories putting informed decision making at risk.[1]

And to be fair, this is a complicated and evolving area of knowledge. We are just beginning to understand what the great Canadian neurosurgeon Wilder Penfield described as the "mystery of the mind."[2] We operate in a relative state of scientific ignorance, increasingly informed by historical standards but woefully ignorant by any future measure. Simply put: we still are at the stage where we are describing different disorders of consciousness and only beginning efforts to explain them. These brain states remain descriptive, not explanatory categories based on knowledge of the actual physiology that produces the condition.

Commenting on the still primitive state of our knowledge one of my mentors, Dr. Jeremiah Barondess, shared a useful analogy to the days before there was germ theory and all infectious diseases boiled down to temperature curves.[3] Before infections were classified into bacterial, viral, and fungal illness and we had a means of looking at them with the microscope, or growing them on a culture plate, *all we had were the fevers.* Back then, in the middle of the nineteenth century, diagnosis was made using a feeble attempt to distinguish one febrile illness from another by its fever curve, a graphic made possible by the advent of the then high-tech thermometer.[4] Well into the early twentieth century, fever curves populated the best medical texts of the day and were studied carefully for insights into infectious diseases that were just beginning to be classified and understood.[5,6]

Early into the twenty-first century much the same could be said about brain injury. Yesterday's thermometers are scanners that image the brain. Yesterday's fever curve beautifully drawn and placed into the turn of the century medical record has been replaced by equally elegant scans emblematic of the current forefront of knowledge. Yet despite this advance of medical technology – and the advent of powerful tools like computerized axial tomography (CAT) scans and functional Magnetic Resonance Imaging (fMRI) – it is hard to accept that we are little more advanced in our understanding of the injured brain than our predecessors were when studying infectious diseases one hundred years ago. We reside in a similar state of ignorance as we begin to classify brain injuries.

Despite the media hype that accompanies the latest "discovery" using these methods,[7] the striking images of the brain remain descriptive and, as yet, do not provide a fully mechanistic account of disorders of consciousness. Neuroimaging cannot predict outcomes and remains inferior to neurological and neuropsychological assessment, in evaluating these patients. While they can provide critically important anatomical and structural information necessary for neurosurgical and neurocritical care, functional studies – assessing metabolic activity of brain regions – as yet do not explain the impact of the underlying injury upon the patient's brain state. Indeed, sometimes neuroimages can be discordant with the bedside examination.[8] In this early stage of their development, neuroimaging methods do more to deepen the mysteries of the mind than to resolve them. They remain a remarkable tool for hypothesis generation and research, topics to which we will return in depth in subsequent chapters.

For now, at least, the standard of care remains the clinical and behavioral assessment of patients based on the clinical history, neurological exam,[9] and neuropsychological assessment, using specialized neuropsychological instruments that test levels of consciousness by bedside assessment.[10] While the formal integration of neuroimaging into the evaluation of these patients will almost certainly evolve as a new standard of care, at this juncture, assessment remains primarily an exercise in clinical assessment informed by diagnostic terminology developed for *bedside assessment*. Let us turn to this terminology.

COMA AND BRAIN DEATH

We start with the comatose patient, Maggie's brain state as Nancy flew home from Paris. Patients who are in a coma are in an eyes-closed state of unconsciousness in which there is no awareness of self, others, or the environment. They can either progress to full recovery, as in the case of a patient who is made comatose by general anesthesia that then wears off, or progress to brain death.

Comas, by definition are self-limited and typically last up to ten days to two weeks. A patient either progresses out of coma or dies a "conventional" death with the loss of their heart beat or by becoming brain dead. In brain death, the lower part of the brain (the brainstem, which connects the brain to the spinal cord) and the higher part of the brain (the cerebral cortex) both die.

Brain death, unlike the conventional – or natural – definition of death with cessation of cardiopulmonary function, is a man-made creation that itself was necessitated by medical progress: ventilators and organ transplantation. Before the advent of ventilators these patients could not survive without their brainstems directing their autonomic functions, like prompting cardiac and respiratory function. Aided by ventilators, these patients could "survive" without intact brainstems. The ventilator would prompt respiration while little nodes in the heart did their best to maintain cardiac function, until they too wore out leading to cardiac arrest and a cardiac death.

But it was really the dawn of organ transplantation that necessitated a new category of death. In 1968, the same year the South African surgeon Christian Barnard performed the first heart transplant, an Ad Hoc Committee at Harvard Medical School put the concept of brain death into the medical literature.[11] Their committee defined brain death as the irreversible cessation of whole brain function, that is both the brainstem and the higher cortical functions.

Chaired by the famed Harvard anesthesiologist and pioneer bioethicist Henry K. Beecher, their rationale was to not let good organs go to waste. They hoped to create a framework to allow organ retrieval when a patient had a catastrophic brain injury, from which no recovery was possible, who nonetheless harbored intact organs that could save other lives. Beecher was quite frank in his assessment at the time asserting a utilitarian rationale for organ retrieval,[12] linking death to the permanent loss of consciousness in what he described as "the hopelessly damaged brain." He wrote that a failure to see it this way would result in the squandering of precious organs in the face of unconscious life. As he saw it, it was a trade-off. Not to retrieve organs from such patients would lead to a:

> desperately radical result: the curable, the salvageable, can thus be sacrificed to the hopelessly damaged and unconscious who consume the time and space and money better devoted to those who could be helped. To pretend that no such alternative exists is nonsense: what one gets the other is deprived of.[13]

Indeed, if his words are parsed carefully, we will see the emphasis placed on consciousness. When it was lost, a physician's obligations to the patient were attenuated, even to the point as to turn the patient into a potential donor.

This powerful inversion of the primacy of the physician's obligation to the patient, associated with the utter futility of brain death and the linked notion of the permanent loss of consciousness, can foster a sense of dis-ease and distrust amongst family members seeking care for their loved ones under stressful situations.

REFLEXES OF A FROG

The usual presumptions of the doctor-patient relationship can become strained when practitioners see the worst while family members still hope for the best. One narrative, whose credulity is stretched by the insensitivity of a physician's assessment, tells of a neurologist speaking with Mary Waters, the mother of Jimmy, a nineteen year old who was hit by a drunk driver while walking in his native Pennsylvania just weeks before he was to deploy to Iraq as a Marine.

Unresponsive from a severe brain injury, the neurologist, with echoes of Henry K. Beecher, recommended organ donation. His mother told me, "And actually I had a neurologist tell me, 'Your son is basically just an organ donor now ... he doesn't have the reflexes of a frog.' "

I asked in disbelief for her to repeat what she had said and she confirmed what I thought I had heard. "Of a frog," she repeated, and continued, "It was the only bad experience I had with this neurologist." She said he told her, "... you should really just consider him being an organ donor. That's the best thing you can do for your son." And she replied, "I completely disagree with you. I'm not making him an organ donor. Go back in there and do the best you can."

When I first did that interview I tried to understand how a doctor could make such an analogy. I thought of pithed frogs from high school biology lab and could only imagine that the neurologist was trying to express his fears that the patient might be brain dead, having lost both cortical function and more "reflexive functions" housed in the lower brainstem. I could appreciate the intent to use an analogy to explain something so catastrophic and tragic, but was appalled by the execution of the effort and saddened by its consequences.

PRACTICE PATTERNS AT LIFE'S END

Jimmy's mother was angered and embarrassed by the neurologist's comment and that it was said in front of her family and in a public space. Mary told us that a stranger observing the scene was so mortified by what she heard that she "left crying because she heard it." So what accounted for this kind of discourse?

Although the comment is insensitive and even inhumane, it was not, I believe, delivered with mal-intent. At one level there was the utilitarian urge, derived from Beecher, to achieve a greater good in the face of what is expected to be a dire outcome. But at a deeper level, the comment reflects how most physicians think about decisions at the end of life.[14]

Most decisions to withhold or withdraw care are made when a patient loses consciousness and the capacity to interact and participate in the decision-making process. End-of-life decision-making data reveals this pattern. In more than 75 percent of cases, do-not-resuscitate or DNR decisions – not to perform cardio-pulmonary resuscitation in the setting of cardio-pulmonary arrest – are made by surrogates after the patient has lost decision-making capacity.[15] It is this loss of consciousness, the ability to interact with the other, that becomes the moral prompt for the conversation.

And this makes sense. Family members and other surrogates appreciate this and begin to make choices about resuscitation or the removal of life sup-port when patients can no longer speak for themselves. As long as the patient can talk there is hope, but when they pass gently into the twilight, every-one appreciates that the darkness of night is near. It is for this reason that the overwhelming majority of DNR decisions are made by surrogate decision makers after the patient has lost decision-making capacity and can no longer direct their own care.

Clinicians confronted with an inevitable death rightly seek to be compassionate and provide proportionate care. Burdens imposed by aggressive medical interventions, like life support, must be balanced by some degree of comfort and support. Here, the physician's task is to demystify the power of the technology he has been touting and acknowledge that it is unable to alter the outcome. This capitulation lessens expectations and helps to switch the goals of care from a curative frame to one motivated by palliation.

In most clinical contexts, the loss of consciousness is the by-product of a long, drawn out process. It reflects the endgame of late stage disease, be it terminal cancer, late stage congestive heart failure, or advanced Alzheimer's disease. In each of these conditions, the loss of consciousness is generally the stigmata of irreversible disease that prompts a reconsideration of the goals of care.[16] Now that a loved one can no longer interact meaningfully, if at all, is continued therapeutic care still indicated? Is the burden of its provision still commensurate with its putative benefit? But if loss of consciousness is a sign of irreversibility, then is ongoing care still proportionate and still indicated?

These are the sorts of questions that are *implicitly* triggering conversations about the reformulation of the goals of care at the end of life, be it a decision to write a DNR order or consider organ donation, as was the case here. To see patients with progressive disease become unconscious is to see these patients at their worst and at the end of a process that usually culminates in death, whether or not a decision to withhold or withdraw care is made.

All this is for the good, except when clinicians misread prognostic signals and mistakenly view the unconsciousness that comes at the start of a brain injury as akin to that which marks the final hours of a terminal illness. Because most of the deaths that are witnessed by physicians in their training have the pattern of unconsciousness preceding death, clinicians have reflexively come to view loss of consciousness as a negative prognostic indicator in all cases of unconsciousness.

And therein is the important difference with respect to a loss of consciousness when it comes to acquired brain injury. Here the analogy to progressive medical illnesses fails. While terminal unconsciousness indicates that death is near, the loss of consciousness in brain injury is bimodal. It could portend death, but it also could be the first step toward recovery. Although this seems like stating the obvious, severe brain injury starts with a loss of consciousness, but does not end there. Patients who are unconscious in a coma can progress, regain consciousness, and recover in part or in whole. A loss of consciousness, in the context of brain injury then is not akin to its occurrence in other contexts. To equate these loses of consciousness is to commit an error in analogic reasoning that fails to account for salient differences in circumstances that redefine the clinical and ethical significance of the loss.

"BUT I HAVE SEEN THE INJURED BRAIN HEALED"

But there is an even deeper meaning embedded in the neurologist's comment. It is an historical resonance that dates to the ancients who debated the significance of brain injury. Theirs was a dichotomous view of brain injury. On one side was the Hippocratic school, which viewed the treatment of brain injury as invariably futile. This was opposed by later Galenics who were less pessimistic and more open to brain injuries viewed as beyond hope by the Hippocratics.[17]

The tension between these two schools of thought lingers to this day (with this author and this volume squarely placed in the Galenic tradition). The importance of this dichotomy was not lost on the aforementioned Wilder Penfield when he was planning the Montreal Neurological Institute, which he founded. In designing the Institute's entrance hall, Penfield captured the tension between Hippocrates and Galen in a beautiful ceiling fresco for his cathedral to neuroscience (see Figure 1).[18]

In an inaugural address, delivered on September 27, 1934, commemorating the Institute's opening, Penfield explained the symbolism of the entrance hall. His remarks were later published as an essay entitled, "The Significance of the Montreal Neurological Institute."[18] Emblazoned on a fresco with "neuroglia cells after a drawing by the great Italian neurologist Camillo Golgi" is "the head of Aires the Ram, which in astrological terms presides over the brain" and four hieroglyphic figures, believed to be "the earliest reference to the brain anywhere in human records." This is encircled by an outer ring in which Galen, refutes in Greek, the Hippocratic aphorism that "a wound involving the brain is invariably fatal."

Galen's refutation of Hippocrates was all the more significant because Galen held Hippocrates in high esteem. His contrarian views were not a criticism of the master from Coos but rather a refinement of our thinking toward the injured brain. Penfield wrote:

> ... Galen called no man master save only Hippocrates, but he took exception to the latter's statement that a wound involving the brain is invariably fatal in the above words which Dr. Francis (*Classicist and Nephew of Sir William Osler*) has translated, "But I have seen a severely wounded brain healed."[19]

Penfield further substantiates the Galenic point of view by invoking the great Sir William Osler. Osler, Penfield's teacher and mentor and the founder of modern internal medicine,[20,21]

> ... said of Galen, "There is no ancient physician in whose writings are contained so many indications of modern methods of research." It is pleasing to have from his pen, eighteen centuries old, the statement

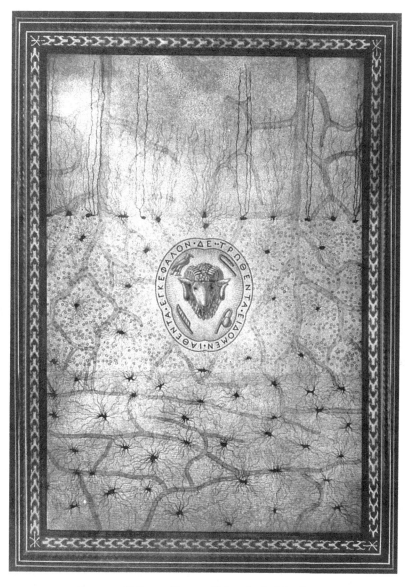

FIGURE 1. Entrance Hallway, Montreal Neurological Institute.
Image Courtesy Montreal Neurological Institute.

that the brain after all is a tissue like other tissues with capacity for
healing; a promise that it too may yield to the physician and surgeon
who come to understand the principles involved.[19]

Penfield was clear about his allegiances. He was a partisan of Galen, not
Hippocrates when it came to brain injury. He did not view brain injuries as
fixed and immutable but rather amenable to treatment and improvement.
This is a view that still needs to be articulated today, especially at the outset
of an injury when the loss of consciousness can be misconstrued as an inevitable
table harbinger of doom.

In retrospect then, there was much embedded in that neurologist's
unguarded comment. We might say it had its ancient origins in the Hippocratic
school and its more modern catalyst in our era's right-to-die movement. And
it is all the more complicated because it might have been uttered under the
guise of beneficence: practitioners now habituated to respecting preferences
at life's end can mistakenly believe that they are acting as advocates whenever
ever they steer families to less aggressive care and on to a palliative course.
While this can certainly be appropriate in many clinical contexts, it is critical
that such direction is not reflexive but based on a reflective process in which
the mere loss of consciousness is not taken to be a harbinger of an inevitably
bad outcome.[17]

So while we cannot excuse the physician's phraseology and word
choice, we can at least understand the forces that prompted him to try and
redirect Mrs. Waters toward the consideration of organ donation. They are
deeply embedded in medical practice, dating back to Hippocrates and Galen
and more recently luminaries like Beecher and Penfield, who viewed brain
injury as immutable or amenable to treatment, respectively, a distinction
that continues to divide the medical profession and society writ large and a
point to which we will return later. But at the center of this schism is the centrality
trality of consciousness and its significance, both symbolic and actual, that
its presence or absence has over medical decision making. As we will see, it
was the loss of consciousness that was a key consideration in the landmark
1976 Karen Ann Quinlan decision, which brought the newly described persistent
tent vegetative state into the public sphere.

4   The Origins of the Vegetative State

A SYNDROME WITHOUT A NAME

The persistent vegetative state (PVS) was first described – and given its name – in 1972 in the prestigious British medical journal, *The Lancet*, by the Scottish neurosurgeon Bryan Jennett, known for creating the Glasgow Coma Scale,[1] and the American neurologist Fred Plum, who less than a decade earlier had described the Locked-in-State with his longtime colleague Jerome B. Posner.[2,3]

Dr. Plum was the revered chairman of neurology at the then New York Hospital-Cornell Medical Center where he was my teacher and eventual colleague. He was an astute observer of detail who had the ability to synthesize information across the neurosciences through beautifully executed prose.[4]

One example of his extraordinary fluency was the paper on PVS he wrote with Dr. Jennett. In the most parsimonious of phrases, Jennett and Plum, described the vegetative state as a state of "wakefulness without awareness."[5] By that, they meant to describe the paradoxical state of what Plum would also describe as "wakeful unresponsiveness,"[6] a state of unconsciousness in which the eyes are open but there is no awareness of self, others, or the environment. It is paradoxical because we arise out of our nightly slumber by opening our eyes and taking in the world. We express ourselves with our eyes. They are the portal to awareness, communication, and humanity community. That is, except for in the vegetative state when the patient is awake but the eyes are unaware and undiscerning. They move randomly about the room with neither intent nor direction like an unmanned sail boat on a gusty day. These usually sentient orbs are now propelled by the primal forces of an intact brainstem that charts no course but simply keeps the body afloat, directing autonomic function like our heart beat, breathing, and sleep-wake cycles.

Jennett and Plum subtitled their paper about the vegetative state as a "syndrome without a name" because they sought to delineate an emerging diagnostic category brought about by medical technologies like the ventilator, which now could keep patients alive who decades earlier would have died. As they put it back in 1972, these "new methods of treatment may, by prolonging the lives of patients with conditions which were formerly fatal, result in situations never previously encountered." And presciently, they appreciated the ethical implications of introducing the "vegetative" concept – a term they felt was well suited to describe their nameless syndrome.

After reviewing a number of alternatives they settle on the *persistent vegetative state*, duly citing the *Oxford English Dictionary*'s definition. To vegetate is "to live merely physical life, devoid of intellectual activity or social intercourse." And to be vegetative is "to live a merely physical life devoid of intellectual activity or social intercourse."[7]

To their credit, Jennett and Plum immediately appreciated that their new definition of persons living a physical life devoid of intellectual activity would arouse both a lay and professional response. Indeed, they noted – even before the publication of their paper – that the accumulation of such cases is "provoking comment both in the health professions and in the community at large" of "ethical, moral, and social issues."

QUINLAN

Jennett and Plum's prescience about the importance of this concept was not misplaced. Just four years after they described the PVS, Dr. Plum was called to serve as an expert witness in the 1976 landmark Karen Ann Quinlan right-to-die case.[8-10]

Like Maggie, Karen was in her early twenties when her young life was irrevocably changed. She had been at a party, consumed some gin and tonics and perhaps Valium. She began to nod off. Her friends later found her not breathing, estimating she had gone some fifteen minutes for two periods without oxygen before she was resuscitated. Drug tests at the hospital were negative, and it remains unclear how and why she had a cardiopulmonary arrest, although like Terri Schiavo she had been on a "starvation diet" to lose weight before she lapsed into coma.[8,11,12] Some speculate that the stress of the diet might have made Quinlan more susceptible to whatever drugs or alcohol she ingested.

Mrs. Quinlan, in her memoir, recounts when she and her family first realized that something was quite wrong and that Karen's opening of her eyes did not signify recovery but some nether state that was counter to all expectations. Like so many other families the Quinlans were confounded by the paradoxical features of the vegetative state, which taunts loved ones with open eyes that neither see nor feel. In a heart-wrenching moment Mrs. Quinlan tells how she and her other daughter sought to reconnect with Karen only to be met with a blank stare. When Karen first opened her eyes, Mrs. Quinlan was initially overjoyed. She soon became dismayed as the paradox of "wakeful unresponsiveness" sunk in. Mrs. Quinlan wrote:

> "Karen!" I half-shouted it.
>
> Julie (Karen's sister) was there – she saw it, too – and she leaned forward and kissed Karen. And then the nurses came hurrying over, and there was all kinds of excitement. For just a few minutes, we thought it was all over,

and that she had come back, and I prayed harder than I have prayed in years and years.[8]

But she didn't recognize us. She was staring right through us. A nurse placed her open hand a few feet from Karen's face ... Karen's eyes didn't follow it. She just wasn't focusing.

> In a way, that was the most disheartening development of all, watching her eyes look into space, or move all around the room, as though she were looking and looking for something – and finally forcing ourselves to realize she couldn't see.[8]

It was a moment to be repeated again and again. The excitement that comes with what appears to be a recovery and the profound disappointment that follows when the opening of the eyes is a contrarian sign. Pat Flores, the mother of George the aspiring baseball player, told us her son first opened his eyes two weeks after his car accident. "With a big yawn, he opened his eyes. And I said 'eureka, he's going to be fine now.'" Years later, with a knowing laugh she confessed, "It looked so normal, the expression on his face, the yawn. It just looked so normal that I thought he was out of it. Everything."

Like so many families that followed in their wake, the Quinlans eventually appreciated that their child was vegetative and the futility of her condition. Knowing this sad truth, they sought to have her ventilator removed. They knew that Karen would have been opposed to life tethered to a machine. Devout Catholics, they sought the guidance of the Church, and as the case became a cause célèbre, the direction of the Vatican. The Holy See issued a statement that it did not make ecclesiastical policy over individual cases and that the matter should be decided with the petitioner's own diocese. Local diocesan authorities supported the Quinlan's quest to remove what was considered an extraordinary measure, and thus nonobligatory, life-sustaining measures.[13]

Notwithstanding the stance of more fundamentalist religious faiths in later right-to-die cases like Cruzan and Schiavo, the Catholic Church's views have remained consistent, drawing the line between ordinary and extraordinary measures. If we return to the case of Sharon Busby, a woman in the vegetative state, we will see how Church doctrine continues to inform care decisions for those families who are observant.

Sharon's mom, Lucy, told us of her family's faith and how she went about making decisions. "One thing we did immediately, within days of learning of Sharon's injury, was to be in touch with our priest. We're Catholic, so from our perspective we wanted to be clear about what our options were in terms of Sharon's care. If we had to make any crucial decisions we wanted to make sure that we were making the right ones in terms of our conscience and our faith and what was best for Sharon. And he [the priest] pretty much came up to the hospital ... and pretty much went over what we had already known anyway but just wanted clarified that ... any decisions that we would make would be based upon our faith and that we weren't obligated to take any extraordinary measures to keep Sharon alive, but that food and water were not considered extraordinary ... and that we should do our best to keep Sharon comfortable and alive and sustain her life, which is what we had planned on doing all along anyway."

A LANDMARK CASE

The Quinlans were clear about their preferences for their daughter, who they had adopted as an infant. Karen had been a vibrant and adventurous young woman known for her spirit and growing independence. This was not how she had wanted to live and they knew her wishes, even at her young age. With a premonition of an early death – she had even bought her sister a $5,000 life-insurance policy so "she would be set for life" – Karen had spoken with friends and family about her preferences.[8]

But her doctors and the hospital objected and the family took them to court. The Quinlan's case was rebuffed by a local court and their brilliant young lawyer, Paul Armstrong, took the case up to the New Jersey Supreme Court on appeal. The highest state court allowed their request to remove Karen's ventilator. Chief Judge R. J. Hughes, a former governor of the state of New Jersey, ruled that withdrawal of life-sustaining therapy was permissible because it would be futile to provide additional care given Ms. Quinlan's irretrievable loss of a cognitive sapient state. The court drew upon the testimony of Dr. Plum, who served as the court-appointed neurologist, to justify their decision.

In his expert testimony, Dr. Plum sought to explain the vegetative state and distinguish it from brain states where higher cortical functions remained intact. He described the elements of brain function as a mix of primitive or vegetative capabilities and higher cognitive capabilities. He explained:

> We have an internal vegetative regulation which controls body temperature, which controls breathing, which controls to a considerable degree blood pressure, which controls to some degree heart rate, which controls chewing swallowing and which controls sleeping and waking. We have a more highly developed brain which is uniquely human which controls our relation to the outside world, our capacity to talk, to see, to feel, to sing, to think. Brain death necessarily must mean the death of both of these functions of the brain, vegetative and sapient.[7]

The inclusion of an ability *to sing* as part of the brain's more highly developed functions was vintage Fred Plum, that bit of color that marks the distinction between the sentient and the merely vegetative. But it also may have reflected Plum's deep knowledge of the case and Ms. Quinlan. An observer of little details and a master of facts, I wonder if he knew that Karen Ann had sung in her parish church and that its priest, Father Thomas Trapasso, thought she had "a pretty voice."[8]

Drawing upon Dr. Plum's testimony, Judge Hughes justified the removal of Ms. Quinlan's ventilator. He took Plum's distinctions as providing the moral warrant for his decision and grounded his opinion in the right to privacy. He maintained that while the state had an interest in preserving life, "... the State's interest *contra* weakens and the individual's right to privacy grows as the degree of bodily invasion increases and the prognosis dims. . . ."[7]

Judge Hughes, a devout Catholic, also took special pains to address the Church's position on the case, not to set a legal precedent, but out of felt concern, "only on its impact upon the conscience, motivation and purpose of the intending guardian, Joseph Quinlan."[14] According to Hughes biographer, John Wefing, this theological digression was not necessary to the legal decision but rather necessary for Hughes "to assure himself of the morality of the decision he was making."[15] That small act of kindness led the Hughes and Quinlan families to become friends after the case concluded, with the Quinlans sitting with the Hughes family at the governor's funeral years later.[14]

Judge Hughes' decision, written for a unanimous court, ruled that removal of life support was ethically justified because "her prognosis is extremely poor."[7] So poor, in fact, that Judge Hughes analogized Ms. Quinlan's condition to a terminal illness like end stage cancer. This underscored the disproportionate nature of ongoing care and set up the expansion of the right to die to conditions other than the PVS. The analogy was part of the justification for the new rights created by his court. He asserted that:

> We perceive no thread of logic distinguishing between such a choice
> on Karen's part and a similar choice which, under the evidence of this
> case, could be made by a competent patient terminally ill, riddled by
> cancer and suffering great pain.[7]

While it was expedient to consider the vegetative state a terminal condition to allow for the withdrawal of life-sustaining therapy in a young woman like Ms. Quinlan, the argument made by Judge Hughes is flawed on two counts.[16] Firstly, the vegetative state need not be terminal absent a withdrawal of life-sustaining therapy. Secondly, it is not a condition in which the perception of pain, much less the experience of pain, is possible.[17,18] Nonetheless, Hughes' argumentation illustrates the thinking at the time and the direness of the diagnosis and perceived burden of the condition.

But beyond the analogy to a terminal illness, the most compelling, and memorable argument made by Judge Hughes was the relevance of a loss of a cognitive sapient state to continued care. Judge Hughes opined that there was no rationale to force an individual to be kept alive in a state devoid of sapience and cognition and requiring round-the-clock care.[7] In such circumstances, efforts to preserve life, without the ongoing consent of a patient or their surrogates, could be seen as futile. In a declarative opinion, Judge Hughes noted:

> ... We have no hesitancy in deciding ... that no external compelling interest of the State should compel Karen to endure the unendurable, only to vegetate a few more measurable months with no realistic possibility of returning to any semblance of *cognitive or sapient life*.[7]

Karen Ann Quinlan's ventilator was removed in 1976 and she lived, breathing on her own until 1985. This came as a surprise in the popular press,[19] but was not unexpected by Dr. Plum.

A SIDE BAR WITH DR. PLUM

Dr. Plum and I were at a reception at Rockefeller University in 2002 or 2003, as I recall, talking about his recollections of the Quinlan case. He told me he knew she would breathe when she was removed from the ventilator.[20] The young acolyte that I was, I asked him how he knew and felt privileged to hear his firsthand account. Not only for his direct involvement in one of the most important court decisions in the history of bioethics, but also my proximity to him as a colleague.

Though he was shorter than me, I recall the sense of looking up to him as he told about an unexpected twist in the Quinlan case. It was obvious in retrospect but took me by surprise. Remarkably, it was not Judge Hughes who ordered that Quinlan be removed from the ventilator; it was Dr. Plum. Admittedly, under a court directed order to perform a neurological examination, he did what he had to do. To paraphrase: "I took her off the ventilator as part of my brainstem exam." And of course he had to. He had to be sure to distinguish brain death from the vegetative state. In the former, there are no spontaneous respirations. But in the vegetative state, a still intact brainstem prompts breathing.

For this reason, to comprehensively assess her brainstem function, and distinguish brain death from the vegetative state, the apnea test is required. In the former the respiratory drive that originates in the brainstem is lost. In the vegetative state, with preserved brainstem function it is retained. To make the distinction, *Dr. Plum had to remove the ventilator* to see if Karen would breathe on her own. I thought it ironic at the time. Most people think it was the New Jersey Supreme Court that ordered the removal of Ms. Quinlan's ventilator when really it was Fred Plum. He rightly interpreted that prerogative as part of his judicially sanctioned neurological exam.[21] Without the demonstration that spontaneous respiration does not occur, one cannot conclusively diagnose brain death.

THE RIGHT TO DIE

Of course, it was the judicial ruling of the New Jersey Supreme Court, not Dr. Plum's assertion of a professional prerogative to make a diagnosis that made history.[7] The Quinlan case – and the right to die – became an important cultural force, much like the nearly contemporaneous 1972 U.S. Supreme Court ruling in *Roe v. Wade*, granting women autonomy over their bodies and their reproductive rights.[22] Each fostered the notion of patient self-determination – the right to control one's treatment, one's body, and the timing and manner of one's death – that became the central focus of American bioethics as it was evolving during the late 1960s and 1970s.[19]

In Quinlan, and other right-to-die cases involving PVS patients, self-determination played out as the negative right to be left alone. The setting was one in which all therapeutic efforts were disproportionate because no benefit would result from the intervention. In such cases, even minimal risks were intolerable because they could not be offset by any foreseeable benefit in patients thought permanently and irretrievably unconscious.

Although the right to die began with the vegetative state, over the ensuing years it would expand to other classes of patients who were not vegetative. And as this happened, generations of doctors would adopt a new normative sensibility in which withholding and withdrawing life-sustaining therapy would be seen as being consistent with good clinical care.[19]

While this evolution certainly represented progress, and spawned the palliative care movement, it was not without a more troubling legacy. The transformation of attitudes toward the right to die came with entrenched views on the vegetative state, which were extended to other severe brain injuries marked by a disorder of consciousness. Because the justification of the right to die was predicated upon the futility of further intervention in the vegetative state, as articulated by Judge Hughes in Quinlan, clinicians have come to view the severely brain injured as a class beyond hope.[23] These brain states, though confused with the vegetative states, are distinct with respect to their prognoses, a difference that makes a difference.

5   A Shift since Quinlan

HOMECOMING

Perhaps to buffer against untoward communication, and to ease the shock of appreciating the degree to which her own child was injured, Nancy was met at the hospital by a couple of girlfriends upon her return from London. Her ex-husband had already left after a long night to get some rest.

Nancy knew Maggie had had a stroke and an operation to remove a clot but neither appreciated the gravity of her situation nor the details of the surgery. As a "really good social worker" and doctor explained, Maggie's stroke was a consequence of a blood clot in the basilar artery in the back of her head just above the spine. It is a crucial vessel that supplies blood to the all-important brainstem, whose essential functions are responsible for reflexes and breathing and all the sorts of things that make someone awake.

The clinical team that met with Nancy were initially circumspect about Maggie's prognosis. At the outset she was being treated for brain swelling that "could kill her." Maggie overcame these early hurdles and the threat to her survival subsided. And as the risk of brain swelling faded, the question of whether she would live or die was replaced by the harder question of the kind of life she might have.

Maggie was at a pivotal junction in her care. She was leaving the acute care heroics of emergency rooms, neurosurgery, and high-tech interventions and transiting into the realm of decisions that would most likely destine her to a life in chronic care, of nursing homes and dependency. Several days after her stroke and into this period of relative stabilization, Nancy began to ask the doctors caring for Maggie about their views of her future. One of the doctors urged her to forgo the pivotal decision to put in her first tracheostomy and feeding tubes that would help her breathe and eat. He told Nancy that, "I needed to look at the quality of life that she would have and what she would want." He also brought up the question of resource allocation and "they talked about even the resources that would be used."

At that juncture, Nancy was asking all the doctors and nurses the simple, but gut-wrenching question, "if this was your daughter what would you do?" This was a question she stopped asking after she gained a better sense of herself. But right then, at that early juncture, she encountered a physician who was frank with his views: "If she was my daughter I would definitely take her off the ventilator." He was "fairly adamant," Nancy recalls. "He felt that her chance of recovering was minimal and that the best, the best recovery she would have would be in a persistent vegetative state."

Based on what her physician had observed of Maggie's condition, it was not outside of practice norms to predict that Maggie would end up in a vegetative state. She remained unconscious in a coma and the extent of her injury was such that permanent unconsciousness was likely.

But it was also a way of telegraphing something more about the reasonableness of ongoing care. The vegetative state's invocation at the bedside was a way to implicitly, if not always fully, communicate that ongoing care would be disproportionate at best and futile at worst. Without saying it, it was this physician's way of suggesting that it was time to let her pass peacefully. And the doctor did advise Nancy that, "I needed to look at the quality of life that she would have. . . ."

Yet there was still the shock of the new terminology and what it meant. Nancy had only a vague sense of what it meant for someone to be in the vegetative state. She was only familiar with it because of the Schiavo case and yet she found herself in a frank and forceful conversation with one of Maggie's doctors about what it would mean. When asked if her understanding of the vegetative state stemmed from the Schiavo debate she responded, "Schiavo, yeah. I didn't ... I never would have heard that term before except for that." It meant "something" to her but only in the "context" of the Schiavo case and its polemics.

PATERNALISM IN A NEW GUISE?

By the time one of her doctors said that the best recovery that Nancy could hope would be the vegetative state, thirty one years had passed since the Quinlan decision. And with the passage of time, a dramatic reacculturation of physicians has occurred. Instead of opposing the withdrawal of life-sustaining therapy, as had been the case in Quinlan, physicians now typically recommend that care be withheld or withdrawn in patients with disorders of consciousness, often asserting that there would be "no hope for meaningful recovery."[1]

Even as the acute care of severely brain-injured patients has progressed during this same period, patients with severe brain injuries have become increasingly vulnerable to treatment decisions that might preclude potential recoveries.[2] Paradoxically, despite the progress that has been made, physicians became quick to judge and to bring their own biases forward in order to provide directive counseling that "engineers outcomes,"[3] paternalistically directing care. At times, such views might even border on the ideological and prescriptive, and entrench prognostic pessimism that may be unwarranted.

The stance of much of the neurological community may be inferred from a paper written in 2007 by Drs. Wijdicks and Rabinstein of the Mayo Clinic providing guidance for the sort of conversation doctors had with Nancy while Maggie was still in a coma. In their paper entitled, "The Family Conference: End-of-Life Guidelines at Work for Comatose Patients," published in *Neurology*, the journal of the American Academy of Neurology, Drs. Wijdicks and Rabinstein suggest that:

> Families should be given an explanation of the success rate and complexity associated with resuscitation, but the physician should avoid needless detail ... have an understanding of the accumulating costs of intensive care if a major advancement of level of care is pursued. . . .
>
> The attending physician of a patient with a devastating neurologic illness will have to come to terms with the futility of care. ... Those families who are unconvinced should be explicitly told they should have markedly diminished expectations for what intensive care can accomplish and that withdrawal of life support or abstaining from performing complex interventions is more commensurate with the neurologic status.[4]

It is a curious paper on both scientific and normative grounds. Scientifically, the title seems ill-fitting because it refers to decision making during the comatose phase of injury or illness. Although there are outcome statistics for coma, prognostication in coma can be especially difficult because of the recency of the injury and the fact that a coma can be rather pluripotent with outcomes ranging from brain death to complete recovery depending upon the nature of the injury and the time since the insult occurred.

Normatively, the paper is also problematic because its recommendations are unqualified in one direction. It seems to advance a proscribed course of action of less care, not more. In a directive, paternalistic tone, the attending physician is instructed to convince those families who have more than minimal expectations for recovery to appreciate the futility of any intervention. And so as not to miss the point of the exercise, this should be done explicitly and families should have their goals redirected to a palliative care course.

I am not against palliative care. I have long been an advocate of palliative care, have taught its tenets to medical students and residents, and authored a volume on the topic,[5] but I have always seen palliation as a personal or family choice, not a course of care dictated by physicians.

The stance advanced by Wijdicks and Rabinstein is all the more troubling because they fail to appreciate that there is, what the medical ethicist Daniel Callahan called, a "troubled middle" where a proper course of action is less clear.[6] At the extremes prognostication is easier. Patients near brain death with *de minimis* brainstem function, and those who are lightening up quickly and regaining some responsiveness can be assessed early on with a greater degree of accuracy. But for those patients in the difficult middle, it can be exceedingly hard to know how to cast their lot. This indeterminacy is heightened during the early days of coma, a transient state whose ultimate prognosis is determined by etiology of injury and the passage of time. To make global statements about expectations in this context, while inadequately engaging the differential diagnosis of coma,[7] is a formulation that seems astoundingly and operatively vague.

A PERSPECTIVE FROM SEATTLE

Dr. Plum, whose work on the vegetative state is often reflexively linked to the right to die, understood the perils of premature prognostication. Plum was interested in the futility of the vegetative state in order to appreciate the utility of treatment for those who might be helped. It was an effort at risk stratification that he learned as a veteran of early efforts using iron lungs on Poliomyelitis patients in Seattle during one of the last epidemics in the early 1950s.[8,9] There too, patients who might be helped were prematurely designated as futile cases. Plum became their advocate. In a memoir of that fight against polio, Dr. Plum is depicted as:

> A scientist with a philosophical bent and an interest in people, he was unquestionably the commander-in-chief, keeping his focus on the patients under his care and on the research going on there that could benefit patients around the country.[10]

He fought for the lives and futures of his patients with a tenacity that would echo in his later advocacy for other patients whose prognosis was unknown and needed to be discerned. Not a sentimentalist by anyone's standard, he was a fierce supporter of patients whose fate remained unclear and might be altered by a more precise diagnosis, careful assessment, or a new technological advance like the iron lung.

His advocacy, and humility in the face of the scientific unknown, comes through in a manuscript fragment I found in the New York–Presbyterian Weill Cornell Medical Center Archives in 2008. I was preparing to give a talk in honor of Dr. Plum at the International Brain Injury Association (IBIA) meeting in Lisboa on the occasion of the first award of the IBIA's Jennett-Plum Award. Dr. Jennett had just passed away and Dr. Plum was too ill to attend. Dr. Plum's wife, Susan, asked me to accept the award on her husband's behalf, and I was honored to make the trip and to speak of his life and work. Along the way, I found a few handwritten pages that succinctly laid out his philosophy and approach to clinical care. Writing in the late 1970s, just after *Quinlan*, Dr. Plum observed that:

> We have studied over a 100 patients ... can identify within 24 hrs. by
> their neurological signs alone who cannot recover above a vegetative
> level ... who will do well. ... This leaves a middle group for whom
> more information is needed but where presenting every effort at
> treatment must be made to know their maximal potential and how
> to judge their early signs. ... .[11]

In this early effort at risk stratification, Plum is trying to distinguish amongst
patients with severe brain injury and prognosticate outcomes. He identifies
the extremes: those who will be vegetative or worse and those who will do
well. And then, most notably for us today, he invokes a precautionary principle for what to do for a middle group whose fate remains indeterminate
and "for whom more information is needed." To his credit, Plum appreciates the limits of his knowledge and is cautious in his prescriptions. These
patients should be given every chance so that "their maximal potential" is
fully appreciated.

A DIFFERENT PRESCRIPTION

When contrasted with the views of Wijdicks and Rabinstein, those of Plum
may seem quaint and a bit cautious. One might reasonably wonder if advances
since the mid-1970s might have made prognostication easier – a reasonable
assumption, but one that is wrong. Prognostication has become trickier
with time. Therapeutic advances, most notably those that remove fluid and
decrease intracranial pressure from within the injured and swollen brain,
have improved outcomes. Craniotomies, where part of the skull is removed
to allow swelling to move out and not down on to the sensitive brainstem –
often described by doctors as the "most important real estate in the brain" –
as well as intracranial pressure monitoring, where tubes are placed into the
ventricles filled with cerebro-spinal fluid, have allowed neuro-intesivists to
regulate pressures within the brain, thus protecting it from the secondary
injuries that occur when the bloated brain has nowhere to go. These interventions, aided by better visualization of brain structures with CT and fMRI
scans have allowed for better care and created a whole new cohort of intermediate outcomes, what Plum called a "middle group." More time and better
information is needed to reach a consensus about their outcomes and futures.

   One neurosurgeon who provided care to Susan Soroka's daughter
Colleen early in her course embodied Dr. Plum's caution in a more modern
guise. Amidst some house officers whose pessimism led the family to "have
names for all of them like Dr. Gloom and different things," the neurosurgeon's counsel was "very neutral." Susan praised the neurosurgeon's restraint
in not making a judgment prematurely. "Everything was wait and see if she
was going to make it through the first twenty-four hours, the first forty-eight

hours." She credited the neurosurgeon with *not* offering a prognosis until that initial hurdle was overcome. What was said, "wasn't even a prognosis, it was just if she was going to live through what was going on, if they could get the pressure down." A more definitive assessment would come later.

Another physician framed prognostic uncertainty to Elinor Quigley in a similarly constructive fashion. When discussing her son Kenneth who had fallen several stories off a ladder onto a concrete slab, he was circumspect and cautious. When asked if the physician was hopeful, Mrs. Quigley responded, "No, he sounded very matter-of-fact, very matter-of-fact." The doctors she spoke to "never gave us false hope." And as importantly, like Dr. Plum's earlier comment, they admitted their relative state of ignorance about prognostication. "They all said a brain injury was something that they knew so little about, that the brain was such an intricate part of the body and they were still learning about it."

And they commented on the seemingly inexplicable variance in recovery that is after severe brain injury, observing, "That some people recovered, some very well and others had a harder time of it." They also expanded the time frame for assessment beyond the acute phase of injury. They told Mrs. Quigley that recovery would take time, "And that the first five years were critical and the first year was very, very critical." Their candor and humility was appreciated by Mrs. Quigley, "They were very good, very, they talked to us, they didn't offer us false hope, they said they didn't know. They thought that the part of his brain that was injured would control a lot of things ... he'd have to learn to do things all over again."

Given the nuance of these more exemplary responses, it is all the more curious to read of Drs. Wijdicks and Rabinstein's unqualified confidence about such early predictions while patients are still comatose and have yet to more fully declare themselves. It is all the more remarkable that such views could be published in *Neurology*, the official journal of the American Academy of Neurology. To be so determinative about outcomes and equally prescriptive, urging families to manage their expectations seems premature at best and paternalistic at worst. If nothing else, these views convey the mistaken belief that all outcomes from a coma are uniformly dire or easily predictable. In such settings, families need more information not less. I am neither sure what is a needless detail when making a momentous decision about the fate of a child or a spouse with a severe brain injury, nor comforted about managing expectations and feeling obliged to withhold or withdraw care and pursue palliative care.

Whatever the balance between curative and palliative care, the hard won right to die – which began with Quinlan – needs to be balanced against the right to care for patients like Maggie with disorders of consciousness.[12] Their individual needs should neither be undermined by ideology nor curtailed by ad hoc case-by-case cost containment. Bringing concerns "of the accumulating costs of intensive care if a major advancement of level of care is pursued," as advocated by Wijdicks and Rabinstein would be discriminate based on financial considerations and jeopardize the opportunity for patient and family preferences to come to the fore and be heard.

When Nancy was confronted by the doctor who urged that care be withdrawn from Maggie, Nancy felt that she was being rushed and bullied. She needed time and the advice of people she trusted. She also needed to think about what Maggie would have wanted. She needed to bring Maggie's now absent voice into the conversation. So Nancy sought the advice of friends and families who knew Margaret well. In lieu of the paternalistic stance of her physician promoting an ill-fitting right to die, Nancy reached out to Maggie's friends and intimates to discover what *she* would want. That seemed more consonant with the true ethos of the palliative care movement, which was never intended to dictate how we die, but instead sought to ensure that patients and families had the requisite discretion and self-determination to make important choices.[13]

6   Maggie's Wishes

Over the next couple of days Nancy spoke with Maggie's friends who remembered an argument she had with her boyfriend during the national debate about Terri Schiavo. Nancy thinks that Maggie must have been especially upset because she came back and shared the details of the conversation with her girlfriends.

Her boyfriend told Maggie that, "if that were me I would pull the plug." Margaret, as her mother would often refer to her daughter, responded, "I would never do that. If that were you I would do everything I could first to make sure that, to give you every chance to recover or survive. ..." Nancy's response to her daughter's views was pragmatic. It would be helpful because, "I mean, it wasn't really about Terri Schiavo" it was about her daughter. "It was kind of this whole unplugged scenario." With a little bit of digging she had discerned that Maggie had a point of view. As Nancy summed it up, "she had an opinion."

But Nancy was not done looking for guidance on what to do next. She recalled that Maggie had written a paper in college about her desire to become a veterinarian. It had included a paragraph on euthanasia and euthanizing animals. Nancy called Smith to see if they could send her the paper, because "I didn't have any other way of accessing it." In the paper, Maggie expressed "great admiration for her mentor" in veterinary medicine "who had euthanized animals." But Nancy noted that Maggie was cautious in her endorsement. She suggested an incremental approach and argued that "before she would make that decision she would give them any number or a different number of ways to succeed ... like, to get better."

In the paper, Maggie argued that, "she would try medication or she would try physical or loving care, or just anything that she could think of." But she would consider the euthanasia option if the animal did not have "quality of life." In Maggie's view euthanasia was a tough choice, "but after trying as many ideas as she could think of she would make that hard decision." The paper's logic and ethical framing of the options was very important to Nancy's thinking about Maggie and whether to continue to advocate for ongoing care or to pull back and let nature take its course.

Like Maggie's need to exhaust all the therapeutic options before making an alternative choice, Nancy felt that there was more to do and that it was premature to pull back on her daughter's care. Maggie's conversations with friends and her written work "really pointed to my decision." Nancy concluded that, "Both of those things were my daughter's voice saying 'I would try pretty damn hard first before I would make end-of-life decisions.'"

INSIDER KNOWLEDGE

It was a tough decision because most of the prognostication was either grim or tempered only by a glimmer of hope. One doctor "said there was maybe a five percent chance that she would have a significant recovery or a meaningful recovery, which might mean that she could feed herself, or possibly have some motor abilities, and perhaps some speech."

But one doctor's counsel stood out as special. It came from a physician who also had a family member with severe brain injury. He approached Nancy and asked if he "could get personal" and share a story about his brother who had a severe brain injury. Tentatively, he told Nancy, "I will tell you my story if you like." She acquiesced and he did. His brother had recovered some basic functions, could feed himself, say a few words but "had temper tantrums like three year olds do and had a lot of behavior issues."

Nancy took it all in, trying to be balanced in her assessment of all the options. Even at that early stage in Maggie's recovery, she had the sense that an alternative view existed about what might be possible and that she should at least hear what her options might be if she continued to provide care. And in this regard, the doctor's comments about his brother were helpful. They were shared not to guide but to inform. Reflecting on the doctor's candor about his brother, Nancy felt "he was not saying what to do; he was just saying that" in his case it was the only thing to do because "his mother was so passionate about taking care of her son." And it was because of his mother's orientation toward care that their family's decision "was the right thing to do."

The doctor was urging Nancy to look inward and see where her own moral compass would direct her. But at the same time, he was not romanticizing the challenge ahead. He was going to be his brother's guardian when his mother passed away and he knew full well it was going to be difficult. These choices were not for the faint of heart. Nancy appreciated his honesty. He told her, "it was going to be very hard and he was just giving me another sort of ... look, but sort of a realistic, stark look. ..." It was a view of the future that was hard to hear but would be vitally important to Nancy and many others.

BACK CHANNEL COMMUNICATION

This sort of insider knowledge of brain injury – the sharing of a family's experience or questioning physician pronouncements about prognosis by nursing staff and other caregivers – was not uncommon amongst the families interviewed and should not go unnoticed. Early on Nancy was influenced by the story of the doctor and his brother. Later she would be guided by the physician assistant who urged her to press on and make the journey to Cornell to participate in our research efforts.

Other families have experienced highly pivotal "back channel" communications that have altered care decisions and often added a contrarian view to physician assertions about likely outcomes beyond the party line of unbridled nihilism. These informal advisors often provide a needed corrective to prevailing views in the clinic that may border on the ideological or assume a level of scientific certainty about outcomes that available data does not support.

Among the many dialogues was one shared by Rachel McIntrye. She remained in the dark about her husband Darren's brain injury and why he remained unconscious after routine surgery. But there was a physician-patient in the adjoining room who helped to interpret her husband's course. Rachel explains, "Nobody knew what had happened, or so they said. I wasn't getting any stories. Luckily there was a patient next door who was a doctor. He was in renal failure, and I got friendly with the family."

The chief of cardiology at another hospital, he told Rachel "to get all the tapes and the paperwork from the OR, that I was entitled to them being his wife, that I want the originals I don't want copies, and to request that they do not throw the tapes away from the monitors from the OR. So I did all of that, and they actually had to sit in the room with me while I reviewed them all, and I allowed this guy to look at them also."

Others had informal intercessions outside of the normal channels of communication. Kathie Manwiller, whose son Dustin was in the vegetative state recalls being helped by a nurse practitioner who took her aside to chat. Until that time she had been confused by the relationship between Dustin's injuries and the vegetative state. He had fractured his occipital bone and had an injury to his brainstem.

In Kathie's view, the vegetative state was, "laying in a coma the rest of their lives. Laying, staring out into space and drooling was what I had in mind." But when she tried to get more information, more clarity – from the doctor "we renamed Dr. Doom and Gloom" – she got less detail and more certainty about the grim diagnosis. "Every time that we would ask specific questions ... the answer would always be, 'we don't know, you never know, nobody really knows enough about the brain and the healing process about the brain and everything.' "

She was frustrated, "They couldn't give you an answer. Like if we were to say, 'well do you think he'll come out the coma?' " The response would invariably be, "We don't know." But there was an inconsistency to the doctor's profession of indeterminacy. She understood "... that really nobody knows, and every single person is different" but at the same time did not understand how he could be so certain that he would end up in the vegetative state. The paradox was that there was so much certainty on the downside of the prognosis and so, "*I wasn't understanding why is he telling me that he's going to be in a vegetative state.*"

It was a nurse practitioner who interceded to provide an explanation and admit the uncertainty that physicians treating disorders of consciousness often have a hard time acknowledging. She provided a more tempered explanation, when it was especially needed. "She came in and it just was after one of my visits with the doctor and I was just really upset and wondering why he would say these things. And she showed me the MRI and was showing me the spots where it showed actual dead brain tissue. I mean, even though right now I feel like I could probably be a nurse, I still don't understand all the particulars."

The nurse consoled Kathie and left open the possibility of a more promising scenario, acknowledging our inability to fully predict outcomes. She told Kathie, "No one really knows, and all you can do is be there to support your son and what will be will be, and there's no reason to get yourself into a state that nothing good's ever going to come of this at this point, because who knows?"

Kathie appreciated the nurse's candor and balanced approach to disclosure. "She was honest too; she wasn't actually saying 'oh it's no big deal.' She said 'yes, he did suffer a very bad injury, there is brain damage, but we can't tell you definitively he'll never do this, he'll never do that, he will do this, he will do that, because really, I don't think we can.' " As we will see, it was wise and prophetic counsel.

Sometimes communication was influenced by some sort of identification with the caregiver, a countertransference that turned the injured patient into an object of shared concern and not merely a hopeless case for which there was an implicit duty to die. One physician-mother, whose son was the same age as Darren McIntyre, also reached out to Rachel.

Rachel understood what was motivating the doctor's concern, "It hit her close to home because she had a son his age ... so she was really much more compassionate." The contrast between the first doctor who "had no bedside manner whatsoever" and the second was striking. The physician-mother "was much more compassionate, and she sat with my sister and I and his mother and spoke really just with tears in her eyes." And like other professionals whose communication was informed by a degree of identification or countertransference, she was also more open-ended about possible outcomes.

She told the McIntyres, "You know, it's only been a few weeks, stranger things have happened to people who are in this state and if you don't try you'll never know."

A final example of back channel communication was between nurses and the physician-mother of a teen with brain injury. Even as physicians "weren't really talking to us," "avoiding us," "passing by in the hallway," and never having a conference with the family, the patient's nurses were making a video of the teen's behaviors (eye opening and laughter) to document what might be indicative of his potential improvement.

When asked, if the nurses took this upon themselves, the patient's mother told us they did and that they received more support from them than the physicians "who would shrug their shoulders say, 'no change, no change, no change.'" This mother, a physician herself, reports that, "They were much more hopeful [than the doctors]. The nursing staff, well the nurses and the nurses' aides all had stories for us of people who they had seen get better, who they had seen improve, who they had seen wake up. And you know, of course we clung to those stories."

While we do not have systematic data on the prevalence of these communications, they do seem to occur at a level that warrants additional study both for their frequency and their utility. If they do occur with sufficient frequency they add a dimension of complexity to an already fraught sphere of communication, potentially undermining the advice and counsel of those professionals charged with breaking bad news and delineating treatment options and prognosis. But if these back channel conversations occur frequently, their prevalence also begs the question regarding why they are needed and why they take place defying usual clinical etiquette if not ethics.

It seems that many of the clinicians who break ranks with colleagues to speak with families more openly – and in their view more honestly – do so because of a sense of moral obligation. Silence would be akin to complicity and they may have the felt need to balance what has been said with less dire predictions. Although their emotional proximity to the patient or their family's plight may create distortions that overestimate prognosis, there is value in diversifying the conversation. This will help achieve balance in the deliberative process and assist with decision making, all the more so if all perspectives could be stated explicitly and those with a contrarian point of view made as part of the medical record.

FELT GOOD ABOUT MY DECISION

Whatever the source, Nancy felt that she benefited from these alternate vectors of communication. She valued the input of the young doctor who brought his personal story forward and then the physician's assistant who urged her to replace the trach tube so she could bring Maggie to Manhattan.

But Nancy was most empowered by Maggie's own thoughts as conveyed through a college essay and comments with friends about Terri Schiavo. Informed by her best sense of her daughter's prior wishes, Nancy felt up to a confrontation with the doctor who was urging that she let Maggie go. Nancy recalls the tone of their discussions, "He and I actually had a respectful argument and he was very forceful." Like those "back channel" communicators, who some might say were more optimistic than warranted, this physician's advice carried distortions in the other direction. Not just in content but in tenor. Nancy was "shocked at how forceful he was."

But Nancy was equally firm because she had investigated her daughter's wishes and had a sense of how to proceed. She recalls, "I was extremely forceful because ... I just felt good about my decision. I had two voices from my daughter that were helping me make the decision." And there was one more thing beyond her daughter's views. It was also the possibility of her progress, "and there were glimmers of hope."

Part of Nancy's reticence about letting go was her uncertainty, "I just didn't feel I could let her go because there was just not enough information." She wanted to hedge her bets. On the one hand, she looked to the future of what might be, if only she would wait. Might her daughter ever think again? Unbeknownst to us, might she even be thinking now, even at this early juncture? And if not, could her broken brain be fixed? But, on the other hand, she did not want to perpetuate a situation that was getting worse.

We routinely asked family members about their loved one's code status, that is, if their heart were to stop or breathing ceased, would they want the patient to be resuscitated. I was really astonished that Nancy had agreed to a DNR order for Maggie as she was getting ready to leave the hospital and go to rehabilitation. After all her resistance to doctors entreaties to withdraw life support by removing the ventilator, I thought she would be as adamant in demanding resuscitation, as some of her doctors were in urging that care be withdrawn. But Nancy made a critical distinction between appropriate actions amidst an unclear prognosis – where Maggie was at the time – and what might be called for if she were to have a cardiac arrest.

She thought it out very carefully. A cardiac arrest would also result in an incremental injury that could make brain function worse and could even cause death. After I confirmed that I had heard her correctly, Nancy told me her feelings about a DNR order. "I didn't have any problem with that because I felt if her heart stopped then that's it, she was dead. ... I didn't feel uncomfortable with that."

PULLED THEM AWAY LIKE DOGS

But beyond the DNR decision, Nancy drew the line, demanding care for her child and resisting what is euphemistically called "organ harvesting."

Prompted by her DNR designation for her daughter, she was visited by a social worker who "said there were people from the organ donation society that would like to speak with me, if I was willing."

Her initial response to the request was positive. "This was during the time where it was sort of touch and go … within like the first two or three days." Nancy "did like the idea that if she was going to die" that something good might come of it. Told that Maggie was "perfectly healthy" and that "her eyes and her liver and her kidneys and her heart" were suitable for transplant, she thought, "wouldn't that be great. …." It was a silver lining.

But as Maggie's condition improved and the prospect of an inevitable death receded into the background, Nancy began to rethink her willingness to turn Maggie into an organ donor.

"But then there was another moment, I think I was making a different decision, maybe it was when I was going to do the rehabilitation route" when the organ transplantation folks returned. "They came back and the social worker kind of pulled them away like dogs, 'Get away from her.' It was sort of a strange moment, because I was so vulnerable that I just was like, 'what are you talking about? Get away from her.' … it was difficult."

Like the surrogates for Trish Meili, the Central Park jogger,[1] and other families I have spoken with, Nancy had come face to face with the enthusiastic "harvesting" of organ procurement teams that occasionally fail to appreciate the ongoing needs of critically ill patients – and the incipient bereavement of families – as they look to a brain-injured patient to provide life-saving organs to others.

A CALL FOR TEMPERANCE

While I laud the intent of the transplant community to save others, I have worried that procurement requests, which are mandated by the Center for Medicare and Medicaid Services regulations,[2] too quickly shift the professional obligations of clinicians from current/real patients to future/potential ones. While organ donation is a noble and worthy endeavor, it should be one that can be achieved while also respecting the rights of patients with severe brain injury, their potential for recovery, and the vulnerabilities of their surrogates. The needs of these patients may stand in opposition to some of the policies pursued by the mainstream organ donation community if we fail to appreciate how easily a patient can be recast into a potential donor.[3]

Federal regulations mandate that hospitals notify organ procurement organizations of the impending death of a possible organ donor as a condition of continued Medicare participation.[4] While the timing of such a notification may be obvious when a patient is manifestly dying, sometimes an impending death can be in the eye of the beholder and based upon judgments about the appropriateness of withholding or withdrawing life support.

Given the complex legacy of Henry K. Beecher and organ donation, and the tight linkage between the evolution of the death and dying movement and severe brain injury, it should not come as a surprise that many patients with disorders of consciousness may fall prey to a view that their death is imminent and that their case be reportable for what is euphemistically described as organ harvesting.

Too often, these patients are viewed as if they were destined to die, even when their prospects for recovery are not exhausted. As an ethics consultant at an academic medical center, I have sometimes seen Organ Procurement Organization (OPO) representatives hover in the ICU, waiting to swoop in – as some critical care physicians have described the process – and claim organs that they viewed as rightly theirs for transplant to others, as if an entitlement.[3]

Hover is a strong word, but Nancy's depiction of the social worker pulling away the OPO representatives "like dogs" is equally powerful. It is an image coming from the mother of an injured child, who is vulnerable to prognostic mischaracterization and the bureaucratic and regulatory forces that seek to increase organ retrieval. Her depiction, and the experiences of others, who report zealous procurement efforts should give us pause and prompt questions about the requisite degree of certainty that should be necessary to deem a patient, with a disorder of consciousness, as imminently dying and thus reportable to the OPO.

Families, who we interviewed, whose loved ones were categorized as reportable, ask with hindsight, sometimes years later, how could such prognostications have been so wrong? Although the level of recovery may be far below what was hoped for, their loved one's longevity belies the designation of imminently dying. Their concerns are justified by scholarship that speaks to our inability to prognosticate accurately in generic medical contexts[5] and the fact that outcomes in brain injury can depend upon decisions made to withhold or withdraw life-sustaining therapies,[6] actions that can be prompted solely by the loss of consciousness, a hallmark of severe brain injury.

Given the possibility of some brain injury patients to be mislabeled as potential donors, it would seem prudent to revisit current procurement practices to mitigate what might be called *premature harvesting* before a patient's prognosis is clearer. Although comatose patients who have herniated or are near herniation (in which the swollen brain presses down into the base of the skull and through the *foramen magnum* where the brainstem and the spine connect) can be said to have a fatal outcome or dire one at best, other patients in coma retain the potential for a range of recoveries.

To accommodate this range of possible outcomes and to decrease the pressure placed on expectant families, I would suggest that we develop consensus views about which patients who are in a coma should be identified for possible organ donation and those who may need additional time or studies to assess more fully. Prognostication for these patients should be sufficiently clear enough to warrant asking the question about donation. But for other patients in a coma, a call for temperance is more prudent and risk stratification is indicated.

Although this recommendation may appear to limit the retrieval of some organs acutely, suggesting this "time out" may increase overall yield by two mechanisms affecting patients and families. Here are two hypotheses that could warrant future empirical studies. The first relates to family attitudes.

Families may view the organ procurement procedure more favorably if the donative question is not immediately admixed with the shock and grief, which immediately follows an injury. The early alienation of surrogate decision makers is not in the interest of subsequent organ retrievals. Many of these patients will remain potential donors because of the gravity of their condition. Better to pause at the outset, avoid inappropriate donations when the outcome is unclear, and preserve the opportunity for more constructive solicitations at a later date.

How and when patients emerge from a coma can convey prognostic information that can aid surrogate decisions about medical care. Delaying donations to this clinical juncture, save for the most catastrophic of injuries or when a patient's or family's wishes would direct otherwise, can more fully engage families in the deliberative process. This brings more integrity to the donative act and helps ensure that decisions are neither forced nor coerced. With additional time and more evidence of an injury's prognostic path, surrogates are more likely to obtain the requisite amount of information necessary to make a considered judgment. Taken together, these reforms help to achieve a level of informed altruism for the donative act, a standard, which is morally good for both the patient's family and the potential beneficiary of a transplant. It ratifies the authenticity of the donative choice for the former, and it ensures that gratitude, not guilt, informs the views of the recipient.

There are also advantages for those professionals engaged in organ donation. A delay in solicitation may also change the dynamic between clinicians and OPO officials who can have contentious, and even adversarial relations with their local procurement agencies, according to a survey of practice patterns conducted by the Office of the Inspector General in the Department of Health and Human Services.[4] Reforming the procurement process in this way, for these especially vulnerable patients, may engender more trust and cooperation amongst clinicians and their OPOs. As significantly, it may decrease a personal sense of dual agency felt by intensive care clinicians who must shift their allegiance from their current patient to a hypothetical organ recipient. Taking these patients off the donative table, at least during a period of heightened prognostic indeterminacy, may lessen these feelings and lead to more cooperative practices benefiting both current and future patients.

COGNITION?

Of course none of these suggested reforms marked Nancy's experience, made all the more difficult because the request for organ donation came at a really difficult time. With the specter of death receding, Nancy was now trying to weigh new information about Maggie's prognosis, information that would indeed haunt her and ultimately bring her to New York for our study.

She was first hearing from her neurologist about a recently described condition, the minimally conscious state (MCS), in which patients are conscious, but liminally so. This was the first hopeful news she had received, so she held fast to it. It was a slim chance and most of the doctors "weren't hopeful" but neither were they "willing to rule out the possibility of ... her being minimally conscious, or possibly have cognition of some kind."

Nancy admits that her memory is hazy of the particulars but the possibility of consciousness was something that she remembered. It was so very important to her, "and so I kind of held on to that." And though she might have first heard of the minimally conscious state later in Maggie's course, she knows that, "they used the word cognition" and I "had to ask them what that meant."

To answer Nancy's question we need to travel back a few years to a little hamlet a few hours from Little Rock. There, a common car accident made uncommon history.

7   Something Happened in Arkansas

Terry Wallis and his friend Chubb Moore were driving their pickup truck in the Ozarks during the early morning of July 13, 1984. There had been drinking and there was a crash. No one knows who was at the wheel, but as Terry's mother Angilee Wallis told us, it was a bad wreck, "one of the boys was thrown from the car and the other was hanging out the window." They were taken to Harrison Hospital and then medevaced to St. John's Hospital in Springfield, Missouri.

During the four-hour car ride to Springfield, Angilee did not know if when she arrived she would find her son alive, "... they just told us that they were really sick boys and they didn't know if they'd be alive when we got there or not. And they did tell us ... that he had a head injury, but *at the time* they had Terry and Chubb confused ... they didn't have wallets on them or I don't know exactly what it was."

Angilee took it that Terry was doing better than Chubb and that Terry's friend was the one with the head injury. She recalls, "... on the way to Springfield I was sitting in the back seat with Chubb's mother and I thought, I couldn't imagine Terry laying even in bed, I couldn't imagine him even being in the hospital because he was always huntin', and fishin', and mechanicin', just an outdoor person. And I was feeling really bad for Chubb's mother because they were talking about how bad he was ... I was feeling, actually feeling guilty because I was so happy Terry wasn't hurt as bad as Chubb was. Even though they said both of them was hurt really bad."

When the families arrived at the hospital it soon became apparent that the boys had been mixed up. Terry was more grievously injured. Angilee was not angered by the error, she was grateful that Terry was still alive, but not yet registering the significance of his having sustained a brain injury.

Ironically, Chubb died during the first week. Terry ended up in the ICU, comatose. His course was fairly typical. He opened his eyes and moved out of the coma and into the vegetative state about three weeks after his injury. His parents were at his bedside, attentive, vigilant, and ever dutiful.

A FAMILY'S EMBRACE

Given the gravity of his condition, Angilee was approached by his doctors about making Terry DNR. Though she "did wonder a lot," she just could not agree to not have her son resuscitated. She put it colloquially, "I just couldn't cut him out." It is a decision that she still thinks about all these years later, "What bothers me so much was ... did I make the right decision?"

Terry had never spoken about end-of-life issues; so ultimately, it came down to her tight-knit family and a question of process and dialogue. "Well I would," she corrects herself, "we would just sit together, the family, and just talk, you know, just talk about it to see what everybody's thinking." That was what "we did, and we still do."

"We would just sit together" is a lovely phrase that speaks volumes about the families who informed our study. They are tight and have this inner focus. The world is within their families, not beyond their walls. It is a kind of preoccupation with loved ones that I have called *familio-centric*, for lack of a better phrase. But there is an enmeshment, a kind of love, that grieves less for what has been lost than values what still remains, finding meaning in disability.

Psychologists looking at couples have examined how the amount of merging of one's self with a partner leads to marital satisfaction or dissatisfaction.[1] The degree of satisfaction is linked to the degree of "self-expansion" or personal growth that one partner gains in their relationship with their mate: new tastes, broader interests, and the like. If your partner makes you grow and be happier, he or she assumes a greater import in your life and hence you are tied more closely to each other.

The parallel here, and the paradox, is the importance that a patient has with his or her family before an injury. If those relationships are self-expanding – to borrow the jargon – there is a strong carryover effect that continues to prize the loved one, even if he or she can no longer fulfill old roles and reciprocate affections. These relationships are marked by loyalty, and deep and sustained concern for the injured patient.

This pattern is different than most families I have encountered in the nearly twenty years I have done ethics consults. In the setting of a profound brain injury, most families demonstrate their fidelity and love by making decisions to minimize the pain and suffering experienced by the patient and the family unit. To be blunt, but not judgmental, they "cut their losses," profound loses that they cannot bear. These families, who are not represented in the sample we interviewed, are the majority of American families, who when confronted by medical catastrophe make decisions to withhold or withdraw care.

While the sociology, or better yet the psychology, of medical decision making is not dichotomous, I suspect that there is a cohort of families who view their choices – and ethical obligations – differently. Informed by past experiences and relationships, they constitute a segment of the population who will need a different approach when confronting severe brain injury. Misunderstood, their demands can escalate into conflicts and disputes over the utility, or futility, of medical care,[2] complicating conversations in the intensive care setting that can be fraught.[3]

But if their style of decision making is identified prospectively, and early in the course of the dialectic that occurs between practitioners and families, their needs can be better met. By reversing the presumption, indeed the prevailing expectation, that a frank conversation will lead to a decision to withhold or withdraw care, practitioners can better place themselves in the place of the "other" and see the case from the vantage point of a bereaved spouse or stricken parent. Seen from their perspective, and from the relational orientation from which their views stem, requests for care, felt "futile" by practitioners, may become comprehensible, though sometimes medically untenable.

However, a family's embrace of a disabled state as a life worth living can point to the need to recalibrate clinical metrics of outcome that fail to adequately distinguish severe disability states, in which the patient is conscious, from death or the vegetative state. Without such discrimination a prognostic conflation occurs that can undermine informed choices by families.[4] These insights can then help physicians and family members find shared meaning about care decisions and lead to contextualized and proportionate care, that is, a risk-benefit approach that fits within a familio-centric value system and is less distorted by prevailing ideology.

This does not mean that practitioners should be compelled to provide inappropriate medical care that is harmful, unproven, or futile. Rather, the goal is to acknowledge a differing value system, intrinsic to some families, without necessarily accommodating it so as to maintain robust channels of communication at critical junctures.

These hypotheses on decision-making styles undertaken by some families warrant additional empirical study,[5,6] but a first step is to appreciate that there is likely a minority cohort that weighs its choices differently. To overlook these families is an error of omission that can lead to pain and ethically consequential actions that can violate the dynamic core of how these families operate, leaving psychic scars that can persist long after bodily ones have healed.

To illustrate the point, all we need to do is recall Angilee's reaction when she was asked to donate Terry's organs, should he die. A family that "would just sit together," as a unit, could not break up that *circle of friends*, to borrow a line from the late folk singer, Phil Ochs. Mrs. Wallis told me, "... it's kind of cold you know. Like I know that's when they have to ask, but when you're right at your worst, and then they say 'if he dies would you want to sign up, would you want to donate the parts?'"

While others anticipated Terry's death, in her eyes, Angilee was still looking forward to getting her son out of the hospital and, yes, back home.

LIGHTEN UP

During the four months they were in the hospital, Angilee was hopeful that the doctors would lighten up on Terry's medications and he would come out of his slumber when they made their rounds. Decades later she is wistful recalling that "I just wanted him to wake up so bad, wanted to just hear his voice." And like so many family members, she wanted him to not feel lost or abandoned, "for him to know that I was there" and as importantly for her to appreciate, "to *know* that he knew I was there."

No one could address her concerns or speak to her desires. The doctors would tell her that "we don't know what he knows, you know, we don't know how bad he is." They did tell her that Terry was given pain medications to provide relief from the swelling in his brain. This worried Angilee who "... actually thought ... right from the start that the coma was *from* medication."

Three weeks after his accident Terry did open his eyes but was not following commands. Presumptively in a vegetative state, he was soon dispatched to a nursing home because "... they started trying to do therapy and stuff like that, and of course he wasn't responding. And then they just, like in two weeks, they said 'he's not responding fast enough so he's got to go to a nursing home.'"

Angilee tried to keep him in the hospital for additional evaluation but the doctors would not have it. Their logic was simple. They told the Wallis family that Terry was "not improving, he's not improving enough to keep him here." And their threshold for improvement was quite high, "they said actually what they try to do is to get" patients "to where they can rejoin the workforce. And Terry was not improving."

One nurse confided, "I'm not supposed to tell you this, but they had put him out on the floor" and tried therapy, but to no avail. He was unreachable, she told Mrs. Wallis, "He's too deep in to be responsive." It was a futile situation. Almost apologetically, she asked Angilee, "You know, what I mean?"

Mrs. Wallis was heartbroken to learn that now no one would help Terry get better, or even try anymore. "I guess that was one of the hardest things, the feeling that they'd given up." There was nothing more to be done at the hospital, "so that's why he had to go to the nursing home."

SOMETHING HAPPENED IN ARKANSAS 63

LEISURE LODGE

In October, after four months at St. John's Hospital, Terry was discharged to
a nursing home, the Leisure Lodge in Searcy, Arkansas. Angilee's sister had
found the place near where she lived. Although social workers "... had called
around, I mean, they were trying as far as I remember, they were trying to find
a place I guess, but mainly it was up to us."

At that time he needed what is euphemistically called "placement" in a
skilled facility because he had a trach. Like Karen Ann Quinlan, his eyes were
open but "he wasn't focusing or anything like that." Although the Wallis
family did not yet know the term, he left the hospital with the blank stare of
the vegetative state, off the ventilator but with a tracheostomy and feeding
tube in place.

Angilee was finally able to find a place closer to her home for Terry
in July 1985 so she "could pop in anytime." She visited regularly, coming
from factory work where she made shirts for the U.S. Navy.[7] On weekends
she would bring Terry home. "I just wanted to keep on talking to him,
taking him home. It just got to be a routine. It is what we did, but I can't
say I really thought he would get better. ... It just got to be a routine."[7]
Thus began a nearly twenty-year vigil that would culminate with Terry's
"awakening" on June 11, 2003 when he spoke his first word in nearly two
decades.

JUST STOPPED DEAD

It began innocently enough.[8] Terry was in the cafeteria with a caregiver and
had finished with lunch when Angilee came in to visit. It was a Wednesday
afternoon, and she had gotten a new job at a shirt factory near town and
came in to make a surprise visit with Terry and check the care he was receiving: "... they had most of the residents back in their rooms, but they had left
Terry and a few of them sitting there, and they were cleaning tables and this
girl, Pam, was cleaning a table and I walked in and she said, 'Terry, who's that
old woman coming through there?' ... she all the time asked him stuff like
that just because, mostly teasing me. And Terry said 'mom' I mean just like
that 'Mom.'"

Angilee did not know what to say and wondered if he had done this
before. She looked to the attendant to gauge her reaction and saw an equal
look of surprise. No one expected this.

"And I just stopped dead, and she just stopped, and I looked at her and
she looked at me. I thought maybe he had done that before and she was surprising me, I mean, that was just a real quick thought. It wasn't though, but
anyway, I looked at her and when I seen the look on her face, on Terry's,
I knew that that was just a big surprise to everybody, you know."

Even Terry seemed surprised. As his mother tried to coax him to repeat himself, Terry had a sense something was going on that was special. Angilee recalls, "We tried to get him to say, and he looked like it just really surprised him. ... His eyes were big, and I don't know." Soon all the kitchen aides had clustered about, all asking Terry questions that could be answered with "mom." As Angilee recalls, "He would answer 'mom,' you know. He would answer the questions because it was always something with mom. ... Of course, no telling how many times he was asked who I was."

When I asked Angilee how she felt when she first heard Terry say her name, she responded by asking me if I had kids, presumably because the feeling she had is only one that a parent could fully understand. When I responded affirmatively she continued, "You know when they say 'mom' or 'dad' for the first time? It just really tickles you, you know, they said 'mom' or 'dad.' Well, this is fifty times more than that. Because you're really, honestly expecting a kid, a baby to say 'mom' or 'dad,' you know eventually they will. But someone like Terry, you're *hoping*, but when it really happens, it's, it's big. Does that make any sense?" It did. I suggested it was something like a second childhood. "Right, Exactly."

A MOM AGAIN

And with that admission came a deeper reemergence, that of the regaining of her own objective self as a mother of a son who could now communicate with her. After all those years of silent vigil, of *hoping that this would happen long after everyone else had given up hope*, Angilee was in the eyes of others, a mom again. His words were as transformative for her as they were for him. That part of her identity that went dark when Terry was silent was reignited when his voice emerged and reciprocal relationships were retrieved from some distant past.

It was a precious retrieval, like an elusive jewel whose rediscovery immediately engenders fear that it could be lost again. And now it was too valuable to be lost again, not after nineteen years.

Angilee's elation came with a real sense of fear that this moment was going to be fleeting, a very thin thread connecting her to her long-lost, but now very present, son. "Of course, I was afraid that it was just a short-lived thing."

"I, I couldn't, I could *never* explain how I felt then. It was kind of like, you know, I didn't believe it, but I heard it. But it, it just tickled me to death. I just didn't really know ... 'cause I hadn't heard that for so long. But ... it wasn't like I thought he was going to continue talking. That's why we kept talking." So, Angilee tried to keep the momentum going.

Even in the early days of Terry's emergence, it became clear that the familiarity and emotional valence of hearing his *mother's* voice had a greater likelihood to engender recognition and a response. "We just kept asking him questions that day. Of course Pam came over and there were several there in the lunch room and I was just sitting down there by the chair, and we was all ganging around the table and just asking him questions, anything he could answer with 'mom.'" Angilee also tried to get Terry to say Pam's name. She stayed there for several hours, and by the time she left was pretty sure Terry did say her name too.

HE LOVED PEPSI SO

Angilee took Terry home that Friday for his weekly visit. She was trying to encourage him to talk but all this was so new to her. Without any help from a speech therapist, Angilee was trying to tutor her son back to fluency, "I didn't really know how to get him to try to say something. But I told him Pepsi, tried to get him to say anything we thought was easy, might be easy for him to say ... he loved Pepsi so well, and he would just make a noise, so I know he was trying to say Pepsi. That was on Friday."

The next morning Angilee was making breakfast and she asked him what he wanted to drink and he surprised her and initiated his own response. "... I thought he'd say Pepsi because I'd been trying to get him to. And he said 'milk.' Which I had not even thought about, even asking him about milk."

On the Saturday before Father's Day, Terry said "dad." By Monday, June 16, he could tell his nurse his birthday, but curiously he did not know how old he was. He asked to call his grandmother and recalled her phone number. The only problem was that it was a phone number from 1984. In fact, for Terry it *was* 1984. In his mind Reagan was still president and his deceased grandmother was still alive.[9] He had lost his sense of time.

Terry was still Terry, but different. He was always a prankster according to his mother and "... now he is all the time teasing somebody about something."[7] But now he was also a bit disinhibited and uncensored. He told a pious Aunt that he was "horny" to the mortification of his mother.[7,9] His sister, Tammy, gently reminds him, "You know you are not supposed to do that."[7]

REALITY CHECK

Within days, Terry's awakening had done more than arouse the sleepy town of Mountain View, it had become international news. Although media accounts described him as awaking from a coma after nineteen years, or being vegetative up to when he began to speak, in actuality, he was responsive at times within the first year of injury. In fact, as Angilee recalls it, within three to five months he seemed to be following things happening in his room.[8]

The family had their doubts that Terry was unconscious because of behaviors that would jolt them from their expectations and leave them wondering if there was more there; that despite appearances, there was a conscious being inside an inert body. His subsequent awakening was a confirmation of all that they thought they had observed over the preceding decades.

Terry's father, Jerry asked that he be seen by a neurologist and was told that an evaluation would be too expensive. "They told us it would cost $120,000 just to evaluate him to see if he could be helped, and we didn't have that kind of money."[10] His father told CNN that, "They said the government will not put out that kind of money on no more chance than he's got to re-enter the workforce."[10]

Angilee noted, "Anytime we would go in, we would turn a light on or off, or try to get him to follow something with his eyes, and ... we thought there were times that he was doing it. But he wouldn't hold; he wouldn't look at it for very long. So you don't know for sure if it was because his eyes would move anyway. So we didn't know for sure if he was doing that purposefully. Because he didn't do it consistently."

Terry did seem to respond more consistently to his grandfather, Andy, with whom he had always had a playful and raucous relationship. Just before Christmas 1984, Terry may have even said Andy's name. "And course he [Andy] was hollering and just like talking to him, we talked to him just like he knew everything that was going on. And Terry did look at him when he said, I don't know, I'm sure he called his name. But Terry did look at him. And then we got to moving things in front of him to see for sure that he was following it, and he was."

In retrospect, Angilee recalls being happy that Terry was responsive but disappointed that the nurses did not believe her accounts because they were unexpected and not reproducible on command, "... he didn't do it all the time and if we would say anything like to the nurses, or anything, like that he responded well or something like that, it was like they thought we were crazy." The clinical staff chalked it up to denial, to wishful thinking: "... they thought that we was seeing it because we wanted to."

Angilee was angered by the indifference of staff to her observations and the lack of a proper evaluation after she had seen patterns of behavior that could no longer be attributed to random chance, but had to be accountable to some degree of intent. After all, she spent more time with Terry than anyone else. How come no one was listening and taking her seriously?

"I read to him, and talked to him, and just, we would just have conversations and sit around him just like, just like he was there with ... like he was talking to us or whatever. But he would turn his head, and I was thinking that it was because he was listening. ... But he would move his head some-times just because, I guess. But when I would see things that I thought he was doing, I wasn't positive ... but I was pretty sure that he was, until I'd see it several times ... he would see a doctor if he was sick, or maybe once a month. But as far as him seeing a neurologist or anything, he didn't." That would only happen when he started talking.

THINK TO LISTEN

Although labeled as permanently unconscious, in retrospect it seems quite likely that Terry had been aware, lying there in a minimally conscious state since late in 1984. A terrifying story from as early as 1993 provides a glimpse of what might have been Wallis's inner experience at that time. Nearly a decade after his accident, and ten years before he began to speak, Terry's nurs-ing home roommate died. According to Angilee, one of Terry's aides was con-cerned that Terry had been disturbed by the overnight events despite the fact that he was still diagnosed as being vegetative and therefore should have been unaware of his surroundings.

"I can remember this, and I can't remember when it was, but it was a long time ago, there was a man in Terry's room, of course you know they changed several times, there was this real old guy in Terry's room, and one of the aides called me from work one morning and told me that she was not supposed to do that but ... that man had passed away in the night, and that it had bothered Terry."

The incident happened more than twenty years ago, so precisely what happened isn't known. Angilee remembers that, "... there was a big contro-versy over the man dying later. He was strangled by the bed somehow or something, because there was this lawsuit come up later." From our perspec-tive, the circumstances of the death – as unclear and as unfortunate as they were – matter less than Terry's response. And vegetative patients should not be responding to their environments.

Angilee recalls that the nurse's "... aide called me from work and told me not to tell that she called but I needed to be down there. Terry was laying there ... it was sometime in the night when the man died, and Terry was laying there with his eyes open wide, he would not go to sleep, I mean, he was making no noise or anything at that time. But I stayed there with him most all day until he finally went to sleep. So I don't know what he saw, but I know that he saw something. And I know that it had, *now*, I knew then it had to be something that was really bad. But how it stuck with him, I don't know. I've wondered about that a lot. Why that would be so traumatic for him for that long, when I know now that his short-term memory is so bad."

One can only imagine Terry's horror of watching the accident and the profound isolation of lying there paralyzed, perhaps understanding what had happened, or just part of it, having no way to share his terror. He was alone with his thoughts, such as they were, because he could neither communicate them nor find anyone who would think to listen.

8   From PVS to MCS

Beyond all the media hype, and faux explications invoking all manner of pseudo-science, how could a patient, like Terry, diagnosed as vegetative for so long, recover so dramatically? There were emerging prognostic rules about such things, and Terry had seemingly broken all of them, regaining consciousness so late in the game. No one came out of the vegetative state after nineteen years. It was *impossible*, and not what the experts had agreed upon back in 1994 when a definitive set of consensus papers were published in the *New England Journal of Medicine* by leading representatives of clinical societies concerned with brain states.

Under the banner of a "Multi-Society Task Force," these expert neurologists, physiatrists, neurosurgeons, and others laid out such parameters about the vegetative state. A central feature of their deliberations was the recognition that brain injuries were not inherently fixed and immutable, but sometimes brain states could, over time, lead to the recovery of consciousness.

They agreed that when a vegetative state continues beyond thirty days, it is described as *persistent* and that permanence sets in three months after anoxic injury (severe oxygen deprivation) and twelve months after the insult resulted from trauma.[1,2] Presciently, the authors of the document worried about being too definitive about predictions, accounting for the possibility of both error and ignorance of our future state of knowledge. To their credit, they hedged just a bit on the question of permanence, making it a more probabilistic statement than an outright certainty. In a brilliant distinction they observed that:

> As originally defined by Jennett and Plum in 1972, the term "persistent," when applied to the vegetative state, meant sustained over time; "permanent" meant irreversible. Notwithstanding Jennett and Plum's precise use of language, confusion has arisen over the exact meaning of the term "persistent." The adjective "persistent" refers only to a condition of past and continuing disability with an uncertain future, whereas "permanent" implies irreversibility. Persistent vegetative state is a diagnosis; permanent vegetative state is a prognosis.[3]

In retrospect, one reason Terry could have breached these categories was diagnostic error. Bryan Jennett, the co-originator of the vegetative state with Dr. Plum, later put it this way, "Some alleged late recoveries might in fact have been late discoveries of earlier recovery."[4]

But if that were the case, why didn't that error become obvious sooner? And if Terry was misdiagnosed during that long winter's night, what was his actual diagnosis? If he wasn't vegetative all that time, what sort of state was he in? So reminiscent of Rip Van Winkle, he fit into a fictional category, but now he needed a scientific one. He needed to be classified as something; that is what scientists do. But where along the continuum from brain death all the way to normal consciousness did he fit?

EARLY INSIGHTS

Looking back over those many years and through interviews with Angilee Wallis, it became apparent that Terry was not vegetative for most of his nineteen years in institutional care but in the minimally conscious state (MCS). Codified nearly two decades after Terry suffered his brain injury, the criteria for MCS were published in the mainstream medical literature in the journal *Neurology* in 2002. MCS was characterized as a "condition of severely altered consciousness in which minimal but definite behavioral evidence of environmental awareness is demonstrated."[5] The MCS is one in which there is definite, albeit intermittent evidence of consciousness. In contrast to the "wakeful unresponsiveness of vegetative patients,"[6] those in MCS may demonstrate intention, attention, memory, track someone in their room, or follow a simple command.

Even more to the point, the pity is that Terry did not have recourse to being diagnosed as MCS because it entered into the medical literature eighteen years after his accident and just a year before Terry put his "vegetative" diagnosis to the test.

Getting more specific about Terry's diagnosis didn't seem to matter because back in 1984, he *had his diagnosis* – the vegetative state. Nothing else was available then. But, decades later, in Maggie Worthen's case, it became the key question. As she got ready to leave the hospital, as her mother worried about her "cognition," the issue was whether she was always destined to be vegetative? Or did she have a chance of regaining consciousness as Terry ultimately did? The comparison between their two cases, if nothing else, dramatically illustrates a striking evolution in how we classify brain states.

As far as it was known in 1984, Terry was fixed in the vegetative state, and it was a brain state he was destined to be in for as long as he lived. Where he had actually been in the years between 1984 and 2003 was a brain state that, as yet, had neither been discovered nor described, although it had been intuited by some investigators. It made clinical sense. Logically there had to be some intermediate state between the vegetative state and fuller recovery. It may have been transient but it seemed likely that there was a way station en route to higher function.

In the decades before Terry spoke his first words, clinicians and scientists, in fact, wondered if patients like him might exist and worried about how to explain them. Bryan Jennett, the Scottish neurosurgeon who first described the persistent vegetative state (PVS) with Fred Plum in 1972, had a very prescient insight while he was formulating the Glasgow Coma and Outcome Scales (GCS and GOS) to assess prognosis after brain injury. As early as 1975, Jennett worried about how patients transition from one state to another.[7] Even as they introduced the notion of empirical assessment of patients with severe injury, Jennett with his collaborator, Michael Bond, urged better classification within brain states.

Jennett and Bond noted that there was a need for more diagnostic precision because diagnostic clarity had a bearing on ultimate outcome. They thought it "... wrong to consider the vegetative state and the severely disabled together because a proportion of those severely disabled in the early stages may improve to a better category of outcome." With this variance in mind, they urged the construction of "recovery curves ... by which to define the interval after which it is unlikely that the outcome category will change, even though there may be substantial movement within it."[8] Their point was to learn how to track the evolution of patients within and across brain states and better appreciate the time lines of feasible recovery.

FROM GLASGOW TO JERSEY

The insights of Jennett and Bond finally took root fifteen to twenty years later when it became increasingly clear that there was another brain state lurking within that group of patients once thought to be vegetative. Clinical neuropsychologists and physiatrists working with patients with severe brain injury in brain rehabilitation programs in the early 1990s get the credit for formalizing this new category, which needed a niche of its own. They had all made the observation that there was a small subset of patients within the broad category of severe brain injury, who were often conflated with vegetative patients, who seemed to defy conventional odds and did a bit better.

Joseph Giacino, a neuropsychologist who led these efforts in pursuit of diagnostic accuracy and was the lead author of the 2002 paper codifying MCS in the medical literature, recalled the origins of the category from the early 1990s. When interviewed, he told me, "For many years, I cannot say when exactly, there was a recognition within rehabilitation that there was a group of individuals who had appeared unconscious, but were not in a vegetative state, meaning they retained some conscious awareness. Their awareness fluctuated; you would see it in some examinations and not see it in others."

It was the same paradox that Mrs. Wallis had observed in Terry. He appeared unconscious but sometimes he demonstrated behaviors that suggested something else. In the early 1990s, Giacino's committee appreciated that these patients were not vegetative and that they retained or, perhaps more accurately, regained conscious awareness. They were inching toward the realization that patients could be conscious but only manifest behavioral signs of consciousness intermittently. It was that hallmark finding, or counterintuition of MCS, that still eluded them.

But they knew enough to be worried. For the brain injury rehabilitation community, there was this fear that patients who showed these signs might have better recoveries than those who did not. The challenge was that they were all clumped together in a single diagnostic category. Speaking of patients who manifested those flickering signs of conscious awareness, Giacino recalls, "There was a lot of concern that this group was not the same as people in the vegetative state, yet no one had encapsulated this other group and the worry was that there may be differences in the way these patients resolve overtime and what their outcomes may be. . . ."

But who were they, and what should they be called? The journey to the current diagnostic category of MCS would take ten years of discourse and debate amongst the brain injury literati. It would require a consensus across a broad disciplinary spectrum of practitioners from acute care and chronic care, who were often academically quite distant from each other, hailing from a wide range of fields including neurology, neurosurgery, neuropsychology, and physiatry, among others. Each of these medical and nonmedical subcultures had seen brain-injured patients during part of their journey, so each had their own limited and potentially biased perspective. Each specialty area also had distinct ways of seeing the world: a more descriptive approach of what functions were observed at the bedside, or a mechanistic one that predicted what capabilities might remain based on the neurophysiology of brain injury. It was literally a bottom-up versus top-down approach. One faction would determine what was manifested at the bedside and another what sort of exam would result from a specific brain lesion.

Initially, the debate started within the rehabilitation community with the precursor phrase, "minimally responsive state," first appearing in a 1991 paper written by Giacino.[9] The paper made a very important contribution to the field when he also outlined a new scale, the coma recovery scale (CRS), to empirically evaluate these patients, building upon the earlier scales of Jennett and his colleagues in Glasgow. Because of this early work and the unfortunate and untimely death of Dr. Sheldon Berrol, who was considered – as Giacino put it – "the grandfather of brain injury rehabilitation," Giacino became chair of the American College of Rehabilitation Medicine's Committee on the Minimally Responsive State.

It was an amazing opportunity for Giacino, who was in his early thirties at the time. His success in that role was pivotal to the evolution of the field and our collective ability to measure patient improvement at the margins of consciousness. Giacino was both humbled by his chance and knew it was career altering. When he took over the committee, "... I was actually very green at the time and amazingly in awe of the fact I had this opportunity because there were people who I looked up to already in this group that were participating and here I am chairing this committee. For me this was a career changer, what it did, it got people thinking more about the minimally responsive state and in fact the committee had gotten named for that condition."

The initial meeting of the Committee on the Minimally Responsive Patient was held on June 2, 1992 at the JFK-Johnson Rehabilitation Institute in Edison, New Jersey, where Giacino worked. It is a small place in suburban New Jersey tucked behind an elementary school. To the unknowing, it looked like a very well-maintained nursing home and not one of the country's premier brain injury centers. But looks can be deceiving, especially in brain injury, and so it was when the committee held its first meeting.

Despite the modesty of the setting, the committee had outsized, almost political objectives. According to committee minutes, which were made available to the author, the rationale for the meeting was not primarily about the scientific challenge of classifying a new brain state but rather addressing a threat to the integrity of the rehabilitation medicine community posed by "coma stimulation" programs. These were questionable ventures that brought brain-injured patients in for unproven interventions, at high costs to desperate families. Because some patients improve on their own and there were no baseline metrics for these natural recoveries, whenever an enrolled patient got better these programs would take credit. Each occasional success would be heralded, attracting more unsuspecting families.

The mainstream rehabilitation community was concerned about these programs, their methods, ethics, and proliferation. An emerging skepticism about them had the potential to tarnish the legitimate work done in rehabilitative medicine. According to committee minutes, there were concerns regarding the "the proliferation of clinical programs serving this population (e.g., 'coma stimulation'), the absence of recognized standards of care and the absence of an organized forum for exchange of information among disciplines working with the minimally responsive population."[10]

Something had to be done and, in response, the committee resolved to define diagnostic nomenclature, establish minimal criteria for clinical programs, and develop guidelines for discontinuing rehabilitation services and communicate their findings through position papers.[10]

CONGRESSIONAL HEARINGS

It is important to note that even while MCS as a category was gestating, it was the product of a complicated pregnancy. Its origins were as much born of controversy, as the much purer questions of science foreseen by Jennett and colleagues. That the proliferation of questionable "coma stimulation" programs is suggested as the first reason given for the formation of the committee is noteworthy.

Brain rehabilitation programs had become a big business by the late 1980s and some critics and consumer advocates were alleging fraud and abuse. According to William Winslade's excellent account of the era, investment bankers saw this field as a growth industry ripe for good returns and for-profit providers proliferated in that deregulated era.[11] They played on the vulnerability of families who were enticed by fraudulent ads of happy patients seemingly making progress. Amidst comfortable surroundings that suggested every option was being pursued, fabricated testimonials simply added to the appeal. Such was the message. The reality was less kind. Nonvalidated "therapies" were offered, without effect save for the improvement that comes naturally with time and chance.

Eventually, the excesses of these *faux* programs were exposed leading to two separate congressional hearings headed by Representatives Ted Weiss of New York and Ron Wyden of Oregon. Weiss, a liberal democrat, noted:

> I would like to think that most people with head injuries receive the best possible care. ... But we have learned that too often they are warehoused in outrageously overpriced, resort-like facilities.[12]

Amongst the revelations: facility staffers confessed to Congress they had been told to falsely document patient progress and to hold on to patients until their insurance was exhausted. "Coma stimulation" – the impetus for the Committee on the Minimally Responsive Patient – was at the heart of this elaborate and tragic charade.

In "coma stimulation," patients who are unconscious are exposed to activities that normally require a conscious and receptive brain. Families were engaged and their loved ones are read to at hundreds of dollars an hour, but the evidence was not there for efficacy. Dr. Nathan Zasler, a brain rehabilitation expert, testified before Congress, "I don't feel ethically it's something I should be charging the payer or family for."[13]

A MINIMALLY CONTENTIOUS STATE

The problem, we now know, is that any intervention when applied to a large enough group will see some patients getting better. This is not because the coma stimulation worked, but because some patients will get better, without therapy, due to naturally occurring recoveries that happen over time. If the elapse of time coincides with the provision of coma stimulation, it will appear that the intervention had an effect. But in reality, such cases are what the logicians would say are "true, true and unrelated." It's true the patient received coma stimulation. It's true they got better. And it's also true that the first statement had nothing to do with the second.

Having made these assertions, it is also true that the coincidence of improvement with time and coma stimulation will be more frequent in patients who inherently are more likely to recover. With twenty years of hindsight, we now understand that those patients would come to be known and described as "minimally conscious." That is why the formation of the Committee on the Minimally Responsive State evolved out of a preoccupation with programs like coma stimulation. Observing a differing frequency of improvement, for whatever reason, pointed to a variance that suggested that there was heterogeneity in the group. This led some to worry that there was an additional diagnostic category buried within the larger cohort of patients described as being in the vegetative state.

If that realization were the entirety of the story it would have advanced diagnostic thinking and suggested a need for empirical work to track patients after injury so as to begin to differentiate degrees (and likelihoods) of recovery. But unfortunately, there were complications stemming from the provenance of the committee and its *raison d'être*. Regrettably, the unkind revelations about coma stimulations were generalized more broadly. They undermined the scientific legitimacy of MCS as a diagnostic category and delayed its receptivity beyond the neuropsychology community, making it something of a minimally *contentious* state. These political entanglements impeded the emergence of MCS as a valid diagnostic category even as important empirical evidence now showed that some patients had a different recovery trajectory, independent of coma stimulation.

A 1997 paper by Giacino and his colleague Kathy Kalmar, showed that patients who were minimally conscious were statistically more likely to engage in visual pursuit than patients who were vegetative (MCS = 82 percent versus VS = 20 percent).[14] Visual pursuit, or more colloquially the ability to track an object with one's eyes, is an important indication of a patient's awareness of his or her environment. While this may seem a small difference in capabilities, it demonstrated that MCS patients were more interactive and responsive than vegetative patients. This variance in ability was also important because it might explain why the responsive subset of patients might have a better outcome than patients who did not engage with their environment as frequently. Giacino and Kalmar also reported that MCS patients had a longer window of potential recovery than VS patients and that they had less overall disability as measured on a disability rating scale (DRS). Finally, their data also showed that a patient's overall prognosis hinged on how the injury occurred. They found that outcomes were better in those patients who had sustained a traumatic brain injury (like Terry Wallis) as compared to the anoxic brain that would occur following a cardiac arrest.[15]

DEFENDING ASPEN

After a meeting in Aspen, Colorado, the group established the "Aspen Criteria" for MCS. Now expanded to include a broader representation of professionals than the original Committee on the Minimally Responsive Patient, this group was able to reach a consensus on the definition of MCS and place it in a mainstream medical journal. Their efforts were codified in a paper published in *Neurology* in 2002. MCS was characterized as a "condition of severely altered consciousness in which minimal but definite behavioral evidence of environmental awareness is demonstrated."[5] But when it came to the question of consciousness there was a twist. "The minimally conscious state is one in which there is definite, albeit intermittent evidence of consciousness."[5] Their point was subtly expressed: sometimes there is no overt behavioral evidence of consciousness, although when the behaviors are expressed, the evidence is definitive, distinguishing such patients from ones who are vegetative. MCS would be distinguished from "wakeful unresponsiveness of vegetative patients" by the demonstration of signs of intention, attention, and memory or the ability to track someone in their room or follow a simple command.

The Aspen Criteria also defined what it meant to *emerge* from MCS en route to additional recovery. If MCS was marked by definite but *intermittent* evidence of consciousness, emergence from MCS was demarcated by being able to engage in more consistent behaviors like reliable "functional interactive communication" and/or "functional use of two different objects." The former might mean the ability to communicate verbally, with the use of yes/ no cards or with the use of an assistive communication device. The latter could be satisfied by complex activities such as picking up a cup to drink or bringing a comb to one's hair.[5] They fit the bill because they indicated a degree of memory about the task and intentionality.

The work of the Aspen Group was truly a landmark contribution. They laid out a nosology, or diagnostic frame that could accommodate and make sense of new knowledge about differing brain states that needed to be stratified. It represented a milestone in the care of brain-injured patients.

But the contribution was not immediately recognized, much less met with universal endorsement from major clinical societies. They were guarded and sometimes even critical of the effort. Giacino was disappointed by the response of organized medicine. He recalls, "I did not just want to publish the paper, I wanted written, formal endorsements from all the major organizations that had a stake. We requested endorsements from ACRM [American College of Rehabilitation Medicine], American Academy of Neurology, AANS [American Association of Neurological Surgeons], Child Neurology Society, the Brain Injury Association of America and the American Academy of Physical Medicine and Rehabilitation. That turned out to be a nightmare. We had to walk though the bureaucracy of each one of those ... organizations and some were layered much more heavily than others." The Aspen Group had some success, "We got sign off from the Neurosurgeons, The Academy of PMR and not surprisingly the Brain Injury Association, as well as the Child Neurology Society."

The greatest embarrassment was that the paper lacked the endorsement of the American Academy of Neurology, the very organization that published *Neurology*, the journal in which the paper appeared. Perhaps vindicated by a decade of medical citations that has demonstrated just how important the Aspen Group's paper was, Giacino is still bothered by the initial snub. He confesses, "At the end of the day, I don't know if people know this, the American Academy of Neurology did not endorse the paper. If you notice in the endorsement statement of the paper, it isn't specifically endorsed by the AAN." Instead they hedged their bets and downgraded their level of support, "What they did was to decide to endorse it as an 'educational tool' to the readership of the journal. They didn't endorse it, the concepts, like every other organizations did."

The picture was made worse by the fact that the paper was accompanied by critical editorials accusing Giacino and his coauthors of conflating consciousness and awareness.[16] Disability advocates from the activist group, *Not Dead Yet*, wrote that the new diagnostic category would demean the disabled by creating a new category that would equate higher functioning individuals with brain injury to those who were permanently vegetative.[17] After a decade of work trying to advance his ideas, the publication was not a time for celebration. Rather, it was a time to play defense.

Even now, Giacino is annoyed about the challenges he and his colleagues had to face bringing the MCS construct forward. "I almost did not get the chance to enjoy the fact we got over this hurdle, that took us really nine years to get to." Even as a decade's effort was going into print, there were immediate challenges. In a notable editorial slight, Giacino "learned quickly that there was going to be opposing opinions that were published *alongside the paper*. This to me was a break from any convention I ever heard, because the first questions I heard was how could these people writing these letters write about our paper when they never saw the paper. If they did see the paper, how were they given a copy of the paper before the authors had submitted it?"

Because the normal protocol is to have letters and author response *after* a paper is published, Giacino complained to the journal's editor. Noting the editorial breach, "I wrote a letter to Robert Griggs [Dr. Griggs was the editor in chief of *Neurology*] basically complaining and saying there is no precedent I know for this. I was given a vague response saying 'under the circumstances this was a unique situation and the letters to the editor would be published simultaneous next to the paper.'"

I wrote one of those letters to *support* the new category in tandem with my Cornell neurologist colleague, Nicholas D. Schiff who had contributed to the Aspen consensus statement but was not listed as an author. I remember drafting it on an airplane ride to the West Coast and gazing out the window, thinking that Giacino and his colleagues had really done something significant by bringing additional diagnostic precision to brain injury. The Aspen Group's work would take MCS and severe brain injury out of the shadows and allow it to gain a solid empirical base. As I wrote the response, I also imagined that I was at JFK-Johnson Rehabilitation Center with these patients and their devoted caregivers who were trying to make sense of their loved ones' injured brains. At forty thousand feet I recalled their devotion amidst the pungent smell of urine that is often the hallmark of long-term care. No one could accuse Giacino and his coauthors of not being advocates for those with severe brain injury and its attendant disability. His career had been one of service.

But that is what was argued in one of the accompanying letters. A decade later, I am still a bit dumbfounded by the reaction from disability advocates who did not see the beneficent intent of the new category and by the resistance of the medical community who questioned the evidence for the new categorization. We rejected both claims.

Schiff and I argued that if we understood the differences between patient types we could do a better job of providing care and doing research. "Opponents contend that in the absence of an evidence base for these criteria, the consensus model used to generate these guidelines represents the consolidation of an ideological stance about the worth of these individuals. But it is also paradoxical. This categorization could be a helpful tool in better understanding the continuum of brain states and designing research and therapies to improve and augment cognitive function."[18]

While we were sympathetic to the concerns of the disability community, in this case represented by Diane Coleman of *Not Dead Yet*, we urged her to redirect her advocacy "to bring therapeutic or palliative care advances to those with brain injury" and to also respect the right "of properly authorized surrogates to make decisions to withdraw life-sustaining therapies in accord with the patient's previously expressed preferences."[18]

INVICTUS

For Giacino, the sadness is still there despite his ultimate success in bringing the field to a new level of rigor and sophistication. "It really put a damper on it for me. At that point we had no idea what was going to happen with this, it could die a week after the paper got published."

Did he feel vindicated with the passage of time? "Absolutely, there is no doubt about that, it's probably a more recognizable term than vegetative state or a better understood term. It's certainly pretty widely recognized, how many people understand it is a different story. Steven [Laureys, a Belgium neurologist who we will meet in the next chapters] has that chart ... of the number of publications on the vegetative state and the number of publications on the minimally conscious state. The curve is dramatically steeper on MCS than it is for VS."

Taken together with the earlier contributions of the Multi-Society Task Force on the Persistent Vegetative State, the Aspen Group had described the missing way station between the devastation of the vegetative state and that of recovery. With the publication of the Aspen Criteria it was possible to chart the course of patients with brain injury from an initial coma to recovery. Giacino and colleagues' work was a singular accomplishment that allowed us to measure a patient's progress.

A ROAD MAP

There were, and are, details to be filled in but the rough sketch was in place after the work of the Multi-Society Task Force and the Aspen Group. With the publication of the Aspen Criteria in 2002, it was understood that if a patient did not regain consciousness after being comatose, they will migrate into the vegetative state, which will become permanent three to twelve months after injury, depending on how they were hurt. If the brain was damaged because of anoxia, severe oxygen deprivation, the vegetative state becomes permanent after three months. If the injury was traumatic, the vegetative state needs to last twelve months before it is deemed permanent (see Figure 2).

Before these vegetative states become permanent, though, the patient can move into the MCS. This transition can be a surreptitious one and will frequently occur after the patient has been transferred from the acute care setting to rehabilitation or a chronic care facility. This creates a host of diagnostic challenges because to the untrained, or less than vigilant eye, it is difficult to distinguish the vegetative state from MCS.

MCS patients differentiate themselves from those in VS by virtue of behaviors that indicate an awareness of themselves or their external environment. The problem is that these behaviors are not reliably reproduced. Theirs

Pathways to Recovery

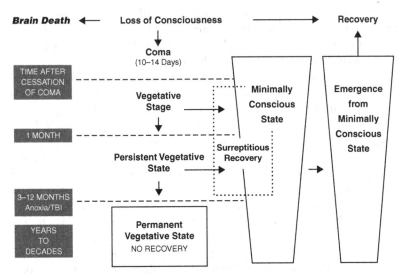

FIGURE 2. Pathways to Recovery. Adapted from J. J. Fins, "Neuroethics and Neuroimaging: Moving towards Transparency." *American Journal Bioethics* 8(9) (2008):46–52.
Courtesy: J. J. Fins, "Neuroethics, Neuroimaging and Disorders of Consciousness: Promise or Peril?" *Transactions of the American Clinical and Climatological Association* 122 (2010): 336–46.

is a light that does not always shine bright but is more like a flickering bulb on a Christmas tree that sometimes becomes lit.[19] That inconsistency is part of the definition of MCS and intrinsic to its biology. But that inconsistency is also part of the diagnostic challenge.

Typically, relatives think they have seem a glimmer of awareness and seek to report it to medical staff, but then the behaviors are not reliably reproducible. As we have seen, staff chalk it up to denial, that these families are hopeful at best or imagining things at worst. They do not countenance the possibility that what they say they saw might be true.[20]

Dr. Zini, Terry Wallis's doctor at the nursing home, did not witness any of the behaviors that Mrs. Wallis saw. After Terry came to international attention, Zini was quoted in *The Guardian of London*, "I felt that he had a blank stare, that he would probably respond to painful stimuli, like pulling on his eye. ..." Zini continued, "I never objectively saw everything she saw, but then neither did he respond to me the way he did to her."[21] Even after Terry started to speak, one hears the echoes of disbelief in Dr. Zini's inference that Mrs. Wallis brought subjectivity to her observations. As he put it, the doctor "never *objectively* saw everything she saw."[21] This is not surprising and worthy of explaining in a nonjudgmental way.

DIAGNOSING COMPLEXITY

Clinical personnel may be disinclined to acknowledge what they have not seen if the findings are unexpected and do not cohere with what is scientifically described for a given clinical context. When a patient thought to be vegetative displays a behavior that indicates consciousness, but does not repeat that same behavior on command, it becomes easier – indeed almost logical – to ascribe the first behavior to chance or to the wishful thinking of family members.

Such diagnostic conservatism is even more likely when a revision in diagnosis challenges medical hierarchies. When a patient carries a "definitive" diagnosis from the academic medical center that tended to their brain injury, who is the chronic care clinician to doubt it? Their views have less standing against the expert opinion of the academic center.[22] Moreover, patients come from the hospital to the chronic care sector with *fixed* diagnoses and with chronic conditions like diabetes, end-stage kidney disease, or Alzheimer's. No one would question the diagnosis of ischemic heart disease for a patient just discharged from a cardiac care unit. Why would they think that a patient described as vegetative had become aware and conscious?[20]

Such thinking would be a radical departure from most of medical diagnostics. We tend to think of medical diagnoses as fixed and these conditions as chronic but these are brain *states* and they may evolve over time. This presents a challenge to the chronic care sector that is designed for stasis and averse to dynamism. Unlike those engaged in rehabilitation, the skilled nursing facilities where patients like Terry Wallis end up are neither prepared for, nor accustomed to, changes in diagnostic categorization so long after acute care has concluded.

Instead, these programs are governed by expectations that additional recovery is implausible and that additional diagnostic or therapeutic engagement would be futile and of little use. This can lead to diagnostic errors of omission, most notably a failure to take note of the subtle state change from the vegetative to MCS. As we saw in the Wallis case, it is often only in retrospect, when the patient emerges from MCS and speaks spontaneously, that this long-standing diagnostic error becomes apparent. Although Wallis's case was noteworthy for being amongst the first misdiagnosed MCS patients to come to wide attention, his fate is not unique. In 2009, Caroline Schnakers and colleagues reported that 41 percent of patients diagnosed as vegetative in chronic care were in fact minimally conscious.[23] Previous studies have suggested a similar and unacceptably high misdiagnosis rate.[24-26]

This is an unconscionable degree of inaccuracy, especially if we compared this diagnostic error rate to other areas in medicine. Imagine an oncologist mistaking one type of leukemia for another,[27] an error that now has therapeutic implications as the subtypes of leukemia have differing prognoses and varying treatments.[28,29] No one would accept such mistakes. But we do accept the possibility of conscious patients lying in nursing home beds being written off as if they were permanently unconscious and in the vegetative state.

The reasons for such diagnostic errors are multifactorial: the pervasive nihilism toward this patient population as a carryover from the emergence of the right-to-die movement; the novelty of MCS as a diagnostic category; the challenge of making the diagnosis when behaviors are intermittent and unexpected; and the impact of the discharge diagnosis on subsequent clinicians.[22]

As Maggie left the hospital, she was not immune to any of these forces, or to a mother's love.

9   Leaving the Hospital

A HOPEFUL DEPARTURE

Maggie was one of the lucky ones. She was ready to leave the hospital and she got a chance to go to a brain rehabilitation program. So with tracheostomy and stomach tubes in place, Maggie was discharged from the hospital and transferred to Spaulding Rehabilitation Hospital in Boston. Spaulding, a Harvard affiliate, is one of the nation's leading programs for brain rehabilitation, and Nancy was hopeful that Maggie might qualify for transfer. Not everyone gets into such rarefied places. They were reserved for those families who knew of their existence and had injuries that might be amenable to whatever rehab they could offer.

At the end of her acute hospitalization, her clinical staff thought that Maggie might be in a minimally conscious state (MCS). (Nancy later recalled that was when she first heard of that diagnostic phrase.) Spaulding had a special program for patients who were in MCS. It was not certain, Nancy recalled, "...but they tested her because they decided that there was a possibility that she would have some consciousness." Spaulding accepted her into their eight-week program.

Nancy was genuinely happy because the transfer provided a glimmer of hope. It meant that the doctors were wondering if she was not actually vegetative. It was a small opening to a bigger future, but hopeful nonetheless. That eight-week acceptance brought joy because it conveyed the sense that the doctors thought that some degree of recovery was still possible. As Nancy told us, "... It was a hopeful thing just for them to accept her into the minimally conscious" program because it meant that the doctors either knew or suspected that she was minimally conscious as opposed to vegetative. Nancy had learned by now that was a difference that would make a difference.

GOOD TO GO

Not all patients are ready or stable enough to leave the hospital and fewer get to go to a rehabilitation center, ending up instead in a nursing home. As Burt Brody, whose wife Jean collapsed in his arms with a brain aneurysm, began to understand placement options he put it this way, "To learn the terms acute and subacute are almost contradictory to what they really are. Acute rehab

83

is that you're in better shape and subacute is that you're in worse shape, and then there's just a plain old nursing home that doesn't do anything other than care for the patient to make sure they stay alive."

But Burt's insights would only come with experience. On the day Jean left the hospital, Burt was called abruptly. His insurance company had denied ongoing hospital care unbeknownst to him. He was told, "There's a medical transport waiting to take your wife to the nursing home ... and you need to come here and sign the discharge papers." The urgency was prompted by the fact that the hospital had just received a fax from the insurance company refusing to authorize treatment at the hospital – for the previous week.

Burt was driving over toward the hospital in a pounding rain storm when their case worker called. Abruptly, he was told, "... your wife is being discharged right now and you need to decide what nursing home you're going to put her in. ... There's an ambulance waiting to take her [the nursing home]. ..."

Burt responded in disbelief, "You've got to be kidding me!" The case worker provided a harsh reality check, telling him that his insurance company had denied a longer stay, "So we're getting her out of here."

Jean had begun to talk and reports from the hospital to the insurance company indicated she was better, so the order was given to arrange the discharge. Burt did not appeal the decision because "at that point ... I had no idea who to talk to. ..." A skilled lawyer by trade, as a spouse, he was frozen trying to do right by his wife. This was real life and not a paper chase amenable to a lawyerly approach, "when this stuff happens you don't go rush and read your insurance policy." Instead, he was experiencing this as it happened, as a husband in which, "you find out how bad or good it is as things happen."

Only later, did Burt find out that he could have fought the discharge. "It turns out that there was an appeals process." If Burt had asked for a review, the hospital would have had to keep Jean for three more days to complete the appeals process, with the insurance company paying for the hospitalization. But Burt did not ask, because, "no one ever told me that."

When Burt arrived at the hospital, the paramedics were already huddled around Jean getting her ready for transport. But when they took her blood pressure it was, Burt recalls, "extremely low, like eighty over fifty." Such values would normally delay a patient's departure, but "... the discharge person said, 'Oh, just give her a bolus of saline and that will bring it up." When the extra IV fluids brought up her blood pressure to a point that it was "not that bad," it was time to go.

Burt remains annoyed by the reckless treatment of his wife. Her low blood pressure could have signaled a serious infection – or worse. Instead of evaluating her more fully, or waiting to see how she would fare after the temporizing measure of additional fluid, once she seemed stable, hospital staff said, "she's good to go." Burt summed it up: "And they just basically threw us out."

NOT 'TIL HE'S STABLE

The same fate awaited Jimmy Waters, whose mother had been urged to turn him into an organ donor. A month after his injury, on Christmas Eve, his family was abruptly informed that he was to be discharged. His mother, Mary, recalls that she was told that, "they were done with Jimmy; he's got to go to a nursing home." She was given a list of facilities to choose from, but no additional guidance.

Mary was concerned because Jimmy was unstable. He had pneumonia and "fevers of 105." So she protested, as best she could: "No, he's not going anywhere, he'll just die, he'll die if you move him." She told the hospital administrators that "he's going to stay here until you get him off the ventilator."

But they did not see it that way. Hospital officials told her, "that's impossible, we can't do that." One doctor threatened her that "if you don't do it, [discharge him] we're going to do it." Mary was "shocked" and said "no you're not, you're not moving him anywhere until he's stable."

The night before Christmas, Mary was by herself. Earlier, she had told her family to go home. Now she was alone and needed helped, so she called a lawyer. She had never done that before but she was desperate, and it had become an unfair fight. She needed to protect her boy.

Once the lawyer got involved, Mary noted an immediate change. She recalls, that the "... next thing you know they couldn't do enough for Jimmy. They were singing a different tune. All of a sudden it was like ... he [the lawyer] said two words: 'risk management.' And all of a sudden they were, 'we're not moving him.'"

It took until March 11, before Jimmy was stable enough to come off the ventilator so he could go to rehab.

WE NEED SOME ICE PACKS

Dustin Manwiller's discharge experience nearly proved fatal. When he was still in the hospital, Dustin's family had to move quickly to find a place for their son. They settled on a facility near their home primarily because it was convenient. They could visit frequently and keep Dustin close. That was its main virtue and they did not have time to seek out an alternative, rushed as they were to meet the discharge plan that had been scheduled.

When he was discharged, Dustin was off the ventilator but still required supplemental oxygen through his tracheostomy. He was still having erratic central or neurogenic fevers, a not uncommon complication following traumatic brain injury (TBI).[1] But the fevers could have also been a warning sign of a severe infection that could not be casually brushed away. Whatever their cause, the high fevers needed to be evaluated and treated.

All of that would start with careful monitoring *that was not available* at the facility. That limitation was an error of omission that only became apparent after the fact. Kathie realized in hindsight that, "it was too early to send him out to a facility where there wasn't monitoring." But when Kathie toured the facility, she did not fully appreciate its liabilities. Eager to be close to Dustin, she rationalized what she saw, "they showed me the gym and I was like alright, that's not what I was expecting, I was expecting more state of the art and you know all this equipment. But we made the decision to move him there. ..." It was all motivated by a desire to have Dustin nearby and keep him in their lives.

"It really wasn't the place for someone in Dustin's condition. There were no monitors in the room, there was no wall oxygen, everything was portable, suction, portable oxygen ... everything was noisy. ..."

The problem was the floor's set up and staffing, "You know, you had to trust that the aide or the nurse was walking down the hall when Dustin needed to be suctioned." And most poignantly, because Dustin was unable to communicate, he was totally dependent upon the consistency, and professionalism, of those to whom his care had been entrusted. He could not call out for help, and even if he could it would have to be over the din. The only way one would know there was a problem that needed assistance would be to have him under constant surveillance, either using technology or frequent nursing visits. Neither was possible at the nursing home. All of this put Dustin at serious risk. Stating the obvious point, that nonetheless needed to be made explicitly, Kathie noted, "There was no way to know he was in any kind of distress unless you actually saw him because he's not going to yell out or anything like that."

It was a disaster in the making and one that happened during his first night there. When Kathie came in the next morning, he was hot and "all red and blotchy." Panicked, Kathie asked the nurse floating on Dustin's floor for a thermometer but she did not speak English. She recalls, "We had no understanding of each other whatsoever, I was trying to tell her 'we need a cooling blanket, we need some ice packs, we need something, his fever is up.'" The nurse responded, "oh no, he doesn't have a fever" and went off to give other patients their medications.

Finally, Kathie was able to get the head nurse to take his temperature. It was 102 and they started packing Dustin with ice to get the fever down. Soon the crisis was abated and the nurse told Kathie to calm down because everything was now under control. She remembers the scene, "Everyone is trying to tell me I got to unwind, I got to let loose." She was told to "understand he's going to be fine, they're going to take care of him" and urged to "go home, go home." Anxious still, and exhausted, but somewhat reassured, she placed her trust in what she heard and went back home for the night.

The next morning Dustin's condition had worsened. His temperature had gone up to 105. This time he was rushed back to the emergency room at the regional medical center. There his fever spiked to 106 and his heart rate galloped along at 165. His blood pressure was barely palpable. "It was so low they couldn't even read it." He was going into shock and circulatory failure.

The situation was dire and it seemed like the end was near. Dustin's uncle, who was a doctor at the medical center, was able to be with his nephew. He told Ken, Dustin's dad, to go home and support Kathie, because they did not think she could stand watching her son die. The stress was taking its toll on her. Through tears, Kathie later recalled that Ken prepared her, saying "his heart can't handle this much longer."

But when Kathie arrived in the emergency room, Dustin rallied. His fever subsided and his pulse quieted. It might have been the medicines or coincidence, but to Kathie it was just unbelievable, "Amazingly, the kid, he's like a horse, this kid I don't know." Laughter had now replaced her earlier tears, "when I got there then they let us both in and I just grabbed his hand and his heart rate went down." She wonders, was it a mother's love? "I don't know if one thing has anything to with another. . . ."

Dustin recovered and the intensity and frequency of his fevers subsided. The crisis was averted but the challenge of placement remained. Soon the social worker appeared again, "Okay, we have to start thinking about where are we going to go?"

In spite of the nearly fatal two-day excursion to the chronic care facility, the family again wanted to go back there. The pull of family made the locale ideal and to place Dustin somewhere further away would have meant abandoning him to a distant institutionalization. On this occasion, their admissions office rejected Dustin's reapplication. They did not want a repeat performance. In retrospect, they knew they could not handle semiacute patients like Dustin still prone to central fevers and hemodynamic instability. It was a hard-won lesson that nearly cost Dustin his life.

DISMISSED AND DISCHARGED

But there is more to learn from Dustin's experience. There is symbolic import to discharge decisions after a severe brain injury. Destined to survive, but deprived of an opportunity for rehabilitation, transfer to a chronic care setting represents new constraints with which patient and family must eventually contend. This should make it a time ripe for conversation, but too often the transition goes unexamined. Instead of speaking openly, care plans are couched in euphemisms. A discharge to chronic care is not attributed to a patient's poor functional status but blamed on a bureaucracy that finds that "your son is not a candidate for acute rehabilitation."

When the conversation side-steps the issues, the act of discharge can speak volumes. An ambulance waiting to take a patient to a nursing home, by its very presence, conveys a prognostic bias that may not have been expressed to the family. Its destination tells the story, even if the patient's clinicians were reluctant to do so. And the nature of that journey becomes all the more significant when the patient is dispatched in a hurry and the family is caught unaware.

A rushed discharge is often attributed to reimbursement issues. And while finances are often the proximal cause, when a family leaves the hospital unprepared, other factors are at play. One can be the unspoken pain felt by practitioners who have devoted inordinate efforts to patient care, only to see their charge do so poorly. For the clinical team, discharge to a nursing home represents a medical failure. And clinicians are uncomfortable when they have to confront their failures.[2,3] So they fail to talk with families at this key juncture in the patient's course. They abandon the patient, and their family, because they feel there is nothing more that they can do because they are frustrated.

Generally, doctors still think of death as a medical failure,[4] but in the care of the severely brain-injured patient, the portrait of failure is more complex. The patient who is discharged to a nursing home means that an adequate functional status has not been achieved. This is one facet of failure. The other is more subtle: the inability to have convinced the family to forgo care and let the patient die, so as not to avoid a life burdened by profound disability.

The clinician who has shepherded a severely brain-injured patient from acute injury, and a near death experience, to an ambulance en route to a nursing home may feel that double sense of failure. In the first place they failed to achieve what is vaguely described as a "meaningful recovery." In the second, they did not preempt the incremental harm of a saved life that is "not worth living" or a "fate worse than death."[5] Burnout, coupled with what has been called "compassion fatigue" can further complicate the countertransference feelings of those caring for patients with severe brain injury,[6] affecting physicians as well as nurses, who can also act "defensively" when confronted by these pressures.[7] One study of burnout amongst 568 Belgian health care workers caring for patients with chronic disorders of consciousness found that rates of stress were high with burnout reported in 18 percent, emotional exhaustion in 36 percent, and depersonalization occurring in 36 percent. The degree of impairment was correlated with the nursing profession and time providing care to these patients.[8]

At discharge all of these forces come together, with placement in chronic care representing a miscarriage of both *techne* and discourse: the inability to achieve a meaningful recovery compounded by a failure to steer the family to less aggressive care and save them from their own their good intentions. The lack of verbal transparency upon discharge both defends against these failures and also sanctions families who did not take the doctors' "good" advice and withhold or withdraw care. Here, actions substitute for words that would prove difficult to say and hear.

Families find themselves the unwitting objects of practitioners' considerable and often unarticulated feelings,[9] as they come to grip with what lies ahead. Although the initial relief of a loved one's survival provides a respite from thinking too much about next steps, discharge makes it impossible to deny the future and its prospects. The ambulance and the gurney that arrives to transport the patient away pierces the security afforded by hospitalization and prompts feelings of abandonment and anger.

With time that anger is directed back at the hospital. But in the short term, families find it difficult to be angry with the doctors and nurses who did, in fact, save their loved one's life. Later they will look back and call these practitioners names like, "Dr. Doom" and speak of their bedside manner with scorn. But initially, they can't help but be grateful. So instead of directing anger at them, the resentment is directed inward.

Such was the case with Dustin's family. Although their motives were beneficent, they blamed themselves for the events that complicated his discharge and questioned their own actions. It did not matter that they had little time to scout out other facilities or to fully assess the facility to which they took Dustin and had no guidance from professionals; they blamed themselves for the care he received there. They remonstrated themselves for putting family convenience over Dustin's needs, even though all they wanted to do was to be able to visit. Nonetheless, Kathie confesses: "it was the one bad decision we made." And later, "I didn't think about what was best for Dustin. I thought I was, but I guess I was thinking about what was best for all of us, the family, we would all be close still. . . ."

LOST A WEEK

Other families report having their loved one sent out of acute care so prematurely that the patient could not benefit from rehabilitation. Elinor Quigley, Kenneth's mother, told us her son was discharged to rehabilitation while still in a coma. She explained, "They told us that he was going to go to" rehabilitation "and they arranged the transfer. . . ." The Quigleys were "very grateful at the time" but were "sad" because he was leaving the hospital. It made no sense to them because "we didn't feel that he was alert or awake or anything."

He hadn't spent any time in the hospital outside of the ICU and now he was going straight to a rehab facility. It seemed precipitous. They couldn't understand why he was coming straight from intensive care to rehabilitation. How could he benefit from their programs if he was still unresponsive? It would be his only chance to get such superb rehabilitation, and they did not want to waste that opportunity when he was incapable of benefiting from it.

Kathy Hansen's family thought she was destined for a nursing home as she was recovering from a brain injury either caused by a fat embolism or anesthesia accident sustained during routine orthopedic surgery. Initially, a social worker told her daughter Heidi, that the only option for her mother was to go to a nursing home. She explained, "There's really nothing else out there for you." But then, as is often the case, a quiet advocate provided the family with more information and another option.

Heidi does not remember his name but recalls, "It was someone else who kind of chirped in our ear." The message was that they should consider a well-regarded rehabilitation center. The family applied and just as Kathy was about to be moved to the nursing home, the rehab center accepted her to their thirty-day rehabilitation program.

But when Kathy arrived, it became apparent that she was not ready to take advantage of her brief stay there. As Heidi recalls, "... we lost the first week." Her mother could not participate in the programs because she was still on the ventilator and worn out from the acute hospitalization. In retrospect, Heidi felt that "... we lost; we considered it a loss because she was being weaned off the vent, so she really couldn't have done anything functionally because her body was just going through so much at the time."

Heidi questioned the justness of her early discharge. "We kind of thought it was unfair, right at the beginning. Because there you are, you just got transported, alright, now they feel you need a day or two there right after moving from the hospital, to get everything situated. ... With that the following day, they start to wean her, and her body's very weak, right, and now they're taking this thing away from her a little at a time, a little at a time."

She questioned the whole process, "... how can you move ahead when you're taking something away from her right off the bat? Her lungs aren't strong enough. So we kind of felt, you know, you lose a week right off the bat ... these things should have happened in the acute care situation. She should have been weaned off there, she should have been sort of ready to go into a rehab center ... the coma emergence program, the rehab part of it, we kind of knew it was sort of a thirty-day trial period. But a week of it was wasted, weaning her off the vent, doing this, all these medical things. ... We lost a week's worth of therapy there that maybe she could have gotten."

And to compound the problem, because Kathy would have to find suitable placement *after* her stint in rehabilitation, the family decided to leave the program early so they would not lose a bed that had been secured at a favored nursing home. Because nursing homes do not get paid when beds are empty, when one becomes available, there is pressure to get them filled, forcing families to make difficult choices.

So the Hansens robbed Peter to pay Paul. They made a choice to truncate Kathy's rehab stay to secure the nursing home bed. It was a tough call. They were at "... the twenty-eight-day mark where the nursing home was holding her a bed [but] they couldn't hold it any longer." The family asked themselves, "We had the choice of getting her the two, three days of intensive rehab which she really needs, or do we risk losing a bed where she's down the street and this is a good place?"

So instead of getting the full benefit of their stay in rehab, Kathy's thirty-day stay – and potentially sole chance for rehabilitation –was functionally reduced by at least a third. As the physician-mother of another patient recalled her experience with a still medically unstable child in rehabilitation, "She was so sick, she started with storming, dysautonomia, and was sick, vomiting, losing weight, getting decubitus ulcers." In retrospect, she concludes, "... she was probably too sick to be in acute rehab, that's what I later felt."

HOW COULD IT BE SO BAD?

The challenges faced at discharge raise the question of why, after so much effort is expended to save these lives, does so little forethought go into the next stage of care and rehabilitation? Part of this is structural, and directly related to how rehabilitation is funded. Health disparities also play a role with non-Caucasians and the uninsured having a significantly lower chance of being placed in rehabilitation,[10] and overall placements are on the decline. Fewer patients with TBI are receiving inpatient rehabilitation since the initiation of Medicare's inpatient rehabilitation facility prospective payment system was enacted in 2002. Comparing admission trends across 123 level I and II trauma centers across the United States between 1995 and 2004, the odds of patients with TBI being discharged to an inpatient rehabilitation facility decreased by 16 percent after prospective payment was put into place.[11]

But most of the challenges reflect the failure of caregivers to provide families with the support that they need at key moments of transition. Jamila Baucom, the daughter of Melva, a middle-aged woman who had a stroke, points out that the opportunity to prepare for discharge is limited. There was a "really small window" between the time when "you should start thinking about" discharge and the moment when the family is told, "she needs to be out." That opening is made smaller by the cool breeze of grief that the family still needs to accommodate. Jamila explains that "... when it's a sudden injury, like completely out of the blue, there's like a certain stage of shock and mourning that happens even if the patient's still alive." Families need to overcome their grief and their relief before they can take on questions about discharge planning. Simply put, "it's like we're not thinking about these things. . . ."

If families are unprepared for the rush of these discussions, when they do occur, little attention is paid to the trauma experienced by family members, as they contemplate being separated from the hospitals – and clinicians – who had just saved their loved one's lives. To sever these relationships and send fragile loved ones back out into the world, where their lives were nearly lost, is to be blind to a family's dependency upon the hospital and the security that its protective cover provides. As Jamila observed: "... I don't think that the staff, the social worker, was helpful in any way in terms of helping us come to terms with those issues. . . ."

A qualitative study of family needs conducted in Canada notes that families of patients with severe brain injury were especially in need of care and assistance upon discharge. When patients were being discharged, families experienced uncertainty, lack of clarity about whether the patient was making progress, as well as transition issues like letting go and making connections with the next facility providing care.[12] A narrative-based study from Australia indicated that families perceive a lack of support and need help in "negotiating the rehabilitation maze" as the transition is made from the acute care hospital and placement is pursued in the community.[13]

Our narratives provide further evidence of need. The families who we interviewed were given little guidance about the available options. They did not know how to distinguish a good rehabilitation program from a bad one, much less discriminate between a chronic care facility, like a nursing home, from one that offers some degree of rehabilitative services.

Burt Brody was typical. He was told by the general hospital that had provided care to his wife, Jean, that "... once you're gone from here you'll have to find a social worker [at the facility] to help you." It was a handoff of responsibility when the literature suggests that family members are especially vulnerable and in need of guidance.[14] All that was done to prepare Burt for this important transition was to give him "a list of all the nursing homes that were in the [local] area with their phone numbers." He recalls, "That was it. They said, 'here's all the information.'" And that was it.

He was left to his own devices. Fortunately, a retired physician friend of his helped him scout out a proper place for Jean. Still scarred by his wife's brain hemorrhage, this skilled lawyer couldn't navigate this next challenge without help. His doctor friend "... helped me, I didn't know what to look for in terms of rehab, and basically he and I went around, and he more than I, interviewed the rehab people." Initially they were disappointed with their options, "First we looked at the nursing home to see is it clean, does the staff seem to know what they're doing, and basically the answers to those questions were no and no." Eventually they found a place that was acceptable: "... there was one place that really had an outside contract for rehab. And the people who were doing rehab were excellent." They had made their choice and rushed as it was, it was somewhat informed.

But families find it difficult to sift through their options. It is hard to assess a program. And to the untrained eye, looks can be deceiving. John Harmon spoke of his experience trying to find a suitable place for his son. "Well, at the hospital they got a list of different places close to home and around the county and [metropolitan] area." Interviews were set up and John went to take a look before sending his son there. On multiple occasions, there was a problem. A facility "... seemed like it would be ok and then it turned out that it wasn't ... he'd end up back at the hospital every time with pneumonia or something."

It became a trauma without end. And the barriers were worse than any of these families knew. As they tried to find placements for their loved ones, concerted efforts were underway to systematically exclude patients from the rehabilitation they would need.

BEYOND BENIGN NEGLECT

Dr. John Whyte, a rehabilitation physician and neuropsychologist who is the director of the Moss Rehabilitation Research Institute in Philadelphia, brought to my attention admission criteria of McKesson Health Solutions, LLC that, as applied by hospitals, often effectively deprives many patients with disorders of consciousness access to inpatient rehabilitation after hospital discharge.[15]

McKesson is a proprietary company that designs care pathways and utilization review for insurance companies.[16,17] One of the cornerstones of their business is the "InterQual criteria." The corporation notes on its website that, "Today, more organizations – payers and providers, public and private – rely on InterQual® than on any other evidence-based clinical decision support criteria."[18] And it was the use and application of this care management program that worried John Whyte.

Under the aegis of McKesson's "InterQual criteria," to be eligible for acute inpatient rehabilitation, patients would have to show sufficient evidence of consciousness and be at a level of "Rancho III and evolving." Rancho III refers to a functional status within The Rancho Los Amigos Scale that is roughly equivalent to MCS.[19,20] (Rancho II would equate with the vegetative state.) *Evolving*, in the context of the InterQual criteria, means that the patient is progressing substantially every day. McKesson justifies these

criteria with the logic that patients need to actively participate in acute rehabilitation to benefit from rehabilitation and that those who are not yet ready
for acute rehabilitation could go to less intensive venues and be referred back
to acute rehabilitation when they were ready.

In theory this makes perfectly good sense. Why would one want to
"waste" scarce resources on rehabilitation when patients are unable to coop-
erate? Why not bring them back into rehabilitation when they are ready to
be treated?

In practice, when applied to many brain-injury patients, this is problematic according to Whyte and his colleagues. Once in the chronic care system, brain-injury patients do not generally regain entry to rehabilitation for
two reasons. First, improvement may require the "coaxing" of a rehabilitation specialist using drugs or other therapies. And second, if the criterion
for admission to acute rehabilitation was improvement, *that improvement
would have to be recognized*, but as we have already seen, these patients are
prone to misdiagnosis when in nursing homes. So even if a patient regained
consciousness and became MCS, there would be a good chance that the
improvement would not be recognized, as we have already seen.

These concerns, taken together, suggest that requiring patients to show
sufficient evidence of consciousness and be at "Rancho III and evolving"
means that many patients who might benefit from acute inpatient rehabilitation may not gain access to these services.

John Whyte and his colleagues of the Disorders of Consciousness Special
Interest Group (DOC-SIG) of the Traumatic Brain Injury Model Systems, a
group of dedicated professionals who run a handful of exemplary brain-injury
rehab programs funded in part by the National Institute on Disability and
Rehabilitation,[21] were concerned about McKesson's criteria and sought to
explain why they thought the company's policies might impair access to
acute inpatient rehabilitation for patients with disorders of consciousness.

So on behalf of the Special Interest Group, Whyte wrote McKesson in
September 2011 sharing his concerns. And since then, multiple e-mails and
calls with McKesson management followed. He pointed out that their criteria
were not evidence based and that they were internally inconsistent. For example, he pointed out that published reports have demonstrated that 41 percent
of MCS patients who have had TBI are misdiagnosed as vegetative once they
arrive in chronic care.[22] He then asked, if that is the case – and the diagnosis
was wrong – how could one know if a patient was "evolving" in MCS?

And even if the diagnosis were correct, improvement or the potential
for additional recovery did not require the high rate of progress that "evolving" might suggest. To be fair, defining the precise rate of recovery is challenging and the problem may lie with the way hospitals or insurance companies
interpret what was intended by the "evolving" criteria.

Alternately, the rate of recovery could be a function of ancillary rehabilitation. That is, patients whose recovery might be occurring at a much
slower, even indiscernible pace might have the potential for more significant
progress if properly diagnosed and helped along with inpatient rehabilitation.
Either way, setting the criterion at *MCS and evolving,* all too often in practice
limits access to inpatient rehabilitation for some patients who might find it
beneficial.

As an alternative, Whyte and colleagues proposed a "front-loaded" system that would allow admission to a brain rehabilitation program after acute
hospitalization so patients could receive intensive evaluation and assessment
as well as therapeutic rehabilitation. This would help patients be more accurately diagnosed and provide them with qualified care when it might make
the most difference. After an interval of care, patients who demonstrated progress could be referred to "mainstream" brain rehabilitation. Those who did
not respond could receive placement in a subacute setting. He advanced this
argument because patients who gain access to acute inpatient rehabilitation
programs avoid many of the medical complications seen in chronic care, have
lower death rates and attain a higher functional status compared with those
who do receive this early intervention.

From a scholarly point of view, the analysis of the DOC-SIG raises
the deeper question of responsibility and causality. How much of the access
to inpatient rehabilitation hinges on the actual McKesson criteria and how
much upon their interpretation by individual hospitals, insurance carriers,
and health care systems that apply and implement these guidelines?

No doubt the sociology and economics of acute care and rehabilitation is complex with both the criteria and their implementation affecting
access to inpatient rehabilitation. How and where these variables intersect
is a topic worthy of additional scholarship, important to start but impossible
to conclude here.

HEADING HOME

Most hospitals assume patients will be discharged to an institutional setting,
but there may be emerging evidence that some families are so discouraged by
their options, that they end up taking their loved ones home, if not immediately then later, as was the case with Terry Wallis.

Cheryl Kursave, the mother of Brandon, a teenager who sustained a TBI
in a fight, decided to take her son home after checking out of the one facility
made available to her. "My son would never, ever go to a horrible place like
that." She confronted the hospital and "... just wouldn't accept where they
told me where he was going to go." Instead of receiving assistance, it's been
a confrontation against low expectations. So, Cheryl pushed back against

their recommendations, "I fought it, I fought a hard battle." To fight against the system and "what they [the hospital] wanted – it's just been a constant battle."

She decided to look for alternatives, "and I opened the phone book, and I went to these nursing agencies" to see if they could provide care at home. But it was new territory for the hospital, which "had never sent someone home with nurses." As Cheryl put it, the novelty of a discharge home "was a new learning curve for them."

Although "every step of every bit of this for Brandon and me has been a battle ... but I brought him home and had the nursing." And he improved: "within a week of him being home he jumped from a Rancho II to a Rancho III." The change from level II to III meant that Brandon had developed the ability to localize a response to sensory stimuli, the difference between being vegetative versus in a MCS. It was a small step, but an important one nonetheless, and ironically one which might have made him eligible under the aforementioned McKesson InterQual Criteria – if anyone had known. But Cheryl was pleased nonetheless. Already Brandon had progressed "further than most people's expectations." Her conclusion: "Him in his home environment, I think it was the right decision to do."

But sometimes home is nothing more than a challenging alternative for care when all the forces that conspire to limit or restrict care coalesce. It is a refuge of last resort when all the other options and benefits have run out. Samantha Berman* and her husband Tom* were challenged by a new baby, home care, and no meaningful benefits – despite the fact that they had private insurance at the start of Tom's injury.

After an aborted attempt to go to a nursing home, which was a sub-acute facility, complicated by a fall, fevers, and a rise in blood pressure Tom ended up back in the hospital. And then his options were exhausted. When he was again ready for discharge, the social worker told Samantha, "They weren't going to accept him back at the subacute facility." She had no alternatives, so her "only option" was to "bring him home." It was a Herculean task and she got little help, "And at that time, the insurance was only offering, two hours per day for twelve ... days per calendar year. So, which was nothing. Nothing, I had a new baby and I had no help with him at that time." The outcome: "So, they sent him home. I have paid, I paid out of pocket."

The fiscal and emotional costs were staggering.

10 Heather's Story

Finding placement for a MCS patient who is severely disabled but still conscious can be difficult for social workers. Paradoxically, it is sometimes easier to find a bed if the patient is vegetative and not in MCS. The "better" diagnosis would require more specialized placement where additional elements of care such as cognitive rehabilitation and physical therapy would be available. The more gravely injured patient, ironically, places less burden on overtaxed facilities.

In one instance, I heard of a case in which a patient with traumatic brain injury, Heather Sykes, was alleged to have been deliberately misdiagnosed, or at least mislabeled as vegetative, in order to facilitate discharge to chronic care. According to her mother, Cynthia (Cindy) Sykes's retelling of her story, she was discharged from the hospital diagnosed as being in the permanent vegetative state, even though Cindy did not believe it.

I met Cindy when we were both speakers at a regional conference on TBI in the fall of 2007.[1] She and an advanced practice nurse partnered up to tell Heather's story.[2] It was a compelling account consistent in many ways with what I had learned from the families I had been interviewing at Cornell. As with Terry Wallis, and so many other families we have interviewed, Cindy thought she saw purposeful behaviors that would give Heather an MCS and not a vegetative diagnosis.

And that is where our experiences diverged because Cindy alleged that her daughter's misdiagnosis was more than the all too common error of omission where an MCS patient is mistaken as vegetative. Instead, she asserted that her ongoing vegetative diagnosis had became one of commission, a deliberate attempt to *misrepresent* her condition, and chronic care needs, in order to facilitate Heather's nursing home placement. If true, it would be an act that some might construe as diagnostic fraud orchestrated to deal with a chronic care system unprepared to accept seriously disabled but conscious patients. It is a sobering and sad story that I share with the generous permission of Cindy Sykes.

PIGEONHOLED

Heather was in her thirties, living in the South, and working as a musician when she was in a nearly fatal motor vehicle accident on the interstate. She was thrown from her car and gravely injured with an initial Glasgow Coma Scale of three, which is the lowest number compatible with life. She was medevaced to an academic medical center where she received aggressive neurosurgical care.

At the outset, things seemed to be going well. Heather had heroic neurosurgery including the removal of part of her skull to relieve pressure on her brain and a remarkably even course afterward. Eighteen days after her horrid accident, she was well enough to be transferred out of the Neuro-ICU to a step-down unit. She had recovered some neurological function and was localizing to pain and tracking objects.

Both of these actions would make her MCS and not vegetative but the challenge was that there were so many turnovers in the step-down unit that no one got to know Heather sufficiently well to make and document these findings. Cindy, a former hospital administrator, made a critical observation. She recalls, "... there were a lot of changes there. The staff was different all the time ... we felt just like they didn't get to know Heather." Cindy and her family "were seeing improvements and changes" but could not get the staff to take note. She tried valiantly to get their attention because they had been advised "... to document what we were seeing because we had been told early on whatever you see have them document it." But she could not get the staff to corroborate what she had observed, "I couldn't get the staff to say she's making forward progress instead of not doing anything ... it just wasn't happening." And when someone did listen, "I really and truly felt they were just patronizing me."

Even at that early juncture, Cindy was fearful that Heather would get labeled as having a deficit she did not have. Presciently, she worried that her daughter would be written off as a hopeless case as if she were deemed vegetative, even when she was not. "So it was very, very frustrating and it was scary because I felt that she was going to be pigeonholed into a spot that we would have a hard time getting out of."

PRESSURE WAVES

Then complications struck. The early smooth sailing was replaced by turbulent seas that nearly took Heather's life. A new fluid collection accumulated inside her brain raising pressure inside her head. This would lead to pressure waves and a downward force on her brainstem. She was about to herniate, a dire development when the brain is literally pushed down onto the spine damaging vital structures like the midbrain and the brainstem. Unchecked, herniation can result in death.

In the short term, the fluid collection caused Heather to have a decline in function. And this reversal led to a resumption of talks about whether aggressive care should be maintained or palliation initiated. Cindy recalls those perilous times: "It was pretty devastating to ... have them basically tell you that we were going to prepare for her to die." Their predictions were gloomy. First the drain that was placed to remove the accumulating fluid would "clot off with blood." And when the drain failed, "her head, her brain, was going to continue to swell and swell and she was going to die."

Along with those graphic, indeed almost gruesome details, her mother was given a grim prognosis. She had "two days to two weeks to live." There was no equivocation. It was all bad.

So Cindy reached out to family so they could come and say goodbye. With a dose of stoicism, she accepted the news: "... we just decided to make the best of it. I called her brothers and said, 'you need to come.'" Cindy paused and cried. "Everybody came, everybody came. They did. And we just ... had family time with her and spent as much time with her as we could."

But as can be the case, the predictions were wrong; Heather "... continued to just hang in there ... the things that they said were going to happen with the brain didn't happen." And the timeline was off too. The drain "didn't fail when they said it was going to fail." And then when it did fail, Heather's own "... pumping system up there, started working on its own." The family was relieved, but again disappointed by her doctors.

Cindy remembers "... thinking this is just absolutely wonderful, something's working right here, she's trying, she's getting there." It was a time for modest celebration, "... we were of course very excited." But again, the medical staff did not share their enthusiasm. They "still didn't give us much hope."

The family's celebratory feelings were short-lived because of an observation made by Cindy's husband, a cardiologist, who had come to visit for the weekend. He noticed that Heather's tube feedings had not been restarted after her most recent surgery. Cindy was very upset by the omission. She thought the feedings had been resumed, as she had been promised and it took a physician's discernment to appreciate that it was otherwise. It seemed like a breach of faith.

The omission raised suspicions, especially because the observation triggered what Cindy called the "stop feeding talk." That is when the team "... suggested that we consider not feeding her anymore because if we fed her she was going to swell more, she'd have more secretions, she was going to cough, she was going to. ..." It was cast as the humane thing to do, to make her more comfortable and avoid the infliction of pain, however she might perceive it. The feeding tube, they were told, "was going to make her more uncomfortable ... she would be in more pain. ..." Cindy was asked, "Did I want to do that to her?"

Cindy was beside herself and huddled with her sister who was visiting. They went to visit Heather together. And then, against all odds, Heather – who had been lying in her bed rather inert – opened her right eye and began to move her hand. It was startling and strained their own sense of reality. Cindy was stunned: "... sometimes you think you see things and you're like, 'whoa,' you wonder whether you really saw it, or was it just you wanted to see something so badly."

The hope was there and the power of wishful thinking ever present. But not this time. When Cindy saw Heather respond, she turned to her sister for a reality check. And instead of that, she got confirmation. Cindy recalled what happened next: "And my sister said, 'no Cindy – I saw that too!'"

Emboldened by what they had *both* seen, the sisters alerted a nurse, "So we're right away trying to get a nurse in there to see what we saw, she's moving, she's doing something." Although this news should have been momentous, it was dismissed. Remarkably, the observation was to be deferred, "They wanted me to wait 'til the next day to talk to the head neurosurgeon about whether we were going to continue care for Heather or not. ...."

Not to be deterred, not after what they had both just witnessed, Cindy pushed back. She told the nurse, "I'm not waiting until tomorrow" and gave her a directive, "I want you to start feeding her." Her rationale was simple, Heather was trying to recover and not getting the nutrition needed to sustain the effort. So the bottom line was clear: "I need to at least give her the chance to show us what she wants to do."

With the sort of pride that comes with taking a principled stand, Cindy shared the outcome, "And so they started feeding her and she started getting better."

A SPLIT DECISION

With the decision to restart feedings, which the family had never agreed to stop, it was now time to make plans to discharge Heather to a skilled nursing facility (SNF). Because occupational and physical therapy had not seen Heather since her initial favorable recovery, her family asked that she be reevaluated to determine if she might qualify for acute rehabilitation. She didn't.

From the therapists' point of view, six weeks after her injury she was neither visually tracking nor following commands, much less responding to touch. At that point, there was no indication of her being minimally conscious and thus able to participate in rehabilitation.

But a week later, things began to change. The doctors who were spending a great deal of time with Heather were beginning to see what the family had first noticed two weeks earlier. Heather was becoming more awake and seemed to be tracking objects in her visual field, at least some of the time.

It was a mixed picture. The family was somewhat hopeful, and the staff was split. The physical therapists were decidedly on the side of recovery. Some of them even began to give Heather therapy on the side, without a doctor's directive, to push her along. They wanted to help foster a recovery and began a rehab program on their own, outside of normal channels, because paradoxically she was not yet well enough to qualify for the very interventions that might foster the requisite degree of demonstrable improvement necessary to secure sanctioned services.

Until that threshold was reached, all of their ministrations were discreetly left out of the medical record where no mention was made of these extracurricular activities. As one sympathetic nurse practitioner put it, there was not a note in the chart about all the rehab they were providing Heather, "It was all on the sly."

IN PALLIATIVE CARE TERRITORY

Even as she inched her way toward improvement, Heather faced a slew of challenges. Beyond the physiological burden of her injury, she faced the stigma of diminished expectations fostered in part by where she was placed in the hospital. For weeks Heather had been on the palliative care service, a venue dedicated to the care of the dying, where the goals of care were pain and symptom management not rehabilitation and recovery. Yet Heather remained there with the palliative care team, which neither shared the family's optimism nor endorsed their approach. A nursing note from the palliative care service, shared by Heather's mother, read the "... family is at the bedside and confident with their decision and to continue treatment is in alignment with the patient's wishes."

For those unaccustomed to reading a medical record, it is important to deconstruct the note's manifest content from its latent meaning. On the surface, it could be construed that the family is confident and has reached a consensus on goals of care. They are dutifully making decisions in accord with the wishes of the patient in line with all the modern-day deference to patient self-determination, one of the cornerstones of bioethics. But if one reads between the lines for the hidden message embedded in the overt language, there is an implicit degree of derision in noting that the family still remains "confident with their decision" about continuing treatment that was not going to make a difference. The note's tone bespoke an unspoken futility. This was not praise of their confidence, but rather a questioning of it.

The final evidence of their true views was a gratuitous comment attributing such preferences to being "in alignment" with the patient's prior wishes, a polite – but pointed – rebuke of the *family's* wishes. It is a proper, yet oppositional note whose semiotics convey a tension between the palliative care team and the family's goals and objectives. The tension between the palliative care team and the family's perspective could be seen in Heather's room. The visitor would see an island of hope amidst a sea of death and despair. It was not draped in crepe and certainly not mournful. Her room was not a Victorian sick room where the dead were laid out. Her bed was not a death bed. Instead the scene was forward looking and optimistic. Heather, the musician, lay there refusing to die. Her bed was covered with CDs of her own music providing the soundtrack for a life not yet concluded though still hanging in the balance. And gathered around was a dutiful mom, a vigilant family, and loving friends who came at all hours to support her and to do range of motion exercises, restorative routines that dying people do not need and do not get.

She got the exercises so she could live another day and not stiffen up. Cindy taught everybody how to do her range of motion exercises, ever assisted by "a couple therapists that took a real interest in Heather." They followed her "everywhere she went ..." and sought to rehabilitate her even as the doctors tried their hand at palliation.

Crying, Cindy speaks of her debt to the therapists. Speaking of these unsung heroines she said, "You know, I am ever grateful to all of them because they went beyond what their superiors were allowing them to do to help Heather." She continues, "And if it hadn't been for them I know that she wouldn't be where she is today." And yet, they could not help directly because Heather was supposedly dying and not a candidate for rehabilitation in that setting. So Cindy adjusted, making the best of the situation. "I basically did all of her range of motion. I taught family, nieces, nephews, whomever I could get, whenever they were there to work with Heather's legs, work with her arms, keep her moving."

But Heather's improvement came with a cost. Cindy had been given a responsibility for the provision of care for which she was ill-prepared and untrained. "I was always so worried ... I was so scared that I was going to hurt her because I'm not a professional and I don't know. Here's these feet that are like this and stiff and hands that you can't pull the fingers out and I was so afraid that I was going to break a bone. ..." Cindy was conflicted about her role and her daughter's needs. It was an impossible predicament for a mother, but ethically she "knew I had to do it," so her daughter could get the care that went wanting. Her response to her quandary? "I just kept on and just prayed every day that it would be okay."

It was the best Cindy could do because the system did not know how to categorize Heather. Heather was in a venue where the expectation was that she would die. Her problem was what might be called "a failure to die" and to adhere to expectations associated with her care venue – in this case a palliative care ward.[3] But like many complicated cases, she had yet to declare herself. She certainly could have died, but that she also could have recovered some was a prospect that was counter to the expectations of those caring for her, categorized as she was by her placement onto the palliative care service.

It was a strange paradox: she was on palliative care and was meant to die, but didn't. One would think that given her family's wishes, she might have been transferred to another service. But she was seen, by her clinicians, as one who was dying and so remained there. Such was the power of the legacies of which we have written – of Beecher, Quinlan, Cruzan, and Schiavo – that she remained there, despite the more hopeful goals of her family.

But it was a hard place to be, in a venue designed for one sort of care even as something else was desired and needed. Every effort was contrarian; every little victory was achieved against the grain. As one nurse recalls, it was "... a real testament to Cindy and Heather's friends that she continued to get range of motion and that sort of thing even up in the palliative care unit, which is usually where we think of people going to die."

But death was neither what Cindy intended nor hoped for her daughter. Over the next weeks, plans were made to replace the cranium that had been removed emergently to relieve pressure. It would be the next step in her recovery, and this too prompted resistance from the palliative care team, which now asked the neurology service to reconsult on Heather's case to better estimate her prognosis.

It was an unusual request as it potentially represented a reversal of roles. Neurologists often make dire pronouncements that lead to decisions to withhold or withdraw life-sustaining therapy. Now they were being asked to comment on Heather's recovery. One nurse, with a bit of disbelief, recalled that now "the neurologists were actually consulted by the palliative care team, because I think the palliative care team really wanted to know what is she doing? What can she consistently do? And how do we classify this?"

The consultant neurologist's views, however, reflected the same indeterminacy of the palliative care team. They observed the lowest level of tracking, but no command following or purposeful movement. Although this would seem to place her on the low end of the MCS, the consultants thought her to be in a persistent vegetative state but hedged. They thought that the prudent thing would be to wait and observe her for one to four months to determine the likelihood of additional recovery.

With this additional input, Cindy pressed to have the skull replaced. Ultimately, with the help of the neurosurgery chief resident, who might have been alone on the medical team in thinking that Heather had a chance, they pushed forward and sought to replace the missing piece of skull. He ordered a CT. There was a fluid collection still outside the skull, which made it impossible to do the cranioplasty. But Cindy persevered, and they put a shunt in to drain the fluid off and let it drain into the abdomen. After a couple of weeks the fluid came off and Heather was able to have her skull repaired. Heather was now finally ready for discharge.

TOO HOT TO HANDLE

Cindy was informed about the discharge process. As a hospital administrator, she was not naïve about such things – she knew enough to be worried. "Well, one of the things that was very frightening was that they wanted her out of the hospital. And I understand, I was at a major medical center in rural Michigan for a long time, I understand managed care, and I wanted her to be in a good place." Out of her state, she noted, "I'm not familiar with any of these nursing care facilities. The first nursing care facility that she went to supposedly had a good reputation and I was petrified to leave her. It was so awful."

One day at this facility, the nurse did not step into Heather's room for an entire shift. Cindy felt Heather was so vulnerable there: "... often times I was alone, and so I would stay 'til midnight because I was afraid that they wouldn't be there to do something or to see something or whatever and it was at that time that her brain started to swell again and I knew something was wrong, I could tell."

And in an episode reminiscent of Dustin's post-discharge deterioration, Heather developed a fever in the setting of indifferent, distracted nursing care. Cindy recalls, "She felt like she was hot to me. I was constantly trying to get them to come take her temperature, take her blood pressure, check her vitals. Please do something, I know something's wrong. And finally she ended up emergently back in the hospital."

Later, Cindy told the social worker at the academic medical center that had referred Heather there, "... don't even ask me to send her back to that place." She was clear about her expectations, "You have to find a better place for her, because I will not sign any papers to release her anywhere." And then making it personal she pleaded, "... tell me from your heart that this is going to be a place that's safe for my daughter to be in."

AN INCONVENIENT DIAGNOSIS

Despite the setback, Heather again recovered and was again ready for discharge. The only problem was that her medical record said she was *vegetative*. Cindy had tried to get her diagnosis changed before her discharge to the *minimally conscious state* but to no avail. Cindy's earlier concerns about Heather being "pigeonholed" into a diagnosis had come to pass, despite her persistent efforts to give her daughter every opportunity to wage a recovery. Heather had done her part, rebounded from tough odds on several occasions, only to be labeled as vegetative when chances were she was not.

Why had it turned out this way? Was it that Heather had defied the minimalist expectations of her assignment to a palliative care bed? Was it the prognostic uncertainty epitomized by the split opinion of medical teams providing her care? Was it just another example of the nihilism about severe brain injured spawned by Quinlan? Or was it something else?

Just after Heather was admitted to the new nursing home Cindy would learn why her daughter had been described as vegetative in her medical record. And it was a disturbing discovery.

Shortly after Heather arrived at the nursing home, the facility's staff called Cindy and requested a meeting the next morning. Expecting a one-on-one session, she was instead greeted by the entirety of her daughter's interdisciplinary team. She recalls it was "... this big team of people: the speech therapist, occupational and physical therapists, and then director of nursing. . . ."

Their message was gratifying and maddening, "... they told me that the patient that they received the day before, my daughter, was not the patient that they were told they were going to get." They were expecting a dying patient who was vegetative who was simply going to need supportive care. But instead they got someone who was clearly minimally conscious. The team put it this way, "... she obviously isn't in PVS, she's responding to her name obviously, when we talk to her she looks at us, she's tracking people across the room, she's moving her limbs, not a lot, but she's moving." Cindy summed it up: "This isn't a patient that apparently they were told was just basically going to have custodial care and be there to die."

Cindy felt misled and betrayed, "And I was upset when I found this out because here I thought that the professionals, the medical team at [the academic medical center] thought that Heather was looking better and I'm thinking, okay, what's happening?"

It was especially so, when she finally appreciated *why* the misdiagnosis had been conveyed to the nursing home. As cruel as it sounded, her daughter's consciousness, Heather's very link to her world and family was being *denied in order to find her a nursing home bed*. As tenuous as that link was, the sad truth was that it was easier to place a patient who was not conscious than one who was, albeit minimally so. The former needed less services and less support and had places to go. Beds were allocated in the system for patients who were vegetative and/or dying, patients whose trajectories were clear and time lines more certain.

But there weren't – and aren't enough places – for those who have indeterminate diagnoses like MCS, whose recoveries are unpredictable and whose level of consciousness demands a degree of therapeutic engagement that is reflective of an ability to interact with others.

It was not even the questionable, though perhaps well-intentioned, practice of physician manipulation of reimbursement rules to help a patient receive necessary and needed care.[4] No, this breach of integrity was solely and simply a matter of placement. Drawing upon her experience, Cindy, the former hospital administrator, speculated, "As time went on I realized that that facilitated them having more nursing care facilities that would take her. If she's going to be laying there, not doing anything, then the nursing care facilities will take her, and they just wanted to get her out of the hospital. So they left her with that diagnosis. ..." Following her logic, it seemed simply more convenient and expedient to do so, even though this deception perpetuated the belief that Heather was unconscious when she was in fact conscious.

This seemingly willful action deprived Heather of the potential to interact with others because her diagnostic label indicated that such engagement was not possible. This portrayal of her condition is far more significant than a bureaucratic ruse designed to secure her a scarce nursing home bed. It represents the denial of the basic right of human community, marked by the potential to communicate with another. This was precluded by the vegetative diagnosis, potentially segregating Heather from relationships with those who cared about her.

BRAIN INJURY, HYPOTHERMIA, AND PATTERNS OF CARE

The legal and philosophical implications of intentionally denying the consciousness of one who has regained it is not just a denial of care but a fundamental miscarriage of justice and civil rights,[5] a topic to which we will return in later chapters. For now, Heather's journey in the acute care setting – and her transit through palliative care and her premature discharge to chronic care while still unstable – speak to the inability of current structures of acute care to identify these patients and to place them in proper rehabilitative settings.

Heather's placement speaks to this point. Paradoxically, while the misdiagnosis got Heather a bed, it was just that, only a bed. Once again, it was a placement that failed to meet her needs and undermined her interests. Her assignment to the palliative care service was predicated upon the presumption that she would die or that her family would withdraw life-sustaining measures. Now Heather was again in a care setting that was ill-equipped to provide her with services that her conscious state would require.

Cindy understood this: "... one of my key things was to get her diagnosis changed. And one of the reasons was so I could get more therapy for her so that the insurance would pay for it and the therapists could start seeing her and she would hopefully move forward." Despite her best efforts, Cindy could not get Heather's diagnosis changed when she left that facility, even though its occupational and physical therapists were *volunteering* their own time to give Heather the rehabilitation they thought she needed, notwithstanding a diagnosis that made her ineligible for such services. These therapists saw something in their patient that the system chose to overlook because recognizing her level of awareness would make her a displaced person between acute, chronic, and rehabilitative care systems.

The consequence of this displacement is that unstable patients who retain the potential for additional recovery can sometimes end up in nursing home beds before they are medically stable. And once there, they can linger misdiagnosed. Either way, through premature discharge or inappropriate placement, patients do not receive the rehabilitation that they need. There are few, if any, settings that can accommodate the acute and rehabilitative needs of patients who have ongoing complex medical issues and a disorder of consciousness.

The problem is that these patients challenge expectations upon which systems of care have been built. But with the advent of medical interventions that are able to temper dangerous rises in intracranial pressure, like intracranial pressure monitoring and craniectomy, patients who previously would have died or become vegetative now survive the more indeterminate state of MCS, an indeterminacy for which institutions remain unprepared.

Outside of a few expert programs, limited to select patients, there is no consistent venue able to provide services intermediate between acute care and rehabilitation for patients with emerging consciousness. As the aforementioned narratives indicate, there is no institutional way station for patients whose mix of incipient consciousness and medical complexity requires more than the usual three weeks of acute care before they are transported from the acute care setting.

This is a growing category, not limited to patients with TBI, who have done better with the management of increased intracranial pressure. This growing demographic must now also account for patients who have sustained anoxic brain injury after cardiac arrest and been treated with *therapeutic hypothermia*, basically the provision of cooled intravenous fluids and use of a cooling blanket to bring down the body's core temperature.[6] Cooling is neuroprotective and helps gird the brain against the ravages of anoxic injury by decreasing metabolic demand and oxygen requirements.[7]

The protective effect of hypothermia is so profound that it has invalidated the long-established Levy Criteria, which dictated prognosis after cardiac arrest.[8] In use since 1981, the Levy Criteria have been overturned for patients receiving therapeutic hypothermia and at present the publications from the American Academy of Neurology now indicate that its earlier guidelines[9] cannot be applied and that clinical judgment must dictate care decisions. Some investigators have warned that current American Academy of Neurology guidelines may be "overly pessimistic."[10]

Brains, and lives, have been saved that heretofore would have been lost. This is a good news–bad news story. Good for all the obvious reasons.

Bad because it has caught the health care system unprepared for a cohort of patients who may need more prolonged intensive care before significant recoveries can be precluded. For example, patients may need ongoing cardiac care for their heart disease as well as neurorehabilitation for their recovering brains that can only be provided in the acute care setting.

Given the U.S. incidence of out-of-hospital cardiac arrest of 383,000 per year[11] and 200,000 in-hospital events,[12] this is not a trivial public health question. Needless to say, if but a small fraction of these patients were to receive therapeutic hypothermia, and this practice is now becoming the standard of care,[13] this new cohort of patients will put a strain on current hospital capacity, where utilization of critical care services is increasing even as the overall number of acute care beds in the hospital sector contracts.[14] This mix of trends will further exacerbate need. Increases in critical care will result in more survival from brain injury and cardiac arrest thus requiring care in hospital beds that no longer exist. This shortage of services will compound the already significant discharge and placement challenges we have enumerated, unless there is a proactive response to this need.

MOHONK'S MOSAIC OF CARE

Patients with disorders of consciousness, from traumatic and anoxic etiologies, will form part of this cohort. And they will need something that does not yet exist, a *mosaic of care* that blends the best of acute, rehabilitative, and chronic care to ensure that their disease trajectory does not strand them between current care structures.[15] Such a strategy was outlined in the 2006 *Mohonk Report* written for the Congressional Brain Injury Caucus, a bipartisan group of legislators concerned with the provision of care to this population.[16] The goal was to delineate a program of care from initial management through acute care and rehabilitation.

Written by leading experts, *The Mohonk Report* underscored the need to share specialized knowledge of disorders of consciousness between settings in order to minimize misdiagnosis and to employ emerging therapeutics. Sharing of expertise would be organized in regional hubs around research centers of excellence that would anchor acute rehabilitation and chronic care facilities. Care would be seamless across venues from initial injury out to chronic care and take place within a network that would have three levels of care institutions. The majority of patients would be in a SNF with the remainder in expert acute rehabilitation centers or scientific research centers of excellences, which would be the investigative core for all the network components.

This capability would help ensure that theory and practice worked together to develop better models of care and innovative therapies that could be readily assessed and disseminated. We anticipated that the Mohonk model would be geographically based with up to five national research cores associated with a larger number of acute rehab centers and SNFs. These networks would conduct a range of studies from understanding the basic science of brain injury recovery to the collection of epidemiological data. They could also be the sites for demonstration projects on medical therapeutics and educating practitioners on how to communicate effectively, and compassionately, with families about disorders of consciousness. *The Mohonk Report* was far-reaching when it was written, although elements of it are starting to be implemented in the Veterans Administration's polytrauma centers, as we shall soon see.[17]

A BAND OF THERAPISTS

Absent the systemic response as envisioned by *Mohonk*, Cindy depended upon the goodwill of a few individuals who stepped forward and assumed moral responsibility for Heather's care, and her future. And Cindy holds these women, her daughter's unofficial physical therapy team, very close to her heart. Speaking with a mother's love she recounts that "... the therapists there took an interest in Heather and they fought for her. And I have to say that they were very ethical, the therapists were. The administrators, however, were not. And so it was a constant battle for them to just be able to treat Heather, and they treated her when they were not supposed to. They would stay after hours and treat her and things like that. And I mean, that's the kind of care I know people can't do, they have busy lives and families and they have to go home to their loved ones too."

Some of the therapists who had worked with Heather were at the conference in and I had the chance to speak with them and Cindy. It was interesting to be with them because the narratives we had collected at Weill Cornell were in so many ways like Heather's story. It was one of the first times I realized that the stories I had heard were not isolated and yet were reflective of practices that were otherwise invisible to distant policy makers. But these women who were close to the experiences of patients and families knew exactly what I meant when I spoke about the neglect experienced by patients and families. They knew the burdens from firsthand experience, which were typified by Heather's story. This was not fiction but a sad reality that they had seen for themselves and tried to repair.

In the dining room of a grand old railroad hotel, they sat at a round table reminiscing as much as celebrating a cause and their advocacy. All mothers, Cindy had bonded with this band of therapists who had engaged in a bit of civil disobedience to do the right thing. They were pleased with themselves and humbled to be recognized as the heroines that they were.

As I sat and listened, really feeling privileged to have been admitted to their sorority, I kept on thinking back to something Cindy had said during her presentation. Reflecting on the many frustrations of trying to secure care for her child, Cindy summed it up as well as anyone could, "And so this is the frustration of trying to help her get to be as good as she can get. So I just pray that things will change and conferences like this with people like you will help those patients. Maybe not for Heather right now, but for a family in the future who is going through the same thing."

Finally, Cindy told us how Heather was doing back home with her in Michigan, about two years after her injury. She had made progress, was self-aware and able to follow commands. And Cindy was pleased with Heather's level and pace of recovery. She told those gathered that she appreciates "... that Heather is going to be different, but I don't think that doesn't mean she won't be a wonderful daughter, friend, sister, and we won't enjoy her for the rest of her life."

Her former therapists delight in the steps that Heather had made since she left their charge. They were neither surprised by her progress nor by the challenges she continued to face. The status quo of chronic care had not changed, even though Heather did. Clinical indifference coupled with bureaucratic barriers still was the prevailing norm.

11 Neuroimaging and Neuroscience in the Public Mind

IMAGES OF CHOICE

Before I left the conference, and my visit with Cindy Sykes, she shared one more observation about Heather's care, which really encapsulated the challenge of prognostication, discerning who will do well and who not. This is a critical task for families as they try and make decisions about care. Having a better sense of possible outcomes is necessary to avoid the heartache of disappointment that comes with unfounded optimism or the lost opportunity for recovery that attends unsubstantiated pessimism. Early during Heather's course, Cindy recalled speaking with one of the doctors at the academic medical center where she was treated who described the predicament. In a confessional tone he shared a secret, most outsiders would not suspect: experts aren't very good at prognosticating, even when they make use of neuroimaging techniques. In fact, sometimes the scans can be very misleading. The doctor told Cindy, "We can look at two patients' scans and one can look very bad and bleak like Heather's, and the other can look very promising, and the two have absolutely opposite outcomes. The one that looked good doesn't do well and the one that looked terrible does very well."

Cindy's response to the predicament was both generous and illustrative of the challenges these families face. Generous in that she felt that both of "... those two patients should have the same opportunity to show their determination against the odds." And illustrative of her experience, the challenge of making choices without being adequately informed about how things might turn out. Without the advantage of prognostic knowledge gleaned from science, one had to give the two patients *both* a chance. It was only fair because their futures were indistinguishable.

But Cindy's caution raised a deeper question of whether or not these families have been deprived of the right to informed consent and refusal. After all, how could they engage in informed decision making without the requisite amount of information they would need to make a choice? All the more so in the face of indeterminacy, that middle group referred to by Dr. Plum in the 1970s, when the outcome *is* unpredictable.

When decisions are devoid of a scientific predicate, the very essence of informed consent – and as importantly, informed refusal – is placed at risk. This was a point made by the great, late bioethicist and psychoanalytic scholar, Jay Katz of Yale Law School. He wrote eloquently of the relationship between science and informed consent arguing that it was the rise of Baconian science – with its notions of cause and effect – that made ethical choices and informed consent or refusal possible.[1] Absent a sense of probable outcome, these decisions cannot be informed save for knowledge of one's ignorance in the face of uncertainty. And while that is better than unreflected upon nihilism, it is still a thin reed to hang momentous decisions upon.

But sadly, that is where the field has been, a state of ignorance in the face of profound uncertainty, not about crude survival data, but rather about mechanisms of recovery and what these factors might mean effectively for patients and their families. Will there be a return of consciousness and, if so, will it be robust enough to allow functional communication and independent living? These are the prognostic questions families ask, and ones we still cannot explain.

Just imagine the relationship between the gravity of the choice and the lack of helpful information. But that is precisely where families have been, unable to access the usual model of shared decision making that is dependent upon some requisite degree of scientific knowledge. Because of this, decisions made by families of patients with disorders of consciousness have been outside of the classic rubric of informed consent, at least as described by Katz and understood by contemporary bioethics.

It becomes obvious. If the clinician asking for consent is herself uninformed, how can she provide the information necessary to secure an informed consent (or refusal) from a surrogate? The answer is that, in many cases, she cannot. Even patients who articulate preferences in advance most likely will not account for prognostic uncertainty in their prior wishes, thus leaving surrogates with only partial guidance. Additional direction needs to come from somewhere and returning to Katz's formulation, that deficit will have to be filled by better scientific knowledge about brain injury, mechanisms of recovery, and biomarkers of differing brain states.

But neuroscience is maturing and coming into the modern era. We are on the cusp of gaining that useful information from neuroscience that will make the provision of true informed consent possible by providing more certain prognostic information that will lead to more informed choices. Much of this knowledge will come from progress in neuroimaging data that will shed light on the brain's structure and function, and even suggest its latent capacity for recovery. This information should prove helpful in suggesting outcomes and proportionate care decisions.

But in the short term these data will also complicate decisions. They will add nuance and complexity to decision making and remove the haven of the simplicity afforded by dichotomous outcomes. It will not be as simple as we had all been led to believe: outcomes are not purely binary. Brain injuries are not just either catastrophic or miraculous. Like all things biological, they exist on a continuum with grey zones in between the extremes.

That wide swatch of outcomes between full recovery and dire disability, what scientists call *variance*, will inform both the ethics and the science of severe brain injury. These actual outcomes will help frame choices for patients and surrogates and direct them to proportionate care decisions that they find acceptable. And as importantly, by embodying the results of mechanisms of recovery this variance will help us understand how to describe, predict, and alter outcomes after severe brain injury occurs.

In short, variance has brought science into the picture, a topic to which we will turn next as we consider the important role of neuroimaging research and its potential clinical applications in the diagnosis and treatment of disorders of consciousness.

TUNNEL VISION

As remarkable as it must now seem, there was a time before there was modern neuroimaging. Indeed there was a time, not long ago, when there were hardly any CT scans: x-ray machines that were able to take pictures in the round and construct three-dimensional images of the brain and other organs.

Although these devices have proliferated, and advanced to include MRIs and Positron Emission Tomography (PET) scans, when I started as a student, The New York Hospital-Cornell Medical Center shared a single CT scanner with Memorial Sloan-Kettering Cancer Center. We took patients on their gurneys through a tunnel buried under York Avenue to have their studies done across the street. As students, we enjoyed the opportunity to leave the floors and take the patient on what we called a "road trip" with IVs and monitors in tow.

Although New York State initially tried to limit the spread of technology by requiring "certificates of need" to justify the deployment of such costly machinery, the information gleaned from these images proved too powerful for it to be kept at bay. There was a felt need that this technology was life saving and nowhere more so than in neurology.

To give a sense of the magnitude of the advances represented by CT scans, one has to remember that just twenty-five years ago neurologists still did myelograms and ventriculograms to visualize the spinal cord and the brain by injecting contrast dye into the spinal cord and the central spinal fluid. The contrast material would light up on a conventional x-ray and neurologists would *infer* what was going on in the brain by distortions in the anatomy that might suggest a misplaced tumor or bleed, abnormalities far from the ventricular system that bathes the brain in cerebrospinal fluid. The technique was not much more advanced than when the Hopkins neurosurgeon Walter Dandy first injected air into the ventricles to visualize the brain in 1918.[2]

Given the diagnostic power of the CT scanner, Cornell's Department of Neurology was able to secure a machine to install right next to the neurology service on the sixth floor of The New York Hospital. It was a great luxury at the time to have a machine at such close range.

We spent a great deal of time at the scanner. I still remember the excitement of going to the scanner to get studies of our patients. We placed them on a hard table that slowly entered the machine's donut portal as pictures were taken. We would sit in the control room behind leaded glass, watch the patient disappear into the donut hole, and listen to the whirling thump as a camera made its circuit around the patient. Then we would wait as now vintage computers struggled to process massive amounts of data to create pictures on our monitors.

By today's standards, the process was exceedingly slow and the quality poor. A cheap cell phone has better image quality than those first machines. The scans were constructed of large pixel boxes whose outlines could barely be discerned. The images were grainy, in black and white, and sometimes blurry if solid materials like bone reflected electrons back in an unkindly way.

But as poor as they were, they were all that we had. It was truly a moment of great excitement when the images appeared on the screen projecting from the top to the bottom, second by second, as a brain came into focus. I remember sitting with my resident waiting for his learned interpretation as we sought to correlate what we thought was wrong, based on the history and an exhaustive neurological exam, with what the scan showed. You just felt that you were on the sharp edge of progress advancing what we knew every time someone was placed in the scanner.

Dr. Plum used to ask us, "Where's the lesion?" With that question, we would have to piece the history and the exam together to figure out how a patient's unique set of signs and symptoms localized to a specific injury in the brain. We couldn't cheat and get a scan first – unless there was a dire emergency – but rather had to go through the thought process of what neurologists call localization.

Imagine our excitement then as the scan emerges line by line and we saw if we were right about what part of the brain had caused a patient's stroke, robbing him of speech but preserving his understanding of our words, or that caused another patient to lose a part of his visual field. The ability to make diagnostic correlations between what we thought was going on and what was actually wrong, which was once the realm of the neurosurgeon – or pathologist, was now something the rest of us could do.

The images of patients in the vegetative state made for powerful correlations, confirming what we had been taught about this dire state, so closely linked with futility and the emergent death and dying movement, which was accelerating in its impact since the Quinlan case. I can still conjure up those images.

In my mind's eye, while still a student, I remember thinking the higher part of the brain, where the cortex had been, was now a gelatinous gel floating above the stump of a brainstem.[3] The thinned cortex coupled with the massively expanded ventricles of *hydrocephalus ex vacuo* suggested profound dysfunction and an immutable, irreversible injury in which consciousness was forever gone, vanished.[4]

CT images of shrunken vegetative brains coupled with the widely publicized report of Karen Ann Quinlan's autopsy results published in the *New England Journal of Medicine* in 1994, which showed that her brain weighed half as much as normal,[5] only added to the sense that patients like her were beyond the reach of modern medical care, and thus, further linked the state to death, dying, and futility.[4]

IMAGES AND ICONS

The status of the vegetative state seemed a settled scientific question with important normative implications. It is not an exaggeration to assert that by this point, the immutability of the vegetative state had become a *truth* essential to the autonomy ethic of American bioethics and the death and dying movement. It was also central to my career as I started to work in clinical ethics and end-of-life at Cornell as a young assistant professor. I founded the Ethics Committee of The New York Hospital in 1994 and began to do ethics consults drawing upon an evolving normative framework informed by the Quinlan case and our knowledge of the vegetative state. It was the same year that the Multi-Society Task Force on the Persistent Vegetative State published their findings on the vegetative state.

A couple of years later, I began to collaborate with Nicholas (Niko) Schiff, a colleague at Cornell and Fred Plum's final neurologist protégé. We spoke at great length about some observations that he and Dr. Plum were beginning to make about some heterogeneity within the vegetative state. It seemed that not all vegetative states were created equally with respect to outcomes, and interestingly, how that iconic brain state appeared on varying neuroimaging techniques like PET, which measured regional metabolic activity in the brain as compared to the static anatomical displays offered by conventional CT scans.

Given the iconic status of images of the vegetative state on conventional CT, I thought it ironic that Plum and Schiff were using *derivative* neuroimaging methods to describe some cases of the vegetative state that did not fully comport with what was becoming a reified set of expectations about it. The same technology that had been so central to the evolution of the almost mythical status of the vegetative state in bioethics –and society in general[6–9] – was now going to be used to challenge assumptions about the state.

As a bioethicist, I was intrigued by the possibility that we had collectively simplified both the science and ethics of severe brain injury. I wanted to participate in an effort to better approximate the truth about these conditions, however inconvenient and naïve such a sentiment might appear in these postmodern times. But the data was compelling and would over the next ten years change how we thought about disorders of consciousness.[10]

NO MAN IS AN ISLAND

Drs. Plum and Schiff began to conceptualize this work with neuroscientists Urs Ribary and Rodolfo Llinas in the fall of 1994 with approval of the Cornell Institutional Review Board in 1995. The first subjects were enrolled in April 1996 including a patient who would become the centerpiece of two papers entitled "Coordinated Expression in Chronically Unconscious Persons"[11] and "Words without Mind,"[12] pieces coauthored with Ribary and Llinas.

The works center on physiological studies of a forty-nine-year-old woman previously employed as a nurse, who at age twenty-nine suffered a series of severe "deep cerebral" bleeds due to an inoperable arteriovenous malformation – or disorganized yarn of arterial and venous vessels – at the base of her cerebrum. She produced spontaneous and isolated words, though she had been unconscious for twenty years.[12] At intervals of twenty-four to seventy-two hours she emitted random words, sometimes in a burst as on one occasion when she said, "down, down, down" or an expletive. All content was divorced from any environmental content or precipitant, an observation noted, not only by the investigators but also, importantly, by the patient's family who had closely observed her for twenty years.

Using both the functional capabilities of fMRI and fluorodeoxy-glucose Positron Emission Tomography (FDG-PET) – which measures glucose consumption within regions of the brain and uses energy consumption as a proxy for metabolic activity – Schiff and colleagues showed that the patient's brain was metabolically as quiet as a normal brain under deep general anesthesia save for isolated "cortical islands" that were more active than average background brain activity. Interestingly, given her random production of speech, Broca and Wernicke's areas, which are central to speech and auditory processing, were lit up as active compared to the rest of her cerebral cortex.

These hyperactive areas – or hyperactive relative to neighboring brain – were also found to be electrically active using magnetoencephalography (MEG), which measures magnetic fields emitted by the brain, unlike a conventional EEG, which measures electrical activity. By using MEG, and providing auditory stimuli to the subject, investigators were able to demonstrate that electrical activity correlated with areas of increased metabolism.

Even before "Words without Mind" was published in 1999, its report in short form as an abstract at the 1996 Society for Neuroscience meeting in Washington, D.C. was perceived as important. Schiff recalls that the abstract's[13] poster presentation "got an overwhelming response ... at least 200 people came through to see it."[14] The abstract shared with the world the startling observation of:

> ... a 49 year old woman continuously vegetative for 19 years who has shown no evidence of attention, recognition, or interaction. Atypically, she occasionally uttered single, understandable words with no accompanying expression or relevance to the environmental stimuli. MRI of the brain revealed no remaining right thalamus and only the anterolateral portion of left thalamus. Varying areas of cerebral cortex remained. Spontaneous and evoked magnetic activity in response to auditory clicks and tones, and somatosensory stimulation were used to evaluate global brain activity. Spontaneous oscillatory electrical activity at near 40 Hz in the brain and its reset to following sensory stimulation in the normal subject has been reported elsewhere, indicating that oscillatory activity near 40 Hz represents a neurophysiological correlate to the temporal cognitive binding of auditory stimuli. In contrast to these normal findings, preliminary data in the unconscious patient indicate a loss of high frequency (gamma) activity especially in the *right hemisphere* and a reduced correlation of brain oscillatory activity between the two hemispheres. The data also suggest the existence of coherent and synchronized spontaneous oscillatory activity around 40 Hz in the *left hemisphere* including partial reset with incomplete synchronization in response to sensory stimulation. These findings suggest that the human cerebrum can express some gamma band activity, words, and an incomplete and disorganized coding of sensory of stimuli in the absence of any behavioral evidence of the conscious state.[13]

Schiff and Plum's and colleagues' data were important for several reasons. Firstly, it demonstrated that there was variance within the vegetative state, further defining the upper and lower limits of that brain state. To that end, "Words without Mind" informed the 2003 Royal College Guidelines as a counterexample of misdiagnosing consciousness in patients, who though they exhibited such behaviors, remained within the vegetative state.[15] The Royal College cautioned:

> In addition to occasionally following moving objects or people with their eyes, patients in a vegetative state have also been known to

utter a single inappropriate word. Behaviour of this kind should lead to a careful search for awareness, but responses like these may occur because small "islands" in the brain have survived but they are no longer able to work together to generate awareness.[16]

But of course, the Royal College's invocation of the paper and its injunction against diagnosing consciousness in the vegetative state also foreshadowed the logical corollary: if one could demonstrate consciousness by neuroimaging then such a state would be incompatible with a vegetative diagnosis. As we will see, in a few years this was precisely what was said about patients who we would come to call *minimally conscious*. These patients were more than a trivial variation on the vegetative theme, they were different and conscious. But that observation would have been difficult to make if someone had not first demonstrated that disorders of consciousness seemed to exist on a biological continuum.

"Words without Mind" also illustrated dynamics of brain organization. It showed that the cortex might be put together in a modular fashion with preserved fragments of cortical function. These cortical islands somehow survived as a beach head despite being awash in surrounding devastation. Words were produced from these islands but in the absence of mind. Mind, or better yet consciousness, would require a bit more than an island or two, as no man is an island. But how about an archipelago? Might that amount of cortical territory bring enough integration about to achieve consciousness?

A nearly contemporaneous piece by David Menon and his colleagues at the Wolfson Brain Imaging Centre at Cambridge sought to answer this question. The team, which included Adrian Owen, a neuropsychologist, as well as the Cambridge neurosurgeon John Pickard, used PET to study the ability of a twenty-six-year-old patient who had become vegetative due to an infectious encephalitis to see whether she responded to images of familiar faces. Four months after her illness, presentation of the images led to activation of the right fusiform gyrus – the area of the brain charged with the identification of faces – with extension of the activation more widely. Eight months after she became sick, she was recognizing faces and speaking in short sentences.[17]

Schiff and Plum engaged the Wolfson team in a friendly debate in the pages of *Trends in Cognitive Sciences* in February 1999, importantly distinguishing Menon's subject, who went on to recover awareness and consciousness, from subjects like those presented in "Words without Mind," who only retained nonintegrative modular function. The latter patient is clearly vegetative. The former may be transitioning out of the vegetative state and into consciousness.[18] Menon, Owen, and Pickard, in their response, ask a crucial question: "whether residual cognitive processing in one or more areas can be integrated enough to provide some level of self-awareness or 'consciousness,' but still have no access to output." Pointing to the import of their work, they raise the ethically troublesome question – and foreshadow much later work on diagnostic error between the vegetative and minimally conscious states – by suggesting that "... our results raise the important (and somewhat disturbing) possibility that patients diagnosed to be in the persistent vegetative state might still perceive and cognitively process at least some sensory inputs relatively normally."[19]

STRUCTURES AND INTEGRITY

As far as the scientific work went, another more expansive paper on variance – or heterogeneity – within the vegetative state soon followed in *Brain*.[20] Although it had taken several years for it to find its way into print, it further questioned paradigmatic thinking about the vegetative state. This paper, on which I served as a coauthor, was notable for showing correlations between type and location of injury in the vegetative state and the findings one might discover on functional imaging. Examining five vegetative patients, we were able to show variance in overall metabolic levels in patients who had been injured by trauma or by anoxia.

As might have been anticipated by the Multi-Society Task Force's statements about the differential onset of permanence in the vegetative state from trauma (twelve months) or anoxia (three months), patients who had sustained anoxic injury had near global – or diffuse – metabolic rates that were about a third normal. In distinct contrast, patients who had sustained multifocal brain injury had preserved areas of normal and near-normal function, surrounded by areas of inactivity.

These swaths of activity, however, did not converge to produce integral function necessary for a modular brain to become a conscious mind. That threshold was not reached even though one of the five patients we presented had quite a bit of cortical territory preserved as active and functional tissue. The putative reason was that damage was done to the all-important thalamus, a walnut-sized body at the center of the brain's function and geography. Located below the cortex and above the brainstem, which caps the spinal cord, the thalamus was the most advanced part of the brain before it was superseded by evolution and the development of the cerebral cortex.

Time has passed the thalamus's supremacy within the brain, but evolution could not erase its connections to the primitive brainstem necessary for arousal and needed by the neocortex for more advanced thought. The thalamus provides the crucial link between these two domains and provides what is both necessary and sufficient for consciousness, allowing the brain to do both bottom-up and top-down processing.

The problem is that the thalamus's unique capability at making connections comes with a price: a vulnerability of being obliterated or severely damaged when the brain is injured and swells. Capped by the skull, the injured brain has only one was to go and that is down. As described in earlier chapters, this process is called herniation, highly dangerous and in its extreme can lead to death. Short of that, it generally leads to the vegetative state pushing the thalamus downward to the base of the *foramen magnum* through which it cannot fit.

A mind without a thalamus becomes a brain incapable of integrative thought and function. In short, it becomes vegetative, incapable of connecting the brain with itself. Those cortical islands, even large archipelagos, cease to function together and never reach the requisite integrative function necessary to achieve consciousness. Without the thalamus, the brain is like Delta Airlines without Hartsfield Airport, its Atlanta hub: the planes are in the air but you can't get there from here because you can't make your connection without flying through Atlanta.

If consciousness is all about making neural connections, then an anatomically precise injury to the thalamus can have an overwhelming impact on integrative (or unified) cortical function. Take the thalami offline and the patient will become vegetative. And what of the opposite point? What if functions performed by the two thalami could be restored or augmented in a damaged or resistant brain? We will return to these questions – importance of the thalamus – in later chapters when we consider the impact of thalamic deep brain stimulation in the minimally conscious state. For now, the important point is the special relationship of the thalamus to consciousness, an interaction that might be open to therapeutic remediation and the reintegration of cognitive function necessary for the achievement of consciousness.

NETWORKS AND NUANCE

This relationship between integration and disintegration can be thought of as a demarcation between the vegetative state and consciousness. An illustration of this is seen in a study from Liege, Belgium by Steven Laureys and colleagues.[21] They used PET scanning and simultaneous recordings of evoked potentials – electrical signals from synchronously firing neurons – to compare the response to painful stimuli measured in normal controls and subjects in the vegetative state. In contrast to the controls who responded to pain by activating an integrated pain network involving mid-brain and higher cortical areas, the reach of the vegetative response was limited to the level of the mid-brain, contralateral thalamus, and primary sensory area. In contrast to the normal subjects who activated the entire pain network – including associated areas that make us *suffer* and ask what does the pain mean and/or portend[22] – the vegetative subjects only had a first order activation.

Their brains were, as the authors put it, *"functionally disconnected"* from secondary somatosensory and higher-level associative areas, illustrating the inability of the vegetative brain to achieve a unity of functional integration necessary for fully processing external stimuli and achieving consciousness.

Laureys's work suggested the salience of network activation as a diagnostic divide between a vegetative and a normal brain. Schiff and colleagues asked the next logical question. What of the minimally conscious brain? Would these patients who were virtually indistinguishable from vegetative patients at the bedside appear differently through the prism of neuroimaging? Would they have the capacity for network activation like more normal patients or lack that ability?

A NARRATIVE STATE OF MIND

In the next major contribution to this nascent literature, Schiff and colleagues published a paper in *Neurology* showing that the minimally conscious brain could muster a far-flung network activation beyond the primary sensory areas.[23] Modifying a passive activation language paradigm developed originally by his coauthor, Joy Hirsch, to do brain mapping before neurosurgery,[24] subjects were read familiar personal narratives by a close relative.

In an interview with the author, Schiff recalls, "Joy Hirsch, who was still here at Memorial Sloan Kettering, and I had been talking for quite some time about trying to do studies on the brain-injured patients that we'd been following. Her graduate student, Diana Moreno, had been working with me since 1996 and had helped me do PET studies on vegetative state (VS) patients and Diana was really excited because she'd been doing all sorts of work in fMRI and she and Joy had developed these stimuli to look at language function in anaesthetized babies. And they found that if they played spoken language ... a mother's voice to a baby, and then reversed it in time, that anaesthetized babies just like normal subjects would activate to both kinds of stimuli and they could see that there were differences and the language systems were intact. So we wanted to do these studies in brain-injured patients. . . ."

The subsequent studies showed large-scale network activation or the sort of functional integration that eluded the vegetative brain. But there was more. Narratives were played back to the subject in both forward and backward modes to see if the responses were different when prompted by language or gibberish. The process was tightly controlled because the narratives had the same signal and the same frequency content when played in either direction.

Appropriate network activation was detected in the MCS subjects in the superior and middle temporal gyrus in the forward speech mode. This result was indistinguishable from "normal" controls. However, it did not occur in the MCS subjects when their narrative, with the same frequency spectrum, was played in reverse and without linguistic content. The implications were startling. These patients who seemed rather inert at the bedside were responding to *language* in all of its glorious syntax, grammar, and prosody.

Appropriate activity indistinguishable from controls was detected in the superior and middle temporal gyrus of MCS subjects when forward speech was played. Activation did not occur when the same narratives, with the same frequency spectrum were played backward, without linguistic content. Although "normal" controls also activated their language networks when exposed to the reverse, perhaps in an attempt to parse out linguistic meaning amidst the verbal incoherence, the response of MCS subjects to language demonstrated that minimally conscious brains were more like uninjured brains than vegetative ones. It was another dramatic demonstration of a growing discordance between what one observed at the bedside and what was actually happening inside the brain.[25]

SCHIAVO

The Schiff and colleagues article was published in February 2005 just as the Terri Schiavo case was about to erupt at the national level.[26] The debate over her diagnosis and medical care, specifically the withdrawal of her feeding tube at the request of her husband, Michael, and legally authorized surrogate decision maker had already played out earlier in Florida in 2003.

At that time, a federal court had ruled that a feeding tube could be removed from the thirty-nine-year-old woman in a chronic vegetative state following anoxic brain injury.[27,28] This decision triggered a quick reaction from the Florida legislature, which passed a bill allowing then-Governor Jeb Bush to make decisions on her behalf.[29] The governor signed the bill into law.

So empowered, Governor Bush ordered that the feeding tube be replaced. His brother, the president, endorsed this action. Ultimately, however, the Florida Supreme Court ruled that Governor Bush's actions were unconstitutional because they violated the separation of powers.[30] This decision was affirmed by the U.S. Supreme Court by its refusal to hear the case on appeal.[31-33] The Florida Supreme Court also found "clear and convincing evidence that she (Ms. Schiavo) was in a persistent or permanent vegetative state" based on the conclusions of neurologists who examined her.[30] This finding was also upheld after additional evaluation by the independent *guardian ad litem*, Jay Wolfson, who had been appointed by Governor Bush.[34]

Despite the certainty of her diagnosis, the debate continued, fueled by partisan politics. And in 2005, the story went national.[35,36] Physician members of Congress including Senate Majority Leader Bill Frist and Representative David Weldon questioned her vegetative diagnosis. Though neither had personally examined her, both were unequivocal in their diagnosis.

Leader Frist, who was a cardio-thoracic and transplant surgeon from Vanderbilt, became the Republican point person in the Senate. He famously said that he had reviewed six hours of video and concluded that she was not in the vegetative state. He had not examined the patient. Although he should have known better as a physician, he was dealing more with "the body politic"[37] than corporeal reality when he asserted, "There seems to be insufficient information to conclude that Terri Schiavo is in a persistent vegetative state. ... I don't see any justification in removing hydration and nutrition."[38] Dr. Weldon, an internist, asserted on the House Floor that "By my medical definition, she was not in a vegetative state based on my review of the videos, my talking to the family and my discussing the case with one of the neurologists who examined her."[39]

It was confusing to all but the most discerning eyes. In some clips where Ms. Schiavo did appear to look toward her mother's voice, it appeared that she was in fact responsive. The only problem was that her glances were random and not causally driven by her mother's call. Taken out of context, the diagnosis could be misconstrued and counterintuitive. It was "hard to get your arms around."[40]

The advocacy of Frist, Weldon, and their colleagues eventually led to passage of a bill, something akin to Florida's "Terri's Law,"[41] requiring a singular – and unprecedented – review of Florida's state court decisions by the federal judiciary. President Bush made a point of flying back from Crawford, Texas, to sign the legislation into law.[42]

The Schiavo case would become high theater and generate volumes of bioethics scholarship about the rights of surrogates to make decisions for those in the vegetative state.[43–45] It would revisit the historic relationship between the right to die and the vegetative state, dating to Quinlan and Cruzan. But this time the debate was against the back drop of a new wave of American fundamentalism, with the White House press office making an appeal to a "culture of life."[46]

Settled questions like the deference generally afforded to the states to govern health care, a prerogative historically advanced by the Right, was now clung to as an assertion of the political Left. So too was the question of whether the removal of artificial nutrition and hydration was the withdrawal of life-sustaining therapy, a point well-established in the *Cruzan* case when Nancy's feeding tube was removed. But no matter, the debate was complex and heated, culminating during the Advent season of Easter with the death of Ms. Schiavo, and Pope John Paul II days later.

CONFUSION AND CONFLATION

All of that was weeks away when the Schiff and colleagues *Neurology* paper was published and referenced in *The New York Times*.[47] Its scientific findings were almost immediately interpreted against the backdrop of the Schiavo case. The argumentation went like this: those who sided with the Schindlers, Ms. Schiavo's parents, hoped to cast doubt on her diagnosis and her prognosis in order to forestall a decision to remove her feeding tube. By raising the question about the unseen capabilities of patients with severe brain injury, the Schiff paper could be used to make the point that Ms. Schiavo might also have unseen capabilities waiting to be discovered if only she too could receive the proper scan. That is, if minimally conscious patients could be seen to respond to language and perhaps process language and *understand* what was being said to them despite the absence of any overt behavioral evidence, might it not be possible that there was more than met the eye when it came to those patients who were vegetative?

The question was a good – and complicated – one, requiring a knowledge of the difference between the vegetative and minimally conscious brains that few had. Because of the paper's scientific import and the historical moment, it garnered front page coverage in the *New York Times*. I thought the data was a game changer and recall being contacted by Ben Carey from *The New York Times* for a comment as I was a collaborator of Schiff but not an author of the paper.

It was an unguarded moment. I had just been called out from seeing patients and was candid in my comments. My remarks appeared on the front page of the paper, "This study gave me goose bumps because it shows this possibility of this profound isolation, that these people are there, that they've been there all along, even though we've been treating them as if they are not."[47] My point then, and now, is that if MCS patients could seemingly respond to speech, it raised the possibility that they could understand us and that they were part of a human community marked by the reciprocity of language and communication.

To this end, the bioethicist, and brain-injury survivor, William J. Winslade who teaches law, philosophy, and medical ethics, captures the centrality of being with another and the importance of language and communication:

> Being persons requires having a personality, being aware of our selves and our surroundings, and possessing human capacities, such as memory, emotions, *and the ability to communicate and interact with other people* [italics added]. These ingredients of our humanity may be damaged or limited – some may even be lost – without forfeiting our claim to personhood. But when they are totally absent, forever and irrevocably, as is the case with the permanently unconscious, we are no longer human beings; hence society no longer has a moral responsibility to sustain our lives.[48]

While I do not agree that the vegetative state equates with the forfeiture of our humanity, as we humans live on in the memories of others and in the acts of goodness we performed while we were able, I do agree that we lose the ability to *act* as persons when we lose our ability to communicate with others. In the context of the study, I took Winslade's perspective not as a way to exclude patients who had lost the capacity to communicate, but to *include* MCS patients who had been discovered, through neuroimaging, to have regained the ability to process language. That capacity suggested the possibility that they could partake in reciprocal relations founded upon the ability to communicate with others.

The data in the *Neurology* paper had profound implications. It suggested that these patients either retained or regained compensated language abilities. And if this were the case, these capabilities came with the prospect that these patients might have more awareness of their situation and their deficits.

Many found this prospect horrifying: to be sequestered within oneself, aware and mute save for the occasional gesture or momentary chance to light off a flare in a scanner. Others saw it as a step toward a more fruitful recovery. But whatever the experience, the state was one of human consciousness that called upon the rest of us to respond. To date, we had isolated these people and placed them in nursing homes to linger, as we shall soon see when we return to Maggie's story.

To my mind these possibilities made it all the more critical to distinguish the minimally conscious from the unconscious vegetative and overcome the conflation error that often clumped all severe brain injuries into one group. Whether the diagnostic conflation was a product of ignorance of other states or motivated by political argumentation, it was critical to distinguish those who could have conscious experience from those who could not.

But this did not happen. The Schiff data on language processing, *garnered exclusively from MCS patients*, was soon generalized to vegetative patients, a patient population to whom the results did not pertain. As the Schiavo controversy flared, I received an e-mail from the Gibbs Law firm, Florida attorneys representing the Schindlers. Opposed to the withdrawal of her feeding tube, they wanted imaging studies to "prove to the court that Ms. Schiavo could benefit from swallowing therapy and advanced testing and medical treatment. To this point [March 5, 2005], all Ms. Schiavo has received is a simple MRI and CAT scan, and this was done before 2002."[49] Joy Hirsch and Niko Schiff received similar appeals. An e-mail from another attorney to Dr. Hirsch made the link to the *Neurology* paper, featured in the *Times* article, explicit:

> I am one of the attorneys working on the Terri Schiavo case on behalf of Terri's parents, Bob and Mary Schindler, who have been fighting in court for more than seven years to keep their daughter alive and to find help for her. The New York Times article this week regarding research

that you and others have been doing in the area of consciousness in brain damaged individuals greatly confirms what we have observed in Terri. I am one of the few non family members to actually have visited with Terri. While I am not a doctor, I am as an attorney trained to make careful observations. It is quite apparent to me, having seen Terri on several occasions interact with her family members, that she is clearly aware of her environment, at least at those times. ... I am writing to you to ask if you or one of the other doctors involved in this research might be able to speak with us to determine if there is some role that you could play in this ongoing family tragedy ... we could use this new research information with the courts in several ways. We could request a court order to permit Terri to come to New York to be evaluated with her parents (she does not interact in any way with her husband). Or we could use the information about the new research to present a medical motion to the court. . . .[50]

Schiff, Hirsch, and I responded to these requests by noting that the work was still experimental and not diagnostic. We might have added that the patients who demonstrated network responses were all minimally conscious and *not* vegetative and that MRI functional imaging in Ms. Schiavo was also contraindicated because she had a metallic deep brain stimulator residing in her right thalamus, the residua of a failed therapeutic trial organized by the Medtronic Corporation dating back to the early 1990s.[51]

MORE THAN A STATE OF MIND

It should not have come as a surprise that the findings in the *Neurology* paper, which was about minimally conscious patients, were linked to the vegetative state. The MCS focus was overlooked by commentators and polemicists because there was a great deal to be gained, at least rhetorically, if one could imply that what was seen with the MCS patients might also be seen in Ms. Schiavo, who was in a permanent vegetative state, some fifteen years after an anoxic brain injury. That sort of diagnostic upgrade could have had a cataclysmic influence on the debate, complicating the right to die, which had its origins in vegetative patients.

Such diagnostic creep was worrisome because it turned an objective diagnosis into values choices, something that Dr. Plum and I addressed when the Schiavo affair was still taking root in Florida. Dr. Plum and I wrote a commentary for the September 2004 issue of *Archives of Neurology* at the time.[52] The title of the piece said it all: "Neurological Diagnosis Is More Than a State of Mind: Diagnostic Clarity and Impaired Consciousness." We argued for the neurologist's professional responsibility in making the differential diagnosis between the vegetative state and MCS based upon scientific and not political or ideological criteria. We made a plea to avoid diagnostic conflation and engage in evidence-based reasoning so as to be able to "... identify patients with some potential for recovery while they are still alive and provide them with emerging rehabilitation strategies and therapies."[52]

In our view, a diagnosis was more than a *state of mind*. It should not become a values choice. It must instead be based on the clinical examination and neurological assessment. The call for objectivity was prescient in light of the intentional diagnostic distortions that would occur once Schiavo made it to a national stage.

THE SUNDAY TIMES MAGAZINE

Sometimes the attempts were, in retrospect, a bit comical. Back in September 2003, the award-winning science journalist, Carl Zimmer, wrote, "*What if there is something going on in there?*" for the *New York Times Magazine* about our work with patients with disorders of consciousness.[53] He spent hours with Schiff, Giacino, Hirsch, and myself and traveled with us to the JFK Johnson-Johnson Rehabilitation Center in Edison, New Jersey. He was precise in his descriptions and careful in getting the science right.

All of us were delighted to be the subject of a Zimmer piece. And so Niko and I were especially surprised when we saw final galleys of his article the Wednesday before the Sunday, September 28 publication date. To our amazement, and shock, the careful piece had been mangled by editorial staff who conflated the vegetative and minimally conscious states, especially in the headlines and pullouts. A memorable header, which had nothing to do with what we had said, read, "New research suggests that many vegetative patients are more conscious than previously supposed – and might eventually be curable. A whole new way of thinking about pulling the plug."[53]

This was as jolting in its tone as it was in its inaccuracy. We had never said the vegetative were conscious. That would be an oxymoron. By definition, once one is conscious, they are no longer vegetative. Neither had we made claims about a cure nor the implications of this work vis-à-vis the fundamental question of a right to die. We had always affirmed the right to die, and I had spent a decade working in palliative care ethics.[54] What had changed? Now we were *also* talking about adequate medical care for the minimally conscious, a marginalized population.

Our collective point in the Zimmer article, and my stance in the soon to follow Schiavo debate, was the need to "preserve the right-to-die and affirm the right to care" for those patients who had wanted it and needed it.[55] This would begin with information to surrogates about the salient distinctions between the vegetative and minimally conscious states and what those differences meant for a patient's lived experience and prognosis. In the context of the Zimmer piece, we were not making claims about the vegetative state but rather about those who were minimally conscious, who merited a bright-line distinction with patients who were unconscious.

When we saw the galleys we went up to Dr. Plum's office for some advice. He had just retired and was now University Professor Emeritus since the start of the year. Dr. Plum had held his University Professorship since 1994. It is the highest academic rank given at Cornell University for a distinguished few whose work had been marked by a "breadth of scholarship."

Although "retired," Dr. Plum was not retiring. He was still a force of nature and told us he was going to call the *Times*. He placed the call as Niko and I sat there. According to my notes, his "regular" contact at the paper was not available and he ended up talking to an interim editor of the magazine section.

We were only privy to Dr. Plum's side of the conversation, but as he later indicated, the editor was making the claim that the distinction between the vegetative and minimally conscious states was semantic.[4] Dr. Plum tried valiantly to illuminate the differences between the brain states, not mentioning that he and his old friend Bryan Jennett had been the scientific originators of the vegetative state. But try as he did, he was not able to convince the interim editor.

As I sat there listening and watching Dr. Plum's face grow red in anger, I thought of the absurdity of a journalist lecturing him about the vegetative state. It occurred to me then it would be like questioning Moses about the Ten Commandments – how iconic the definition had become and how central he was to their formulation. But historic memory is short, and the editor was unimpressed. She told Dr. Plum that the differences were unimportant. She did not actually know enough to appreciate the subtlety of the distinctions.

The article went to press – or was released as the printing was already accomplished – without any changes. It was an unfortunate error, especially for families with vegetative patients who did not read the fine print and were misled into thinking that there was hope for their loved ones. It also distorted our work and efforts to be precise with our own diagnostic discernment. In response, we wrote a letter to the editor pointing out the errors and demanding a correction. I was joined by my colleagues, Drs. Giacino, Hirsch, and Schiff. A few weeks later, the magazine issued the laconic correction:

> October 19, 2003, Sunday: An article on Sept. 28 about people with brain injuries or impaired consciousness referred imprecisely to the condition of Daniel Rios, one patient studied, a year after a blood vessel ruptured in his brain. He was minimally conscious, or had some level of awareness – not vegetative, or showing no signs of consciousness.[53]

The correction was a pyrrhic victory and a more important lesson: the work had ceased to be scientifically neutral. Neuroimaging had given both scientists and commentators another means to refract new knowledge. Emerging data could be used to understand the brain's complex biology or spun for ideological purposes, guaranteeing the work high visibility.

GAME CHANGER FROM CAMBRIDGE

If ideology challenged the integrity of scientific findings, new data soon challenged established diagnostic paradigms the following September, when Adrian Owen from the University of Cambridge published a paper in *Science* featuring a twenty-five-year-old woman who was diagnosed as vegetative five months after sustaining a traumatic brain injury.[56] Contrary to all expectations, her responses to verbal stimuli were "indistinguishable" from normal controls: she demonstrated integrated neural networks when placed in the scanner.

She was asked to imagine herself playing tennis and walking through her house and challenged with linguistically ambiguous sentences. The tennis prompt elicited significant activity in the supplementary motor areas. The imaginary walk through her house led to activation of the parahippocampal gyrus, posterior parietal cortex, and the lateral premotor cortex. The parsing of similar words activated the middle and superior temporal gyrus bilaterally as well as the left inferior frontal region. All of these regions would have been employed by normal subjects who were moving, navigating about their home, or disambiguating similarly sounding words.

These were startling results in a patient who was clinically *vegetative* by the usual behavioral criteria. Given the report's scientific importance, and its political implications in the wake of the Schiavo case just a year earlier, it garnered front-page coverage in the *New York Times*,[57] and a response from partisans on both sides of the Schiavo debate.

Defenders of a right to die worried that the deconstruction of this iconic state would undermine patient self-determination at the end of life. One heated exchange on the Medical College of Wisconsin (MCW-Bioethics) LISTSERV – a discussion group of bioethicists – featured the ideological critique of a proponent of the right to die asking a neurologist who sought to explain the results, "why bother?" He worried that this would erode the hard right to die by opening a Pandora's box of new knowledge.

In response, I expressed concern over this dismissal of emerging knowledge. Diagnostic precision was something to be prized because the history of medicine is full of examples of how more specific disease classification has led to treatment improvements.[58] This becomes clear if we consider the case of acute myelogenous leukemia, which until recently had been fatal. Now there are eight to ten subtypes, many with their own genetic signature and with variable survival rates. This progress was a consequence of diagnostic discernment. As the great physician, Sir William Osler wisely said long ago, "the determination of structure with a view to the discovery of function has been the foundation of progress."[59]

Opponents of the decision to withdraw care from Ms. Schiavo pointed to the latent capabilities of Owen's subject, which had been unmasked by new imaging technology. If it were possible for one vegetative patient to respond this way, would it not be reasonable, or even logical, to ask if Ms. Schiavo had the same capacity? [60]

And politics aside, it is a good question. Why should one vegetative patient respond one way and another differently? To address this we need to carefully review the differences between the Owen subject and Ms. Schiavo, both etiologically and temporally as well as biologically. On both counts they were distinct, a point inferred from *Science*'s "special note" about the Owen paper, which cautioned that the paper, "should not be used to generalize about all other patients in a vegetative state, particularly since each case may involve a different type of injury."[61]

And to that distinction, it is critical to note, in contrast to the anoxic brain injury suffered by Ms. Schiavo, the Owen patient had sustained a traumatic brain injury, the more favorable etiology prognostically. More critically, when the debate ensued in 2005, Ms. Schiavo had been in the vegetative state for some fifteen years. The subject of Owen's study had been injured only five months earlier. So combining etiology and time course, and invoking the definitional criteria of the persistent and permanent vegetative states of the Multi-Society Task Force,[62,63] we see that the Owen subject had not yet reached a state of permanence. Migration into the MCS was still possible. That possibility had passed years ago for Ms. Schiavo whose vegetative state was permanent.

It appeared that the Owen subject had been in the midst of this transition when she was imaged at five months. That is, her brain had become responsive to the outside world, in this case auditory stimuli, which were able to generate *integrated* network activations. The problem was that her body, as yet, had not caught up and become able to mount a motor response. That is, she could imagine actions but not execute them behaviorally. In fact she had no behavioral repertoire beyond the autonomic functions of the vegetative state.

Five months into her injury, this subject's potential for incremental recovery beyond the vegetative state had yet to run its course as she had not yet reached the one year mark after traumatic injury. And by eleven months, as reported in supplemental materials on the *Science* website when the paper was published, it was reported that she was able to fixate her gaze on a mirror held at a forty-five-degree angle on the right side of her face.[64] This advance was very significant because it indicated that she was able to behaviorally respond to her environment indicating, that she had entered the MCS eleven months after injury.

Beyond these generalizeable considerations of time and type of injury, the biological distinctions between the cases were vast. The Owen patient had a large structurally intact brain with a range of preserved physiological responses described in their report. Schiavo had no detectable electrical activity and a global loss of volume and at autopsy had depletion of brain cells in all regions, consistent with a diagnosis of the vegetative state.[65]

NONBEHAVIORAL MCS?

But what of the Owen patient's state at five months? How should it be described? Overtly she appears vegetative by behavioral criteria. But by neuroimaging, she seems to be responsive to external auditory stimuli, activating widely distributed networks, a response inconsistent with the vegetative state. In some sense it was akin to the question of genotype and phenotype in genetics. One might have the genotype for a late onset condition but, as yet, not have manifested it phenotypically.[58] The same notion of latent and manifest content could be at play when a patient first demonstrates a neural flare on imaging and later develops the ability to mount a behavioral response. How could this intermediate response be classified?

Just after the Owen paper was released, I wrote a piece coauthored with Niko Schiff for the *Hastings Center Report*, in which we asserted that the most accurate way to describe Owen's subject was to add the concept of a *nonbehavioral minimally conscious state* to our growing nosology describing patients with disorders of consciousness.[66] By virtue of her network responses to auditory stimuli the patient could not be vegetative within a precise biological construct. But she was vegetative in the prevailing framework in use, which relied on behavioral manifestations and not imaging data to make diagnostic statements. The definitional work-around was to label such patients as being in a *nonbehavioral minimally conscious state*.

The notion of nonbehavioral MCS could imply a number of things. The first that she was not *yet* able to demonstrate a behavioral response, a fact affirmed by her subsequent ability to visually fixate to the mirror presented to her face. In this way, the nonbehavioral MCS could be seen as a transit point between the vegetative state from which she originated and her progression into "classic" MCS – and perhaps beyond – based on behavioral criteria. When I heard of the subject's status some twenty-two months after her injury, I learned she had improved to the point of being able to smile and respond to questions with a simple yes or no.[67] By this progression, her nonbehavioral MCS was but one transit point en route to a recovery of a higher functional status.

In addition to this "transition argument," a patient might conceivably progress only as far as a state of nonbehavioral state. That would also be expected, if as with all things biological we acknowledge that outcomes are on a continuum. A patient might make it to the point of having recovered the ability to produce mental imagery without being able to translate that cognitive work into motor output. Absent neuroimaging technology, which would be the only way to identify patients like her, this could be seen as a paradoxical step – of uncertain significance – above the vegetative state, in which there is mental responsiveness as evidenced by imaging flares but no behaviorally demonstrable signs associated with the activity seen on neuroimaging.

Unchecked, or delimited by a known epidemiology of the vegetative state, this raises the prospect that all vegetative state patients could theoretically have been misdiagnosed and might, in fact, be minimally conscious. Although there is a pervasive risk of confusing the two states, there is some reassurance from collective data of all the major centers doing this work, that none of the patients entered a state of nonbehavioral MCS after the time frames first advanced for the outer limits of the vegetative state by the "Multi-Society Task Force Report." That is, this move to some degree of recovery – the transition– will come earlier, not later in the disease process. Such was the case in the report by Owen whose subject was first noted to be in this state five months after injury, well within the twelve-month upper limit of the "Multi-Society Task Force Report."

Another way of thinking of the *nonbehavioral* designation is to read it as *neuroimaging criteria* for the MCS. While I am convinced that neuroimaging will play a role in the diagnosis of these patients, the consensus from a meeting held at Stanford University in 2007 on neuroimaging and disorders of consciousness did not endorse diagnosis by neuroimaging criteria.[60] It was felt that this would be premature and a potentially dangerous use of neuroimaging outside of a research context. We worried that clinicians would jump to neuroimaging tests without the requisite diagnostic thinking necessary to make sense of the results.

Even now, the technology is young and still not ready for clinical prime time. A "positive" scan could suggest that a patient was responding to external stimuli, but could also be noise versus actual signal. Conversely, the lack of a response does not necessarily mean that the patient was not minimally conscious. The technology could be insensitive to a brain response because of the intensity of the signal or the timing of the flare in relation to the actual brain activity. This delay or latency could potentially bury responses in the subsequent cycle of stimulation and response.

As should be well appreciated by now, two similar scans at different stages of the disease process can have very different diagnostic and prognostic meanings; what distinguishes the results are the probabilities of what is expected in the scan. The problem, or cause for excitement, continues to be that much of what we see on neuroimaging is a surprise. That is why this still remains the province of research and not the domain of the practitioner. Medical practice is meant to be predictable. Research by definition is not. It is an exploration, guided by hypotheses to be true (or not), but reined in by conforming theories with empirical results. But if medical practice is meant to be predictable, how can the care of patients conform to established *predictable* norms when the very nosology by which we classify them is under an evolving critique?

A TYPOGRAPHY OF IGNORANCE

Here the challenge for the practitioner is to be open to new knowledge and not wedded to the old. While the old may provide comfort in its static view of the brain with a disorder of consciousness, stasis is not called for in the advance to new knowledge. But neither is overconfidence in our emerging science. We need an appreciation of the limits of what we know and skepticism about what we think we have learnt.[68] Oliver Wendell Holmes Sr., the Harvard anatomist and father of the jurist, said it best in a volume aptly titled, *Border Lines of Knowledge in Some Provinces of Medical Knowledge.* Published in 1862, his words still resonate with our evolving science of the mind:

> Science is the topography of ignorance. From a few elevated points we triangulate vast spaces, enclosing infinite unknown details. We cast the lead, and draw up a little sand from the abysses we shall never reach with our dredges.
>
> The best part of our knowledge is that which teaches us where knowledge leaves off and ignorance begins. Nothing more clearly separates a vulgar from a superior mind, than the confusion in the first between the little that it truly knows, on the one hand, and what it half knows and what it thinks it knows, on the other.
>
> That which is true of every subject is especially true of the branch of knowledge which deals with living beings. . . .[69]

12 Contractures and Contradictions

Medical Necessity and the Injured Brain

Maggie left Worcester Hospital for Spaulding, a leading rehabilitation center in Boston, on May 17, 2006. The good news was that Spaulding offered her three hours of therapy each day, five days a week. Even better, it was paid for. But it did not start off that way.

Maggie was covered by her father's health insurance plan, which he had through his work for a tribal casino in Connecticut. The problem with the move to Boston was that Spaulding was out of state and out of Paul's insurance network. This is not an uncommon problem for people seeking rehabilitation for brain injury, whose options are often limited by geography, either because of limits within private networks or by state-based Medicare plans.[1,2]

Maggie's challenge was that the care that her family wanted her to receive was from an out-of-network provider. But unlike most cases in which an appeal would be presented to an insurance company, Paul took her case to the tribal counsel and they made an individual decision in favor of providing for her initial rehabilitation at Spaulding. Nancy was not sure why the tribe decided this way but speculated that it may have been "... because Paul had friends in the Indian community, or maybe they decided because it was a disability and they were compassionate."

Either way, I found their deliberations interesting. Maggie was not an abstract case from an unknown family, but the daughter of a friend and a colleague who needed help, who needed a hand. It was a communitarian response of mutual support in which each member of that counsel could personally imagine the ordeal that this one family was facing and how they collectively might temper that burden. The counsel's proximity to the people involved in the case, who would be affected by their decision, brought both integrity and compassion to the deliberations.

Perhaps their process could be a model for a community-based appeals board. It had the virtue of bringing the individual to the fore and keeping decisions from being bureaucratic and anonymous, a problem that becomes a barrier to care.

SPAULDING

Once she arrived at Spaulding, Maggie got an hour of physical, occupational, and speech therapy each day. Speech therapy also focused on getting her off her tracheostomy tube. Her nurses and therapists also got her out of bed and sitting up in a wheelchair.

Nancy was happy to be there. Not only did it portend a future for her daughter and the possibility of rehabilitation, but the people at Spaulding seemed to be plugged into the needs of families. The specialized staff there appeared to understand what families go through when their lives have been turned upside down by the shock of having their precious child or beloved spouse stricken with a brain injury. In contrast to acute care providers who focus on the physical and relegate psychosocial concerns to a second tier of importance, the conversations at Spaulding were far more balanced; as staff provided rehabilitation they also attended to the psychological needs of families still trying to navigate the many choices ahead.

A keen critic of the care her daughter had received, Nancy was favorably disposed to the facility, "And then at Spaulding they were actually quite good. ..." They empowered families by providing information that would allow for more informed choices and fuller engagement. Nancy was grateful for an informational booklet, computer access, and a "research person ... [who] ... would do research for you and collect information for you that you could read." There were also family meetings and a "psychiatrist who worked with the patients but also worked with family members. So that was quite good because they at least had people to talk with families about their issues."

MEDICAL NECESSITY

The bad news was that Maggie showed little improvement during her eight-week stay. So as good as Spaulding's outreach to families was, the one issue that Maggie could not overcome was one that policy makers call "medical necessity," or "improvement standard," *an obscure federal regulatory concept that does as much to influence patient outcome as the biology of injury.*

The problem was that Nancy was not getting better fast enough to qualify for the state-based insurance support that would take over once Paul's benefits ran out. Nancy explains that, "... because she was so minimally responsive ... she wasn't going to get more intensive physical therapy because she wasn't going to progress the way [the insurance company] would pay for."

And then the tutorial about medical necessity: "You know how there's those rules about you only get physical therapy if you progress from one level to another in a certain number of days. So obviously someone who is minimally conscious is less likely to succeed in those categories even though they might need physical therapy. *Those benchmarks don't work for people who are not conscious. But they're still used."*

Nancy's explication is entirely correct. Simply put, medical necessity is the basis upon which care is paid for by Medicare, the insurer of last resort when someone becomes severely disabled. By statute, Medicare will pay for what is "reasonable and necessary for the diagnosis and treatment of illness or injury to improve the functioning of a malformed body member."[3] Reasonable and necessary is thought to refer to questions of amount, frequency, duration, and efficacy of the proposed treatments.

But it is not so simple. As Nancy W. Miller, a lawyer specializing in health law characterizes the situation, "The problem is that determining medical necessity is not always easy. The dilemma is due to several factors, the first of which is definitional. There are almost as many definitions of medical necessity as there are payors, laws, and courts to interpret them." And to make matters worse, indeed capricious, the Center for Medicare and Medicaid Services (CMS) has authority, derived from the Social Security Administration "... to determine if the method of treating a patient in the particular case is reasonable and necessary on a case-by-case basis."[4]

And the determination of progress in the minimally conscious state is especially complex. One parent of a child in MCS made the astute observation that for progress to be deemed reimbursable, behaviors had to be performed consistently. So if a patient seemed to understand the meaning of a joke and laugh appropriately one day, but then did not repeat that behavior, that first appropriate response would not be viewed as evidence of potential progress of comprehension and an effort at expression. Because it was a sporadic manifestation it would not count. As the parent of one patient sardonically put it, if she were to write a memoir of her experience with brain injury and bureaucracy, she would entitle it, *"No Points for Laughing."*

This makes no sense because such episodic demonstrations of behavior *are part of the definition of the minimally conscious state.* At the very least determinations of progress need to be consistent with the biology of the patient's condition suggesting that efforts should be made to write a proper International Classification of Disease Code[5] (ICD) specific to MCS.[6]

Returning to the challenge of medical necessity, these determinations can even be made retrospectively, denying a facility reimbursement for care already provided and recouping interest payments for the unjustified payment. Such decisions put in-patient rehabilitation facilities at risk and prompt a defensive stance when it comes to admission policies. It also puts facilities at odds with families and their staff in ethically suspect dual agency roles in which their advocacy for what is best for the patient is informed by risk avoidance against retroactive denials of payment.

Generally the risk of providing care and incurring costs only to be potentially not reimbursed, or even worse to incur penalties, leads facilities to be very conservative in their admissions and benefits policies. Although the goal should be the promotion of health and recovery, it often becomes one of institutional solvency where risk aversion leads programs to deny admission to patients who might benefit from rehabilitation.

Maggie failed to *demonstrate* the overt improvement that would be a necessary predicate to grant her ongoing rehabilitation. After eight weeks at Spaulding, she was deemed as not worthy of rehabilitation at worst, or beyond its reach at best. No matter that the eight-week limit to care has absolutely no grounding in the biology of how the brain is injured or recovers. It boiled down to what insurance would "reasonably" cover. It might have been possible to advocate for more time, but it would take a fight. The norm was just eight weeks and then discharge, although exceptions had been made for others. Nancy weighed her options and decided, at that time, the fight was not worth it.

TO THEM IT'S MONEY, TO ME IT'S MY HUSBAND

But other families have taken a more assertive stance against denials of care. Andrea Gratton, the wife of Wayne who was in a motorcycle accident resulting in his being in the MCS, told us of how his insurance company sought to have him transferred to a less costly venue by threatening his rehabilitation program with nonpayment. Andrea astutely observed that payors exert greater "pressure" on facilities "... than they do me when they want to stop doing it." It is a coordinated exercise in denial directed at both the facility and the family. As Andrea notes, "... they do start pushing the facility saying 'we will not pay beyond a certain date and you have to find another.'"

When Andrea asked her social worker a question about what care was covered, her worker would respond by invoking guidelines from a private consulting firm that produced the Milliman Care Guidelines. She had neither heard of the company nor their guidelines which are used to control medical costs for providers and run corporate benefit programs. As Andrea recalls, "I got very little out of the social workers. ... I had a question about something one time, and I asked, what the Milliman Care Guidelines were. Because the hospital was saying, 'because of the Milliman Care Guidelines. ...'" In her view, they were what "insurance companies use to determine how long a patient should take to recover from certain illnesses." She was a quick student, learning that, "Milliman is a company that collects data from hospitals about different illnesses and how long it takes to recover. And they set up guidelines for hospitals and insurance companies."[7]

Another insurance carrier tried to deny the Grattons ongoing coverage but Andrea appealed the denial. With the help of Dr. Carrie McCagg at JFK-Hartwyck, an internist with a great deal of experience and expertise in the care of brain injury, they ultimately gained an extra six months of rehabilitation. But it wasn't easy. Dr. McCagg had to write a letter and "... there was lots of correspondence back and forth asking for medical records, additional stuff, the rehab center actually did a videotape of my husband to let the insurance company actually see him and how he was responding to therapy. He wound up being denied it the second time and we appealed again."

The problem was that, "the insurance company was just saying they didn't want to pay for him anymore, that they thought he wasn't recovering fast enough, that his recovery was too slow." And how did their carrier know this, whether he was recovering at a proper pace? According to Andrea, "They were using the Milliman Care Guidelines."

But there was a clinical illogic to their deployment in brain injury, because the pace of recovery can be so variable. Andrea thought it was double-speak. She had been told by her husband's doctors from the start that everyone was different. And now he was being held to a single reimbursement standard. It made no sense and seemed unfair. Andrea protested their use in assessing Wayne's course and coverage. She told me that the guidelines should not be used because their application contradicted what she had been told, "... from the very first day he was in the ICU unit they told me that every brain injury is different, every patient recovers at a different speed, no two people recover the same way. So how could they apply a guideline and say that without knowing the patient himself?"

In response to Andrea's argument, "... they [Blue Cross Blue Shield] just said 'we go by the guidelines.'" Andrea appealed this initial denial and filed a second appeal, "that went to a committee made up of doctors and nurses and lay people supposedly, but since we did it over the phone I have no idea who was on the committee." Although the skeptical reader might wonder why Andrea did not ask for the names of those on the committee, that would miss the point of the profound power imbalance that accrues when appeals are made: a distraught wife, grieving the loss of her husband's health and well-being making a claim for more care from experts who are likely employed by the very payors whose policies are being adjudicated. No wonder she did not jot down their names.

But Andrea still held her ground, making the important rhetorical point about what she had been told by Wayne's doctors in intensive care, "We did interviews with the doctor over the phone, and I point blank said, 'when he was in the ICU I was told that he not only injured his brain, he scrambled his wiring. That he had what the doctor explained to me as a functional disconnect. And that because of that functional disconnect, he was going to take longer than another brain injured person to recover. So how you can say he should have gotten better in six months, when brain recovery is twelve to eighteen months so to speak, what they know of it, and I was told he was going to take longer than that.' "

Through her tenacity, Andrea secured an additional six months of coverage. She has seen Wayne continue to improve, noting somewhat defiantly, that "I don't know if it's progress to anybody else, to me it is!" She remains optimistic and antagonistic to insurance companies who have denied her what she believes her husband still requires, "To them [insurance companies] it's money, to me it's my husband. And I continually hold out because the father of someone I know had an accident, over five years ago, and he's doing things now that they told him he'd never do. They told he'd never be able to plan ahead, he would never be able to think forward and do things, and he's planning two-week road trips."

But her optimism has come at a high cost. Even as she appeals her most current denial from her new insurance company, which is invoking a prior insurer's decision as a precedent, Andrea is paying out of pocket for much of Wayne's care. Thus far she has spent $100,000 just for the rehabilitation. His drug cost was $400 a month and the rehab was more than $600 a day. Doctor bills are included in the rehabilitation tab but as of our interview in October 2009, she has spent $170,000 of her own money.

I asked where someone gets that kind of money. She acknowledged she is in debt but, "I still owe them let's say $100,000 ... I've paid them $60,000, plus the medications, I've already paid all that." Her most recent invoice was $98,000 for the prior year, although someone in the finance office "offered to charge us only the Medicare rate, which is $435 a day as opposed to $600."

A small act of kindness amidst an anonymous bureaucracy.

REGULATING PRACTICE

Whether in-patient rehabilitation will be provided and/or reimbursed hinges upon criteria first laid out in the 1985 Health Care Financing Administration Ruling (HCFAR) 85-2, the predecessor agency to CMS. CMS coverage determinations are made on a case-level based on the severity and needs of the patient irrespective of his or her underlying impairment. Though at an institutional level, to qualify for in-patient reimbursement funding, a facility historically had to admit 75 percent of its patients from a list of thirteen broad medical conditions specified by CMS. Brain injury and stroke are on this list. This expectation, known in rehab circles as the "75 percent rule," has recently been decreased to 60 percent. Failure to achieve these percentages can lead to forfeiture of reimbursement and/or reimbursement at lower acute care rates.[8] These fiscal incentives can influence admissions policies and eligibility for patients whose rehabilitation is paid for by private insurance, as the required patient-population mix within an in-patient rehab facility is an amalgam for all patients, public and private.[8] Scholarly data indicates that longer rehabilitation lengths of stay correlate with commercial insurance or Medicaid as the primary payor in one univariate analysis.[9]

There are eight core criteria in HCFAR 85-2 by which rehabilitation has been adjudged by federal courts to satisfy the requirement for being reasonable and necessary for a particular patient. Two criteria are particularly challenging for patients with severe brain injury. The first is "the patient must be likely to achieve a significant practical improvement." The second is "the patient's goals must be realistic."

This first expectation presupposes a degree of certainty about the outcome that is still beyond the realm of prediction for many patients with severe brain injury. Even the "must be *likely*" casts the outcome as probabilistically favorable, information that cannot be gained with foreknowledge but only through experience and the wisdom that comes from the provision of rehabilitation, or rigorous clinical trials designed to assess the effects of postacute rehabilitation. The latter has been suggested by a team of investigators who study the relatively more straightforward question of rehabilitation for lower extremity joint replacement. Even in that simpler realm, there is a need for evidence to inform reimbursement policies.[10] Simply put, medical necessity applies a *somatic time frame*[11] to cognitive injuries that do not obey conventional temporal expectations.[12]

This is especially the case in brain injury where the natural history is neither known nor fully predictable. If a patient receives rehabilitation after hip replacement, the pace of recovery and likelihood of outcome is pretty well understood. A failure to progress beyond a certain point is predictive of a poor likelihood of benefiting from more rehab. The pace of recovery from brain injury neither adheres to somatic standards nor always manifests itself in evidence at the bedside. As we have seen, what is observed – or not observed – by overt behavioral criteria may belie the recuperative process occurring within the injured brain.

Now it can be said with a high degree of certainty that a patient who is permanently vegetative by all available diagnostic criteria (behavioral assessment and investigational approaches in neuroimaging) would not meet medical necessity. Rehabilitation would be neither reasonable nor necessary for such a state. Permanently vegetative patients can be said *not* to satisfy this first criteria about "practical improvement." The problem is, however, that patients who appear vegetative on cursory evaluation may in fact be minimally conscious, and these patients may achieve a "practical improvement," if given a fighting chance.

But herein lies the real challenge. They need to be given the chance, the therapy and the *time* to recover and *demonstrate* that practical improvement is taking place. But this option is often truncated by an attitudinal bias that, as we have seen, takes refuge in the second criteria that makes the normative assertion that, "the patient's goals must be realistic."

At the heart of any of these complicated cases, amidst the devastation wrought by a brain injury, hopes for recovery can seem far from realistic, and instead, families are left grasping for futile interventions with precious little yield. This perspective, combined with the misdiagnosis of minimally conscious patients as vegetative, too often gives hospital administrators and utilization reviewers the rationale to deny ongoing rehabilitation or admission to the only facilities where these patients have a chance. And it is done all under the cover of an ill-defined concept like medical necessity.

IS MEDICAL NECESSITY ETHICAL?

Ethically, the invocation of medical necessity raises questions about what is owed to patients in need of rehabilitation. Disability scholar Kate M. Stinneford and physiatrist Kristi L. Kirschner ask the provocative question if the obligation to rehabilitate is greater than treating disease, "Medical necessity questions in rehabilitation are further complicated by teleological questions: What are the proper ends of rehabilitation? Are rehabilitation services strictly 'medical'? Are they meant to restore function, to cure, to improve the quality of life? Should they allow the person to return to life in the community rather than an institutional setting? If not strictly medical, should rehabilitation services be covered by health insurance?"[13] These are all good questions that should be asked, if nothing else, to examine the values that are implicit in medical necessity but remain unexamined. All we have are the lived experiences of families of brain-injured patients who perceive it as unfair and unreliable and a barrier to care for their loved ones.

Without necessarily knowing what is meant by *medical necessity*, family members invoke its rather malignant influence throughout our interviews echoing the questions raised by Stinneford and Kirschner. A case in point is posed by Rachel McIntyre, Darren's wife, when she implored us to fix a problem that did not have a name. At the end of our interview, she asked if she could add a few more comments to our time together. Plaintively, she asked, "Sorry, another issue is that I just have a huge issue and … I don't know if you guys can do anything about it in the future, but in reference to therapy for patients like Darren, anyone with brain injury and how they, they're not consistent in a quick enough time frame, they're automatically reduced and reduced."

She encapsulated the problem with medical necessity, the failure to improve quickly enough to remain eligible for ongoing rehabilitation. With the wisdom of experience, she articulated the consequences of neglect and she points to the contractures and the contradictions of withholding rehabilitation. "And it's not good for physical therapy especially because he starts to have contractures and whatnot. And it's not fair to them. And I know a lot of it has to do with the health care system, medical insurance, and I know it's not just brain injury, I think it's anywhere basically that you need rehab therapy."

Like Andrea Gratton, Rachel points to the hypocrisy of mixed messages heard by families: a mantra of patience coupled with an impatient benefits plan. Reflecting on what she heard in the ICU, she recalls, "... they sit there on day one and tell you how long a brain injury recovery process actually is and they drill that into your head. And that's all fine and good and we have to understand that. But why can't they say, 'okay, well you know what, they deserve from day one, five years of therapy.' Five years, not twelve months, or after six months we're going to reevaluate, nine months we're going to reevaluate, twelve months you're cut off."

Then comes the recognition of the illogical and the insensitivity of a system that fails to appreciate the struggle of families like hers. There is moral indignation in her voice, "I just think that's horrible, it's ludicrous because who knows ... how bad of an injury they actually sustained and how long they're actually going to need in their recovery process. I mean, yes there are a lot of people who unfortunately do not come out of it and that stinks, yet even ones that do have a lot more contractures and whatnot because they're not rehabbed properly. The therapy that they should have received they weren't [getting] and I think that's just wrong to the patient. I don't think it's right. And I wish to God you could go to ... somebody who makes these health care decisions and say, 'you know what, what if that was your loved one there?' But unfortunately until they're in that situation they don't look at it as such, and it's sad."

STATE OF DENIALS

Andrea and Rachel are not alone. Consider the experience of Burt Brody, the husband of Jean who had sustained an aneurysm. When Jean progressed to be able to talk, Burt thought she might finally qualify for acute rehabilitation, satisfying the medical necessity requirement. She didn't, however, because the pace of her progress was too slow. Without other options, Burt decided to take Jean home. He was pressured by insurance coverage and serious concerns about his ability to pay the bill. His coverage hinged on the pace of Jean's progress. It cost $16,000 a month for nursing home care, but that was at risk if Jean's pace of recovery did not quicken, "And my insurance company is paying that reluctantly and saying, 'you know, unless she gets better really quickly we're going to end this soon.'... I wanted to do what I could for her, but I don't have that kind of money. I'd run out of money very quickly if she had to stay there and the insurance company decided not to pay for it."

It was a hard decision for a man who loved his wife and wanted to give her every opportunity to recover. And it left him critical of how care is structured for patients like Jean whose access to rehabilitation depends upon the advocacy of loved ones who must contend with medical necessity and levels of rehabilitation that obscure both patient need and potential. Although others would see it more charitably, his parsing of the rehabilitation landscape conjures up an Orwellian *Newspeak.* Despite the euphemisms, he explains that, "Acute rehab is that you're in better shape and subacute is that you're in worse shape." And however each level of care is demarcated, the unspoken goal is to classify so as to limit services.

Other families have yet to break the code and are surprised when time in rehabilitation runs out. It came as a surprise to the family of Kenneth Quigley, the man who fell from a ladder onto a concrete slab. His mother, Elinor, got a call from her daughter-in-law that "... 'they're going to move him.' And I said 'they're going to move him where? When?' And she said 'they're going move him to a nursing home.' And I said 'how can they do that?' And she said, 'I don't know but we have two [nursing homes] we have to look at, and they want him moved by Monday.' This was a Friday that they told her this and she called me. So we had to go out and we had to find a nursing home. I didn't know then that I could have fought that, I didn't know that then, but evidently the insurance or whatever he had was only going to pay for so much and he had to be moved." Over the six weeks in rehabilitation Kenny had made "very little progress."

There's a strange bureaucratic tautology to the very notion of medical necessity: a physician can provide medical care so long as it is needed with need manifested by demonstrable improvement with the intervention. Elinor explained how this odd strategy played out for her son's care. Rehabilitation was seemingly only for those who were prepared to receive it, not an intervention in and of itself that might facilitate additional progress possible. Although patients ready for rehab should certainly get it, it did seem problematic to withhold it from those who still might benefit. As Elinor observed, "Well, rehab is very limited. Anything that Kenny has achieved it's been through my sister, through myself to bring him to the next step. Because they'll take him so long and then say 'oh well, unless he can advance.' And so then we work on him so we can get him to the next step and they take him again. But they're working on the same things we've worked on. We're the ones that got him sitting up, we're the ones who got him on his feet, and then they take over and they'll do it for so many weeks, and then 'oh well, we can't go on because he hasn't progressed.' But they've only done what we've done, they haven't tried to take him further, the next thing is up to us to take him to the next step again. It seems like the ones that we've dealt with, outside of one group that are no longer there, do not take the initiative. They do not show you, they do not. Once the therapy is over that's it, they don't want anything to do with you. I know it's not them, I know it's the insurance, but it feels like you're left in the dark."

It is a bit of a paradox that insurance benefits for rehabilitation are set ahead of time, and if the patient does not meet the preset goals, their benefits are terminated. Betty Wexler told us how she sought rehabilitation for her daughter, Sarah, after she recovered from meningitis. They got her into a convalescent home across the street from the hospital where Sarah had once worked as a clinical dietician. She was accepted there because people knew her and it was comforting for the Wexlers who live in Connecticut that their daughter, though marooned in California, was amongst friends.

But there was the perennial problem of adequate rehabilitation. "In retrospect it was not very good because we had great troubles getting her any physical therapy. In fact, that was a weakness in all of the places where physical therapists are because of insurance. They do the minimal unless they can set a goal that can be achieved in "x" number of treatments, they can't see the person. I'm taking her privately now to other physical therapy."

Sometimes the eligibility requirements can, truth be told, be *mindless*. Consider the challenges faced by Heather Sykes when she returned to Michigan from Virginia. Her mother, Cindy, tried to get her into a quality rehab program. The problem was that Heather had reached the maximum coverage on her private insurance. The truck driver who had hit her car was not liable, so her mom sought a Medicaid waiver for her.

But the approval process was Kafkaesque: in order to get more rehabilitation to get to the point of being toilet trained, Heather needs to already be toilet trained. Cindy told us, "... there's a lot of criteria involved in that, and unfortunately, the place that she's at, some of things they want her to do in order to get into the program is the toilet, bowel and bladder control, and things like that."

Hoping that Heather "would probably laugh at it at some point," Cindy apologetically told of her daughter's challenges with toileting and ultimately, qualifying for more and better rehabilitation. She recalls, "I've been trying to get her on the toilet myself, and it's a struggle because you have to stand her up, pull her pants down, sit her back down...everything doesn't work in the right sequence. And so a couple weeks ago, she said she had to go, indicated she had to go, and so I said ok, so I get her in the bathroom and I said, 'Heather, you have to stand up.' She sat right on the toilet; I said 'you got to stand up so I can pull your pants down.' And she was vocalizing, she wanted something, and she was reaching over for the toilet paper. So I took some toilet paper off the roll, well she put it in between her legs, wiped herself with her clothes all on, and then after she did that, she realized then that she went to the bathroom and she didn't have her clothes off, and so she was wet."

And then the pathos that is self-awareness and embarrassment. Heather did her best, tried to do something that was once so easy and that now consumes all her energy, only to fall short. Her mind knew of her body's failure, *itself a sign of progress*, but from a bureaucratic point of view it was representative of failure.

Her mother's voice captured the sense of disappointment, "And she was so upset and frustrated ... she wants to do it so badly. ..." But her daughter's determination would not be sufficient without the help of others. Her progress will be stalled, "... if everybody isn't on board with it." And they are not. Then, almost wistfully, if only, "... she were in a TBI facility they would be working with her. But unfortunately she's not." It is simply an absurd way of making decisions about care and coverage.

Many of these families convey a sense of betrayal, that they have been treated unfairly by an irrational set of rules that do not cohere with their lived experience. They have all been unwitting students of the economics of brain injury, and yet others more distant set the curriculum. Some have more or less control over these decisions, but even when the powerful and well-off are struck by brain injury the consequences can be devastating on an emotional level, even if fiscal disaster is averted.

Perhaps Mary Waters, the mother of Jimmy, put it most simply – and said it best – when she was notified by her insurance company that her son was going to be transferred out of rehabilitation. Bottom line: "you have to make progress or you have to go home because it cost $40,000 a week being there."

HOME CARE

One mother, a physician who wishes to remain anonymous, has taken her teenage daughter, who is minimally conscious, out of chronic care because she perceived care there as inadequate. With a generous state-based Medicaid benefit, the help of family, and other resources, she has been able to do a version of home-schooling for her daughter.

Worried that rehabilitation was inadequate and the priorities were skewed, she brought her child home. She observes, "the biggest obstacle to recovery for her is that there is nothing, or very little, given to brain injured people. I feel they're given ... maximal care but minimal therapy. You know, just sort of range of motion therapy it seems like, everybody wants us to do range of motion. ... I felt like there was no cognitive therapy at any point. At all."

After progressive reductions in therapy because of medical necessity, premature discharges to chronic care facilities when her daughter was medically unstable and scouting out adult facilities for her child that "seemed absolutely horrendous to us, like nursing homes," the patient's mother and her three older sisters decided to take her home.

Her mother acknowledges that "it was a huge, huge, huge undertaking" but adds that it was something her daughter "deserved." To them it was a felt obligation, a responsibility that could not be delegated with impunity. After contending with renovations, transportation issues, and the hiring of nurses, they now have it down. They tell prospective nurses that, "we are rehabbing [Elaine],* this is a rehab center, this is her personal rehab center, this is not a nursing home, she's not chronic care, she's in chronic care but she's not, we're not tending the vegetable garden here, we're not just watching her 24/7. We're talking to her, or playing music, or reading to her, or touching her, or stimulating her."

Proudly, she adds, "So we've revolutionized the nursing care, customized to Elaine, which I think everyone should have. And she's responded to it, she's doing so much better!"

BONDS OF FRIENDSHIP

Most families do not have this home care option, made possible by geography and personal circumstances. Consider, Stephen Carrier, the bond trader at Deutsche Bank. He told us that the greatest barrier to care was insurance coverage for his wife, Mary Beth. As he recalled, "Well the insurance was huge. It seemed every couple of weeks there was a threat to be discontinued. ... I actually had to discontinue twice and had to appeal several levels and was able to get it overturned." Even with private insurance he was under this threat. But he had good colleagues at work who were sympathetic.

Unlike many families affected by brain injury, his position at work gave him a greater opportunity to argue on behalf of his family's needs in the face of insurance denials. At the outset, he was ambitious, "Initially, I needed to get my company to change their entire plan because their plan was, as soon as something became chronic they would pay for any type of facility rehab or whatever for 120 days per year and that was it." And he was successful, liberalizing the time limits. But the challenge of medical necessity still remained. The lengthened benefit coverage was still predicated upon the demonstration of medical necessity and ongoing improvement. Modestly, he recounts that, "... for whatever reason I was able to get them to look at it, and they lifted that cap so it became unlimited ... ," although ongoing coverage was still "... subject to progress being made. ..." But there was some room for interpretation, "since it was so new, there was a lot of disagreement between the insurance company and the facility about what 'progress' was."

Despite the eventual limitations on provided care, Carrier appealed to his peers and got them to place themselves in his shoes, assuming the proverbial veil of ignorance and imagining that their seat around the conference table was the one with a brain-injured spouse. With a bit of moral suasion he "talked to the head of benefits for Deutsche Bank U.S., and just explained the situation. And frankly what I think happened was I was a similar age as a lot of the executives here and I think everyone looked at it and thought if that was them with two kids at home and in a high stress job and suddenly you lose your wife, you know, what you do? And I think a couple of key guys just went to bat."

Others were similarly sympathetic, sometimes to their own peril. An insurance case manager went beyond the pale for the Carriers in the face of their adversity. Grateful for these acts of kindness, both corporate and individual, Stephen notes, "... there's been some incredible things that have happened. I ended up with a case manager at the insurance company that ended up getting 'reassigned' over this case because she, her forbearance was so incredible. I mean, she kept approving things, and, I mean ... she actually talked to Mary Beth on the phone one day. I mean it was just a hello, but she took that as huge progress. And like I said, at some point she got reassigned. So I think she got put in a box for it."

When I practiced primary care medicine and encountered a drug or service denial for one of my patients, I would try to get someone on the phone and try to make them feel responsible for the fate of the human being who had been entrusted into my care. I would follow up with a letter but I would make the call with the patient or their surrogate in the exam room listening.[14] This way, the utilization reviewer or admissions officer on the other end of the phone would know that there was someone, a real person, affected by the decision they were going to make. It was a microeconomic response to a macrosystem that can be too capricious and utilitarian for individuals, especially when the rules that govern decisions are not informed by science and the clinical facts, but ill-fitting bureaucratic contrivances. Simply put, I tried to make it personal for the one empowered with the authority to make life-altering choices for families and for them to assume some degree of responsibility for their decisions. To use Mr. Carrier's language, the goal was to get these decision makers to step out of the confines of their role, their box as it were, and empathize with the patient or family member sitting in the room with me. It did not always work, but it was often necessary to get these people out of the protective space of their role to appeal to the humanity that they ultimately shared with the patient or family making the appeal.

"MEDICAID DIVORCE"

In his early advocacy, Mr. Carrier achieved what I tried to do in my practice. He had made his wife's case something personal and it worked, at least for a while. Later he would have to sacrifice a marker of his love to sustain these efforts for Mary Beth and their kids. When private insurance was exhausted and it came time to switch to Medicaid, Mr. Carrier was advised by his lawyers to get a divorce to preserve his assets for his family. When asked about Medicaid, he told us, "... I had to get a divorce to do it. Which was another whole obstacle. And that's something that back when she was at Spaulding, so this was you know six to eight weeks after her injury, one of the social workers called me in and said, 'you know, you really need to think about getting a divorce to protect your assets.' And again, whether it's shock or whatever, I was like, I couldn't believe it."

At the start he resisted. As he told us, "... I wouldn't do it, and I didn't do it for the longest time, it just seemed wrong to me. And I'm not necessarily religious, but it did seem like the wrong thing to do." Eventually he was persuaded by the fact that, "enough people had" convinced him. He had lots of advice and had "talked to enough people, mostly the social workers in the rehab community."

Ultimately, it was a reluctant choice because "... unfortunately this country doesn't allow a catastrophe like this to take care of someone without wiping out a family." He justified his decision by coming to believe that he was doing it for his children, "And frankly I was, I guess the way I made myself go through with it and feel better ... I convinced myself that I was doing it for the kids. You know, I have two kids to put through college and I have a decent amount of assets I've accumulated over time and to have it all go, took this route. So it was not easy ... it wasn't a guarantee either."

With some sadness, he recalls, "... finally I did get a Medicaid attorney and in order to get her to qualify she couldn't have any assets, so we did a 'Medicaid divorce,' her parents were her guardians, and I had to set up a trust for her, but all of our other assets were able to stay with me in a family trust." He was legally well represented and was able to enlist the support and cooperation of his in-laws who were given custody for their daughter, "The attorney that I found, and it was from a list of Medicaid attorneys ... was a great guy, very compassionate, and [he] found someone who would represent my in-laws, who when I mentioned this were very supportive. In effect they said to me when I finally said something was 'well, we wondered how long it would take.' So they fully expected me to do it."

Medicaid divorce prompted by severe brain injury is an increasingly common strategy used by families to protect assets. Mr. Carrier observed that it has become routine enough so as to not be adversarial, "Well it's common ... but it's not common. It's a route that a number of people take, and the agencies on the other side don't find it unusual. You know, they don't look at it and say 'well you were divorced a month ago and now she's getting' ... even the opposing counsel were very onboard with the whole thing."

It has even come to the attention of the *New York Times* columnist of "The Ethicist," Randy Cohen. Cohen maintained that shifting assets in this way is ethical. In response to a reader's query, Cohen noted that:

> ... it is through divorce, paradoxical as it sounds, that you can best honor your marriage vow to cleave to your husband for better or worse. Preserving your small savings will be enormously beneficial to you both.

He rightly observed that the contemplated action is "not the exploitation of a legal loophole but adherence to the regulations governing Medicaid." His proviso: "Done with respect for the law and compassion for your husband, such actions, divorce included, are prudent and ethical courses of action."[15]

I would agree and make two additional points. The first is that the decision comes at an emotional cost for the spouse who is initiating the action. Severing the bonds of marriage under duress, even if it is for "better" and not "worse," can feel like abandonment or an abdication of responsibility.

Burt Brody plaintively describes the challenge of severing the relationship between husband and wife precisely as the injured spouse improves. Talking about his beloved Jean, he told us how he reaffirmed his vows in the face of ongoing adversity and sustained improvement: "There are numerous occasions when I'll wake up in the morning and she's got tears rolling down her cheeks and she mouths out to me, 'why me?' ... I hold her, tell her I love her, and tell her I'm going to find whatever help there is out there and I'll never abandon her. Because I took our marriage vows very seriously ... I won't cheat on you and ... I won't abandon you. I say 'the last breath I take will be taking care of you.'"

He describes the paradox of improvement and heartache, "I think that the better she gets, actually the harder emotionally it is for me." He begins to cry as he tells us, "I think I've figured out I've got more to lose now."

Burt has gotten his wife back from the thralls of injury and now, "The better she gets ... I have a wife who can tell me she loves me. I have a wife who last night at the hotel obviously wanted to say something to me, and I said, 'what is it?' And she said, 'I want a good kiss right now.'" He pauses, "I don't want to lose that."

Burt's reluctance to sever his marriage vows and to lose Jean as his wife points to the pain that may accompany Medicaid divorces. As logical as they may be and as essential to the family's future, the emotional cost is not to be discounted for the loving spouse who makes the decision to fulfill his or her vow by breaking them. A paradox to be sure, and one that points to the need for reform of Medicaid regulations for catastrophic medical events, laws that compound tragedy with pathos.

And a second point about Medicaid divorce is that of shared surrogate decision making between the former spouse who had been entrusted with medical decisions before the divorce and the parents who are now going to assume that role. Conflict could ensue if the spouse's relationship with in-laws were suboptimal before the injury. In the worst kind of estrangement, the spouse could even be excluded from care decisions.

Absent a collaborative relationship with his wife's family, Stephen might have had have no ongoing role in Mary Beth's care. Fortunately, that was not the case in his relations with his in-laws, but it could be an outcome in more contentious relationships. If we imagine a family dynamic like that which affected Terri Schiavo's parents (the Schindlers) and her husband (Michael Schiavo), it becomes clear this is a not a solution for everyone. Fortunately, for Mr. Carrier, this was not the case.

He is grateful for his in-laws who have stepped in to make this work, "And again, it's only because my in-laws, my relationship with my in-laws is so good that I'm still very involved. But no, they *could* say 'don't listen to him.' And in fact the case manager that we had at [a long-term care facility] that we had for a while had difficulty getting that. And so she *wouldn't take any direction from me*, or she would double check with my mother-in-law. Which we worked through, and it was fine, by then nothing was bothering me. But yes, I've given up that right to make those decisions."

A final point about Medicaid divorce is that if it is legal and viewed as ethical under the circumstances, it is unfair that the legal advice that would be necessary to entertain such a step is not uniformly available to all families who might reluctantly pursue this option given the alternative. Although the importance of structuring assets in the setting of disability is seen by some attorneys as an important professional responsibility with practical consequences for families,[16] many of our respondents were never given this choice.

FOR RICHER, FOR POORER

And Glenie Donato is a case in point. She preserved her marriage but became impoverished in the process. She may not have had a choice because her husband was far more aware than most other subjects in our studies. Amongst all the families we have interviewed, she is perhaps more resentful than most, possibly because her husband Angelo was aware of the care he did and did not receive and its burden on him and his family. Angelo had a brainstem stroke, much like Maggie did. But unlike her, Angelo could reliably communicate.

His responses suggested that he had fully preserved cognitive function, resembling a patient in the *Locked-in-State* (LIS), a condition in which there is essentially normal cognition but sparse motor output save for blinking and head movements. These are actions transmitted using the cranial nerves above the area of injury or disease that blocks output through the spinal cord. Extraordinary memoirs have been written by individuals who were locked-in and mistaken for vegetative. The most recent was the elegiac *The Diving Bell and the Butterfly*[17] by Jean-Dominique Bauby, the former editor of the French edition of *ELLE*. He wrote that exquisite volume by creating an alphabet based on the number of blinks produced by his one operative eye.

Janet Tavalaro wrote another memoir of her time at the Goldwater Hospital on Roosevelt Island in New York City. She too had been mistaken for being vegetative, and was only later discovered to be in LIS. Memorably, she drafted a poem describing her entrapment in a nonresponsive body in a volume fittingly titled, *Look Up for Yes*. She has breath but no voice, silenced by the precise localization of her injury in her brainstem:

> When I awoke
> I was still in the same old hoax.
> My body was the same:
> Wanting to move.
> I had no voice, only a hole for breathing.[18]

Angelo had a bit more motor output than a classic locked-in patient. More impulses got through his brainstem and he could nod a bit and weakly shrug his shoulders. And like Bauby and Tavalaro, he was keenly aware of his environment and the depth of his isolation.

Even as his professional caregivers made erroneous judgments about his capabilities, he engaged in communication with his wife by blinking and using a letter board. As Glenie became increasingly aware of his abilities she became ever more frustrated with the care he was receiving. He was getting better but no one seemed to take note of it, and if they did, he was not moving fast enough to qualify for therapy that might facilitate his recovery.

Like many of the families we have interviewed, Mrs. Donato figured out that Angelo was aware and quite *there*. Case in point: Glenie was writing on his letter board and "every time I stopped writing I would put the board on his lap." She believes she had done this five or six times when Angelo's eyes widened indicating he wanted to spell something. And with no loss of sarcasm, he spelled, "keep knocking the board into my crotch and I'm putting you back on my list," referring to his roll-call of people he was mad at.

Proudly, she reports, "So this is how aware he is, he knew I kept dropping it on his lap. But I'm the only one who sits there and communicated with him." Since then, he wished Glenie a happy anniversary, "... the day before our anniversary, he said, 'happy anniversary for Friday.' So, you know, I can't get through to anybody that this is how aware he is and he needs to get things to help him be able to communicate. It shouldn't be such a process to help somebody."

We asked her when she knew he was aware and quite present and she told us, "I have actually been. Even before the spelling board, [I] knew he was aware by asking him questions and him nodding before I knew he could spell. Everyone else wasn't quite aware of it. But I was absolutely sure of it when he started to spell."

She had taken on these "professional" activities, untrained as she was, because the professionals had ceased to ply their craft. Motivated only by her love of Angelo, she carried on, mimicking what she had seen done. She had to step in because the therapists "had stopped his speech therapy five days a week, they were doing flash cards and stuff like that. And then they told me they weren't doing it anymore."

So Mrs. Donato improvised, "I started writing on a board, asking simple yes and no questions, getting yes nods and no nods. And that's when I realized, it's probably been three months, four months" that he has been aware. But there was a problem: she was the only one who recognized it.

She had made these observations because she had spent more time at the bedside than the doctors, nurses, and therapists, who were more hesitant to grant that he was aware and actually reading. She got through and therapy resumed, but at a lower level than she would have liked. Angelo was relegated to simple picture-flash cards instead of promoted to actual reading. This frustrated Mrs. Donato who was "... a little annoyed at the fact that he read the word but they were still continuing with flashcards for numerous weeks." She tried to be patient, but her tolerance waned. Finally, she said, "... listen, he's actually answering words. And I write down things, and he reads everything I write. And if he doesn't know, he can shrug his left shoulder." She convinced the powers that be and an alphabet appeared.

Mrs. Donato still does not understand the logic of undertreatment and treatments delayed. All the more so because the delay of treatment made him ineligible for continued treatments. The denials "cost me my insurance because they won't cover him now." It is a complicated tangle of issues all with dire consequences for the fiscal well-being of her family, "... the physical therapy stopped, the insurance stopped. He's not on Medicaid yet, he's been shipped around with Medicaid, they want information and there's information I've given them and they ask for it again and again, it's going on a year this month."

Although she applied for Medicaid in November, "it's going to run out this November and it's still not approved." The consequences of all this? "I had to sell everything he owned. If he dies I don't even. ..." She pauses to admit her desperate circumstances, "I had to cash in his insurance policy. If the man was to die today I don't even have the money to bury him. I owe [one facility] money ... because the insurance didn't cover everything there. I owe [another facility]."

Mrs. Donato is a proud woman who will have to both sell her husband's home and at the same time give up the dream that he will ever leave the facility. "It gets harder because I know he's most likely never coming home. Part of me knows, that's never going to be ... that I'll probably have to sell *his* house."

Crying, she shares her estimation of the status quo: "The system just sucks you dry, in order for him to get help I have to get rid of everything he owned. It's hard." And doubly so, because she is selling Angelo's hard-earned home, losing another legacy while he lies locked-in a facility that he can ill-afford.

Glenie tells us plainly, "It's hard to give away what's not mine to give away. I had to sell his business, it's not mine it's his, he worked all his life for it. They had to take everything away. No building, his annuities, they even made me cash in his life insurance, I don't even have enough money to bury the poor guy. So it's not just the ailment and the brain trauma that effects the family, it's financial burden that comes along with it. "

She will be impoverished once this is all said and done, and it is impossible to not be sympathetic and want to help. A middle-class couple struck down forever by a stroke of very bad luck. It is blatantly unfair as Glenie sums up her situation, "You know, I mean, the financial burden is horrendous. ... And I'm not rich to begin with, you know ... I have a son who's seventeen who just started college, I have a job that just pays my mortgage." And then there is that phrase I have a hard time forgetting, "*I have to become poor in order for them to help him.*"

PACE OF PROGRESS

In spite of her financial challenges, Mrs. Donato's greatest frustration is with medical necessity. Like so many of the families we have interviewed, she is annoyed that coverage remains tied to the pace of the patient's progress. In Angelo's case, physical therapy was stopped because it was claimed he was not cooperating even as she saw some progress. Mrs. Donato disagreed but without avail, "I see some improvement. They stopped his physical therapy, they just do occupational therapy and I would rather see the physical therapy back. I don't understand their logic for not doing it ... they were saying ... he's not making an effort to roll ... try to get from the bed to a chair. Angelo might never get from the bed to a chair. His whole left side does not move at all."

More hopefully, as if making a case for more therapy, she tells us what *he can do*, "He can do thumbs up, if you say give me thumbs up he can give me thumbs up. He tries to roll his hands over, he can wiggle his fingers goodbye, he can rock his foot. He shrugs his shoulder."

But the answer is still, no, "... according to them, their words to me were from the therapist is that they can't do physical therapy forever. Now, I was like very upset over that. Because why can't you do physical therapy forever? If the brain is so complex, what he might not do today, he might do three months from now. But if you don't continue to do it with him he's not gonna do it at all."

All cogent points, which she capped off with a trenchant question: "*You know what I'm saying?*"

Then more philosophically, she asks, "... you know, they keep telling me brain trauma, the brain is so complex. And I'm thinking then why stop the therapy? He may not do it right now, but in a month he might do it. And the therapist gave me the answer, 'we can't do this forever.' And I kind of thought, yeah, you can be in therapy forever. I've seen improvement ... they have restrictions, they have goals to hit. And he doesn't hit their goals at whatever time."

But there is a wrinkle to those goals and that is the relationship between time and recovery. The problem with cognitive rehabilitation and physical therapy in the setting of brain injury is that rehabilitation might well be occurring sight unseen. That is, the brain might be getting better without necessarily exhibiting a change in overt behavior to show for it. It might be that recovery *prefatory* to motor output is taking place – sight unseen within the brain – that will be necessary for the more robust recovery to come. But of course, this is problematic because the lack of a behavioral manifestation might also indicate that no progress is being made. In this way, prefatory progress would be indistinguishable from an outright lack of progress at the bedside.

Other possibilities exist too. Progress can be slower than what might be expected for a somatic injury given the complexity of the biological system that is under consideration. If we think that it takes decades to educate the human brain, does it not follow that it could take as long for an injured brain to recover? And of course, the lack of overt recovery may be because the patient has, in fact, reached his maximal potential.

The problem with our rehabilitation system is that it is not positioned to distinguish between these alternatives when a patient's progress seems to stall. Instead of piquing curiosity about why a patient ceased to progress or failed to improve, the general response is to curtail services and call it a day.

This response may be human nature and the force of our collective acculturation. But it is also in contravention to a 1999 National Institutes of Health consensus panel on traumatic brain injury, which advocated that "Persons with TBI should have access to rehabilitation services through the entire course of recovery, which may last for many years after the injury."[19] Instead of the patience urged by this consensus statement, patients and families have been victimized by a temporal discordance fostered by our expectations for quick recoveries. This is then enforced by a punitive reimbursement system that rewards adherence to constructs like medical necessity which fail to acknowledge variance in the pace of recovery. All of this with dire consequences for patients and families who are desperate for a bit more time and more care.

WHITHER MEDICAL NECESSITY? AND FOR WHOM . . .

As this book goes to press, there may be some hope that medical necessity, as currently enforced by Medicare, may undergo some helpful modifications for patients with chronic conditions and disabilities, with the Obama administration agreeing to revise coverage guidelines.[20]

It all started with a nationwide class action lawsuit challenging the legality of medical necessity. The suit, *Jimmo et al. v. Sebelius*, argued in Federal District Court in Vermont, lodged a complaint against the Department of Health and Human Services and then-Secretary, Kathleen Sebelius. The plaintiffs made the:

> allegation that the Secretary has adopted an unlawful and clandestine standard to determine whether Medicare beneficiaries are entitled to coverage, resulting in the wrongful termination, reduction, and denial of Medicare coverage for beneficiaries with medical conditions that are not expected to improve. Plaintiffs seek to certify a nationwide class and request, among other relief, an injunction or *writ of mandamus* enjoining the Secretary from applying this alleged unlawful standard.[21]

The government, according to recent press reports, has agreed to a settlement that would revise the alleged current standard, which requires evidence of patient improvement. The new – more liberal– criteria would pay for care and services if needed to "maintain the patient's current condition or to prevent or slow further deterioration" and not require additional evidence, or prospect of, further recovery for coverage.[20]

The willingness of Medicare to settle this case, with such a dramatic reversal of policy, is an acknowledgment of medical necessity's nefarious effect on the lives and welfare of patients with disability and chronic care needs. An editorial in *The New York Times* opined that, "the proposed settlement will reverse this irrational and unfair approach to medical services."[22]

At the time of this writing, the state of the settlement is yet to be determined, but if the agreement is accepted by Christina C. Reiss, chief judge of the Federal District Court in Vermont, the change in policy will have a laudable effect on countless beneficiaries, including those whose claims were

denied before January 18, 2011, when the lawsuit was initiated. These beneficiaries will be able to have a re-review of their claims and previous denials.
Future beneficiaries will have more access to needed care.

This is unimpeachable progress, but several questions remain about the
new criteria for medical necessity as it relates to patients with disorders of
consciousness. First, will the preservation of the patient's current condition
be good enough when coverage is adjudicated? Because the value of life with a
disorder of consciousness is a state so discounted, will assessors view its con-
tinuance as akin to a deterioration? All the more so because these patients
sustain complications like bedsores, urinary tract infections, blot clots, and
pneumonia because of poor quality of nursing care or the intrinsic challenges
of immobility and their inability to manage respiratory secretions?[23]

Another worry is the state of entrenched attitudes toward this population, which this volume has sought to describe. That perception will lead
many to think that these changes in policy do not apply to this subgroup. An
example, drawn from Terry Wallis's medical history, is illustrative. Although
the neuroimaging requested by the family in the 1990s would have been paid
for, Mrs. Wallis and her husband were both told that it was either not a covered benefit or that it would not matter.[24] The benefit was there for the test,
but the lingering, entrenched attitudes toward patients like Terry prevented
them from being used for the benefit of the patient.

The somatic challenges of caring for this population will inevitably
lead most observers to see deterioration, not the new-normal of stasis as the
benchmark. And if that is the case, then this progressive change in Medicare
policy will constitute an advance for others with chronic care and disabilities and leave those with disorders of consciousness further isolated and
underserved.

REHABILITATION AND THE AFFORDABLE CARE ACT

Cautious optimism is warranted about the fate of the Obama administration's negotiations over medical necessity because it will happen against the
backdrop of the implementation of the more far-reaching Patient Protection
and Affordable Care Act (ACA), the landmark legislation passed by Congress
and signed into law by President Obama.[25] At the time of this writing, the
Supreme Court has upheld its key provisions and full implementation is
in the future.[26] But it is not too early to voice some preliminary concerns
about how this law came into being and how this transformative legislation
might affect patients with severe brain injury.[27] First the provenance of the
legislation.

As remarkable as it must seem, coverage for rehabilitation was *not*
included in the initial frameworks for the ACA. *Rehabilitation was an*

afterthought, included only after lobbying from organizations like the Brain Injury Association. Advocates worked with the administration to get rehabilitation services included in the purview of coverage as one of several stipulated key categories that were deemed as essential health services that would be covered.

They also worked to articulate an appropriate definition of "rehabilitative" services and "habilitative" devices, making the assertion that these services and interventions should be categorized as medical care and thus covered as available care just like acute interventions. Additional concern was voiced about the exclusion of certain specialists, like neurologists, from benefit packages because these physicians often serve a primary care role for this patient population. These concerns are ongoing at this time.

One could get mired in the details of the legislation and the semantics about what is and what is not covered, but for our purposes it is best to focus on the outright exclusion of rehabilitation from the ACA and the *timing of this oversight*. That rehabilitation had to be lobbied for, after the brain injury sustained by Congresswoman Gabrielle Giffords, is astonishing, but true. Even after her injury, and the attention paid to her life-saving surgery and the exceptional rehabilitation she received at Houston's The Institute for Rehabilitation and Research (TIRR), rehabilitation was not in the original bill.

The Brain Injury Association of America,[28] Representative Bill Pascrell,[29] chair of the Congressional Brain Injury Caucus, and Pia Carusone,[30] Congresswoman Gabrielle Giffords's Chief of Staff, all appealed that rehabilitation be included in the legislation.

Ms. Carusone's wrote to Kathleen Sebelius, the Secretary of Health and Human Services, on the congresswoman's official stationery and made a heartfelt appeal for the inclusion of rehabilitation in the ACA. She wrote just three months after the January 8 Tucson shooting that nearly took Representative Giffords's life.

The letter is worth quoting in full because it demonstrates the fundamental disconnect between policy and politics. Despite the concern voiced for Ms. Giffords and her hoped-for recovery, the rehabilitation upon which her progress would depend was relegated to an afterthought when it came to policy. Bravely carrying on in the absence of the congresswoman, Ms. Carusone wrote Secretary Sebelius on April 2, 2011:[30]

Dear Secretary Sebelius:

In the past three months, our office has become intimately familiar with traumatic brain injury rehabilitation. During this difficult time, we remain grateful for the comprehensive, quality medical care that Congresswoman Gifford is receiving at TIRR Memorial Hospital to restore her physical, cognitive, and psychological functioning – and concerned that all brain injury patients receive quality, comprehensive care. As you work to define "rehabilitative and habilitative services" as part of the essential benefits package of the Patient Protection and Affordable Care Act, I hope you will consider the care Congresswoman Giffords has received and work to accommodate the needs of all individuals with traumatic brain injury (TBI) to receive the same full continuum of medical treatment.

The March 2, 2011, *USA Today* article, "For Brain Injuries, A Treatment Gap," explained that most military service members and other Americans who have sustained TBIs lack access to the same high standard of care from which Congresswoman Giffords currently benefits from under the federal workers' compensation as a federal employee injured on the job. According to the piece, access to care can depend upon the type of insurance plan you have, if any; where you live; the expertise of treatment providers in your insurance company's network; the willingness of your insurer to flex benefits; and the knowledge and skills of those advocating on your behalf.

As Congresswoman Giffords's family and staff have learned, comprehensive rehabilitation is vitally important for *all* individuals who sustain TBIs. When someone sustains a brain injury, acute surgical care at a trauma center or hospital is only the first step in recovery. Post-acute rehabilitation of sufficient scope, duration, and intensity is necessary to regain lost skills and learn new compensatory strategies. Once active treatment ends, individuals need access to ongoing management toward off medical complications and slow the progression of neurologic, neuroendocrine, musculoskeletal, and psychiatric diseases induced by brain trauma. With proper treatment, we know that individuals, like Congresswoman Giffords, who sustain even the most severe injuries can live healthy, independent and productive lives.

We have been deeply moved by the outpouring of support for and attention to Congresswoman Giffords's recovery, but we remain cognizant that over 1.7 million other Americans will sustain traumatic brain injuries this year. We believe it is imperative that all Americans with TBI have access to the same full continuum of medical treatment that Congresswoman Giffords has been so fortunate to receive. We urge you to ensure that all Americans have access to such care by defining it as part of the essential benefits package included in the Patient Protection and Affordable Care Act. Thank you for your service to this country.

Sincerely,
Pia Carusone
Chief of Staff
The Office of Congresswoman Gabrielle Giffords

It is remarkable that this letter had to be written at all given the bipartisan concern engendered by the congresswoman's injury. Even more so when one considers the attention paid to TBI associated with the war in Iraq and Afghanistan, described by Representative Pascrell, co-chair of the Congressional Brain Injury Caucus, as "the signature injury" of these wars.[31] Sympathy for the congresswoman and hundreds of thousands of wounded warriors and veterans touched by brain injury because of the war should have rallied policy makers to the cause of rehabilitation. But it did not. It is an omission that begs an explanation.

One possible rationale is simply cost in light of the concerns over the depth of the deficit. Nobel Laureate Joseph Stiglitz and former Assistant Secretary of Commerce Linda Bilmes estimated in 2006 that TBI costs related to the War in Iraq would be $14 billion if the war lasted until 2010 and $35 billion if it had ended in 2015, conservatively assuming that surviving soldiers would have a forty-year life.[32] President Obama declared an end to combat mission in Iraq in August 2010[33] and the fighting continues in Afghanistan. While these projections were contested before the House Committee on Veteran Affairs by members of the Bush administration as overestimating potential expenditures,[34] the cost of ongoing care for returning wounded warriors will be significant. A 2012 estimate of service members and veterans affected by TBI in 2012 suggests that 230,000 individuals have been affected.[35]

Another reason for the omission is society's collective desire to dichotomize outcomes related to severe brain injury. As we have seen, outcomes are either thought to be dire or miraculous. Seen this way, there is nothing much to do. The former category is beyond repair and the latter is without need of assistance. In both scenarios rehabilitation is either pointless or unnecessary. But, as is apparent from these narratives, the reality is that most patients' futures fall somewhere in the middle, where any semblance of hope is predicated upon ongoing assistance.

When Representative Giffords entered the House in August 2011 for the first time since the shooting she was welcomed as the returning heroine that she is. *The New York Times* reported Representative Debbie Wasserman

Schultz, friend and colleague of Giffords as saying, "The room just exploded" as her vote was cast on the electronic ballot. "We've all seen her empty light and we all wanted to see her name light up." Giffords's presence was a balm after a tough legislative session, "Everybody's heart was so grizzled and hardened," she said. When she walked into the room, "everybody's heart just melted."[36]

And with the applause comes the unspoken desire that all is and will be well. To think otherwise is unspeakably sad and it is human nature to defend against it. So, the impulse is to dichotomize and see her battle as over, as a success. But though it is a success, her struggle is a work-in-progress that will need ongoing care and rehabilitation for years, if not decades to come.

Sarah Wheaton, writing for *The New York Times*, captured the difference between Ms. Giffords's outward recovery and the challenges that remained when Giffords returned to the scene of the shooting in January 2012 to lead her former constituents in the pledge of allegiance.[37] Tempering the triumphalism of such events, Wheaton offered the views of Giffords's husband. She reported that, "The man next to her, fighting tears, offered his own remarks. 'For the past year, we've had new realities to live with,' said her husband, the astronaut Mark E. Kelly. 'The reality and pain of letting go of the past.'"[38]

THE AFFORDABLE CARE ACT IN PRACTICE

As its name would suggest, ACA seeks to make medical care accountable and affordable, primarily by enhancing efficiencies that will improve access to primary and preventive care and lead to an overall decrease in costs. These efforts are supplemented by efforts to minimize fraud and abuse. The law will also seek to improve the quality of care provided and enhance consumer protections, through better regulation of insurance companies and a major reliance on the electronic medical record and information technology.

The cornerstone of these efforts are accountable care organizations, groups of physicians and hospitals who cluster together to improve care. These groups of providers are tied to each other organizationally as well as fiscally because they are reimbursed based on an incentive schema that rewards performance and the achievement of efficiency measures. Experts agree that this new way for paying for care – with its assumption of risk – will alter historical revenue streams.[39,40] And while this revisionary reimbursement model could lead to greater reimbursements, projections indicate that academic medicine will receive less, not more funding – even when the provision of care is "efficient."[41,42]

What does this mean for patients with severe brain injury? In short, ACA is a mixed bag. The Brain Injury Association of America's useful analysis of the ACA reveals both positive and negative dimensions of the law.[28]

On the positive side, dependent coverage is extended to twenty-six years, a genuine benefit considering the demographics of TBI with its profile affecting the young and active amongst us. Extending coverage after eighteen will help mitigate vulnerability during a phase in life when the incidence of brain injury is high. Another benefit is broadened Medicaid eligibility to 133 percent of the Federal Poverty Level (FPL) as well as tax breaks and credits for families whose incomes fall between 133 percent and 400 percent of the FPL. There are also provisions for affordable coverage for pre-existing conditions and six months of insurance coverage for "high-risk" patients, potentially meeting the needs of those who have sustained serious brain injury. More benefits include additional consumer protections; coverage with federal non-discriminatory rules; and the gradual elimination of insurance caps limiting yearly and lifetime coverage.

On the negative side is ACA's reliance on efficiency measures; care that is inefficient or wasteful will not be covered. This makes sense because what constitutes efficient care is known but becomes deeply problematic when knowledge of disease trajectories or pace of recovery are still unknowns. Efficiency models assume a knowledge of what would constitute appropriate and timely care, a knowledge threshold we have yet to pass for patients who have disorders of consciousness, whose trajectories of recovery we are just beginning to understand.[42]

But at this juncture, we can neither predict the timing and pace of emergence from MCS nor describe its mechanism. Given this state of relative ignorance, it is impossible to say that care is efficient or not and plot a patient's status against a timeline that determines how the pace of progress is gauged. Notwithstanding the expectations of legislation like ACA, *MCS brains recover by biological standards not reimbursement criteria.*[43]

VETERANS ADMINISTRATION POLYTRAUMA CENTERS

But there is a ray of hope from a pioneering program from the Veteran Administration's (VA) Polytrauma Centers for veterans and active military members with disorders of consciousness.[44] Directed by skilled professionals whose work has been dedicated to patients with disorders of consciousness, these programs represent a response to the aforementioned *Mohonk Report* [45] and, as such, a model for providing care to these patients.

The VA has four polytrauma centers in the United States that have created a specialized programs of care tailored to the needs of patients with disorders of consciousness. Unlike shorter, conventional rehabilitation programs, patients are admitted to these Emerging Consciousness Programs (ECPs) for ninety days, during which time their ongoing medical needs are met along with requirements for rehabilitation. These programs use an interdisciplinary approach and have periodic assessments to mark the patient's progress and level of consciousness and functional status. Special care is taken to avoid iatrogenic medical injury or harm by failing to tend to medical urgencies and priorities that, as we have seen, are often ignored when patients leave acute care settings for conventional rehabilitation, leaving patients less able to make progress. They are also mobilized in order to prevent medical complications like bedsores and blood clots. In addition to these preventive interventions, patients receive trials of "neurostimulation" using advances in pharmacology as they become available. Progress is tracked through multimodal assessment utilizing bedside examination tools as well as neuroimaging and other technical modalities.

As importantly as what is done with patients is what ECPs do for families, who when patients leave these programs will need to be sufficiently informed about their loved one's condition to make informed choices about ongoing care. Steps are taken to make sure families understand the patient's injury, prospects for recovery, and potential barriers to care while the patient is admitted to the ECP. Families participate in educational seminars and engage in meetings with staff addressing medical, psychological, and social work issues throughout the patient's stay. Most notably, families are given an online "Polytrauma Family Care Map"[46] to coordinate their stay within the ECP. The map breaks the course of admission into workable stages to help families adjust to the new and evolving realities of having a member with severe brain injury.[47] Discharge planning is also a major focus of ECPs and efforts are made to prepare both patient and family member for discharge to skilled nursing facilities as well as to home. When the latter occurs, it is done so with sufficient support, "a large safety net and requisite family training."

Regrettably, the VA's superb program is the exception and not the norm, especially in the current climate of reform, dominated by the ACA. Implicitly acknowledging the potential impact of ACA on its ECP program, the VA issued a statement after the Supreme Court upheld the law to assuage fears of beneficiaries and families. Dated July 13, 2012, it read:

> The provisions of the Affordable Care Act (ACA) upheld by the U.S. Supreme Court will not affect the current role the Department of Veterans Affairs (VA) has in the lives of America's Veterans. We will continue to provide Veterans with high quality, comprehensive health care and benefits they have earned through their service. VA health care does not change as a result of the ACA.[48]

As the VA statement suggests, provisions in ACA will create tensions much like those seen with medical necessity, but on a grander, more pervasive scale. Although incentives that reward "quick" recoveries will be balanced, to some extent, by consumer protections that are new to the ACA, these protections will likely fall short of ensuring care for those with disorders of consciousness. This will prove problematic because the climate of care, under ACA, will become of expediency and not patience, a virtue when it comes to the biology of brain recovery.

PATIENCE IS A VIRTUE

For the MCS population, patience is a very special virtue when it comes to predicting when recovery might occur. The Australian investigator Michele Lammi and colleagues have shown that emergence out of MCS to an ability to communicate reliably is *unpredictable* and occurs in a rather open-ended fashion two to five years after injury.[49] More recently investigators have shown that improvement in functional status with traumatic injury can occur within the first five years.[50]

Such a long timeline should not come as a surprise to readers of this volume, now familiar with cases like Terry Wallis. It does, however, challenge conventional expectations about recovery, which holds that the longer one is sick the less likely recovery becomes. A maxim true for most maladies has its notable exception here. Contrary to popular expectation, and with apologies for the *double negative*, it turns out that time is *not* a negative predictor of recovery once a patient is minimally conscious.

Instead, it is a patient's ability to engage in object manipulation that predicts recovery of functional communication.[51] As Lammi observed, an MCS patient's prognosis is not dependent on time in that state.

> The low correlation coefficients between duration of MCS and the outcome measures suggest that prognostic statements based on length of time a person is in the MCS cannot be made with confidence.[49]

Observations like this one take families and clinicians by surprise and also prove problematic to how we structure treatment beyond what is conventionally called acute care.[52] We typically think of the next phase of care as *chronic* care a word etymologically linked to time. As the *Oxford English Dictionary* reminds us, "chronic" is defined as "of or relating to time" and secondarily "lasting a long time, lingering, inveterate."[53] Inveterate? It works as a synonym if we presume that these brain states are immutable, unchangeable and yes, chronic. But the data suggests – and as we will see in the biology of MCS – something quite different.

Nonetheless, we describe the reemergence of functional communication in these patients as a *late recovery*. Knowing what we know about the normative patterns of recovery and our growing experience with patients described by Lammi, we need to ask *late by whose standards?*

If we don't ask these questions we will fail to realize that our chronic care system was never designed for MCS patients, but rather for patients with degenerative conditions like Alzheimer's dementia. MCS patients have been placed in this care sector because there is nowhere else to put them. So there they linger, as if they were inveterate, their prognosis conflated with elderly patients with dementing illnesses that are progressive and herald decline with the advance of years. Though they may share a disordered state of consciousness, the MCS patient's prognosis has advanced, regaining awareness, while the Alzheimer's patient progressively loses awareness of himself and others as his conscious grip on the world fades away.

Unless we appreciate their differing biology, we will continue to see MCS as a condition worthy of chronic care and not more active therapeutic engagement. And if we label recoveries late or otherwise, before basic prognostic information is available, we fall prey to the mistaken notion that recovery should have happened sooner. This further stokes the notion that the absence of "early" recoveries is evidence that these patients are never going to get better and that brain injuries are static and immutable. As I observed in a paper written in 2009:

> These perceptions are increasingly scientifically untenable and only serve to run out the clock for hope and expectation. Would it not be better if our expectations for what might be possible were concordant with the actual tempo of recovery experienced by patients with these disorders? And would it not be even better if we actually knew the biology behind these mechanisms of recovery?[52]

In Chapter 13, we will take some time to consider these questions.

13 Minds, Monuments, and Moments

TEMPUS FUGIT AND MCS

During the summer of 2010, I presented a lecture at the Third International Conference on Disorders of Consciousness at the *Campus di Baronissi Facolta de Medicina e Cirugia* just outside of Salerno, itself an important seat of medical knowledge in medieval Italy.[1] The conference took place about an hour's drive from the spectacular Greco-Roman ruins of Paestum, the Latinized name given to a settlement named for the sea-god Poseidon. Now several kilometers inland, Paestum was fittingly once on the Mediterranean. The passage of millennia has landlocked the ruin and deprived the modern tourist of glimmering seascape vistas that the ancients once enjoyed. Today, the visitor can only imagine that the sea lies just beyond the next archaeological mound.

The conference's proximity to Paestum was fitting because the most famous of its findings is the ancient *Tomb of the Diver*. On a series of white slabs, from which his coffin is made, the tomb depicts the passage of a young man to the afterlife. En route, he attends a symposium, embarks on a procession, and – most remarkably – dives naked into an awaiting pool from the Pillars of Hercules (see Figure 3).

The image captures the diver in mid-flight suspended in a moment. Despite the image's flat relief, its ancient artisan depicts time as a fourth dimension. By freezing the young man between life and death, he is "forever overhead" as the archaeologists S. DiGregorio and M. T. Granese note.[2] DiGregorio and Granese describe the diver's portrayal as "the unmeasureable interval between and unrepeatable before and unimaginable after."[2]

AN ETERNAL PRESENT

When I heard their account of the diver, I was reminded of Augustine's conception of an "eternal present" in which the deity is similarly suspended in all time. Like the diver's moment, this too is an "unmeasureable interval" because it is an infinite convergence of past, present, and future. In an attestation evocative of the description of the diver, Augustine writes of God:

> In your "today" you will make all that is to exist tomorrow and thereafter, and in "your today" you have made all that existed yesterday and for ever before.[3]

(Bk I.6)

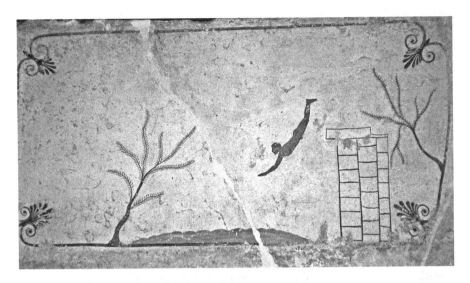

FIGURE 3. Greek Tomb Painting, 5th century BC.
Photo Credit: HIP/Art Resource.

I had last thought of Augustine's theology when thinking about Terry Wallis, except that his eternity was 1984, the year he was injured.[4]

Despite Terry's emergence from MCS in 2003 and his spontaneous communication, he remained stuck in 1984. Like the diver from Paestum, he was locked in time.

Terry has continued to live in an eternal present since then, although his speech has become more fluent and he is laying down new memory. For example, he now knows the song "Bad Boys, Bad Boys, what you gonna do?" – which, I like to joke, may or may not represent an improvement. But it is important because this song, *which did not exist in 1984*, shows that his brain is learning and making new memories. And even more notably, it appears that his brain is also undergoing structural changes decades after his injury.

Neuroimaging studies using advanced diffusion tensor MRI imaging techniques performed at Weill Cornell showed evidence of structural changes in Mr. Wallis's brain.[5] Diffusion tensor imaging (DTI) looks at the directionality of fibers in the brain and can provide a detailed map of brain structure.

Over an eighteen-month interval two DTI scans of Wallis revealed *dynamic* changes in his brain that were interpreted as related to possible axonal sprouting and pruning reminiscent of what happens in the maturing or developing brain.[6] What was seen were proposed to be new connections between remaining neurons in his severely damaged brain.

It is not known if these neuroimaging changes were responsible for his ability to speak, but they are suggestive. In tandem with his improved functional status, the neuroimaging findings show that while Terry was temporally locked in an eternal present, his brain injury was not immutable, his recovery was moving forward.

But despite Terry's forward progress, to him, it remained 1984 and in his mind Reagan was still president. As his mother related to me a couple of years ago, he and his family watched President George W. Bush deliver the State of the Union Address at their home. Terry turned to his mother and asked, "Mama, who's that?" Mrs. Wallis said, "That's President Bush." Terry responded, "What happened to Reagan?"

On another occasion, I called the Wallis family to check in with them and to secure their ongoing permission to share their story. They graciously allowed me to continue to talk about Terry and his progress. In our conversation, Terry's mother told me that Terry's daughter, Amber, had graduated from college the night before. Since 2003, Terry has had difficulty reconciling that Amber was his daughter and not his ex-wife, who she evidently resembles. Amber had been born after Terry's accident and Terry confused her with his former wife because in 1984, he was still married and had no children.

So it was all the more remarkable when Mrs. Wallis told Terry about his daughter's graduation and he demonstrated a newfound temporal sensitivity. He was able to acknowledge the passage of time and appreciate the maturation of his daughter. His comment is pregnant with insight: "Amber's graduating college? She's not a kid anymore. She's a young lady."

Although Mrs. Wallis tells me that it's "still 1984, most of the time," Terry's appreciation that Amber was getting older suggests the return of a temporal sense, at least on an inconsistent basis, now *almost three decades* after he was injured. As of September 2012, she reports that though Terry still thinks he's a teenager, "he's more aware of time now." When his parents ask him what year it is, he won't answer, because he has a sense that his answer may be wrong, which is an improvement over the status quo. And when he is told what year it is, he protests and "refuses to accept it" saying that he could "not be that old."

TIME TRAVELS

Terry Wallis is not alone in his temporal dislocation and his slow march of recovery. The brain-injury literature recounts other cases. In a case cited by William Winslade in his prescient and early volume, *Confronting Traumatic Brain Injury*,[7] a psychologist describes his temporal disorientation after regaining consciousness:

During this period, I had no awareness of time. *I existed in a world of the here and now.* I was not even aware that such a concept of "time" existed. I knew who "I" was but did not think of myself as being a child, a boy, or a man...One day, however, my "mental clock" began ticking again and the concept of time began to become significant.[8]

Cases like these raise perplexing questions about time and personhood. Can you fully be you stuck in an eternal present, not knowing whether you are "a child, a boy or a man"? Imagine the thought experiment of self-awareness devoid of temporal reference points.

Although neuroscience may be on the way to answering this age-old question, the humanities have already weighed in on the issue over the course of millennia. Augustine saw the eternal present as that which divided the human from the divine, a conflation that is somewhat obscured in the eternally robust, yet dying, Diver of Paestum. Like the "eternal present," the diver's permanent state of transience is discomforting. In more modern times, Martin Heidegger would write in his aptly titled masterwork, *Being and Time,* that we achieve our potentiality as "Beings" only after fully assuming a temporality and appreciating our broader place in history.[9]

Fundamentally, we need to be aware of the march of time for an authentic understanding of our "Being." Humans are not meant to reside in an "eternal present," "suspended overhead" – or as the psychologist put it, "a world of the here and now." We are destined, instead, for a temporal grid with a past, present, and most importantly a future. As the Spanish philosopher and bioethicist, Diego Gracia Guillén has observed, it is this anticipation of the future that marks us as uniquely human.[10] This is a process of becoming, of transitioning out of the present. But it is an evolution that is not solely dependent upon biology. It is also dependent upon context and the dire expectations applied to this population, expectations that truncate our imagination.

Regrettably, there are many barriers to care that are encountered in patients with severe brain injury. They are the consequence of failing to appreciate that recovery occurs over an unfamiliar time course, and that when these patients improve they do so in a manner that can be counterintuitive and still unpredictable. Part of the challenge is that we assume that each of these brain states have true diagnostic standing, that is, they are fixed diagnoses and not still syndromes with quite a degree of variance.[11]

I believe that this is where we fall prey to temporal errors. As the reader will recall, a diagnosis is defined as the identification of the nature and cause of a disease. With modern diagnostic thinking deeply informed by Koch's classic postulates about disease and causality,[12] the modern practitioner is habituated to search for such causal relationships between pathogenic agents and resultant illness or injury, much like the infectious disease specialist is trained to isolate the specific microbe responsible for a pneumonia or meningitis in order to confirm a diagnosis.

In modern-day clinical practice, we have come to expect cause and effect, and our differential diagnosis is constructed around a theory or hypothesis about how the patient became sick or injured. When our differential diagnosis is scientifically constructed – and informed by the history, physical exam, and laboratory data – it becomes less speculative and more likely. We are more able to link cause and effect as they relate to current and future states ultimately being able to predict the course of a disease, its cure, or conclusion. And the more tightly hewn the diagnosis, the less variance around its outcomes. In short, at that juncture, the emphasis moves from a differential speculation about a range of possible explanations to a more definitive diagnosis.

PROGNOSIS BY A DIFFERENT CALCULUS

For all these reasons it is not useful to view disorders of consciousness as reified and static diagnoses, but rather as *syndromic* works *potentially* in progress. Instead, it is heuristically useful to view them as temporary or evolutionary states (until proven otherwise), whose persistence, permanence, or evolution toward recovery is defined by etiology, intervention, and time course. Their outcomes play out on a temporal horizon that both portend progress and set limits on recovery. Indeed, it is nearly impossible to discern the implications of a "vegetative" examination without knowing how long a patient has been in that condition and the etiology of the offending insult. What outcome becomes possible vis-à-vis recovery is determined by evaluating the patient's current state against a time gradient. At this juncture in the evolution of our knowledge, it is often best – except at the extremes of brain death and the permanent vegetative state – to place the emphasis on a differential speculation rather than on a true diagnosis, heeding the advice of David Berlinski who remarked that, "under the mathematician's hands, the world contracts, but it becomes more lucid."[13]

By this truncation, I mean being attentive to the range of diagnostic possibilities that might be plausible in the classical sense of differential diagnosis, but also differential as understood in differential calculus. The analogy to advanced mathematics is germane because calculus provides insights into change with respect to time. A differential equation thus could help us understand how a diagnosis changes over time. It can describe a trajectory of a patient's state through time and link diagnosis to *prognostication*, which can be understood as a diagnosis played out over time and, as the bioethicist and medical sociologist Nicholas Christakis reminds us, is a "moral duty."[14]

Until we better understand mechanisms and are more precise about prognosis, the metaphor of a differential equation may provide a helpful framework to fulfill Christakis's moral duty and describe brain states that can be dramatically different over a time course. Indeed, in their temporal dimensions, a disorder of conscious can be understood more as a *prognosis than a diagnosis*, where a prognosis is understood as the *differential* statement of:

> *prognosis is a function of the change and rate of change of the diagnosis over time*

or

$$P(x) = f\,(D(x)/dt)$$

In this equation, Dx/dt marks the slope of a curve, which is a disease trajectory over time.

DIAGNOSIS, PROGNOSIS, AND THE VEGETATIVE STATE

This relationship between diagnosis and prognosis, though a bit obscure, was in fact a point made in the 1994 landmark "Multi-Society Task Force Report" on the vegetative state published in the *New England Journal of Medicine*.[15,16] The authors of that document, which included leading neurologists of the day, implicitly invoked temporality when noting that the persistent vegetative state (PVS) was a *diagnosis* but that the permanent vegetative state was a *prognosis*. They observed, as previously noted, that:

> As originally defined by Jennett and Plum in 1972, the term "persistent," when applied to the vegetative state, meant sustained over time; "permanent" meant irreversible. Notwithstanding Jennett and Plum's precise use of language, confusion has arisen over the exact meaning of the term "persistent." The adjective "persistent" refers only to a condition of past and continuing disability with an uncertain future, whereas "permanent" implies irreversibility. Persistent vegetative state is a diagnosis; permanent vegetative state is a prognosis.[15]

As is apparent from this quote, time infuses our nomenclature. Both adjectives, *persistent* and *permanent*, are defined in part by a time course and their place in time. Persistence in the 1994 report refers to the past and an uncertain, limited future duration. There is a contingency to the condition as seen in the definition of *persistent* in the *Oxford English Dictionary*, which defines the term as "persisting or having a *tendency* to persist."[17] Here again, invoking *persistence*, our nosology is marked by the hand of time that will either cause something to endure or have a tendency to decay.

James Bernat, a Dartmouth neurologist, attended the Multi-Society meetings and served on the task force. He has reviewed the minutes of deliberations of the February 29 to March 1, 1992 meeting in Dallas when the persistent-permanent appellations for the vegetative state were discussed and shared some observations.[18] He notes that:

> Fred Plum pointed out that he and Bryan Jennett chose the term "persistent" as a descriptive term to merely state that the vegetative state had existed without improvement for a month. He also explained that "vegetative" is a biological concept but "persistent" is not.[18]

Importantly, Bernat describes the consensus reached about the distinction, especially as it portends to an irreversible state of consciousness lost, and the importance of having a nomenclature that provided some prognostic guidance:

> All members agreed that "persistent" is distinct from "permanent" because the former term describes only that a clinical state has existed for a period of time without implying that it will continue unchanged in the future whereas the latter term implies a clear prognosis of irreversibility. ... The members discussed the point that "persistent vegetative state" was an inherently confusing term because, above all, everyone wanted to clarify prognosis and that the mere presence of a vegetative state for a month was not the most clinically relevant fact.[18]

Bernat observed that, "Interest was expressed by some members, particularly Ronald Cranford, in coining a new term 'permanent vegetative state' to identify those PVS patients for whom we could determine irreversibility." Cranford, who was a strong advocate of a right to die, may have been motivated by his views on this issue to be more definitive about permanence, but this initiative did not gain traction. It faltered because of a seminal distinction by Bernat. In Dallas, Bernat pointed out that a "persistent vegetative state' was purely a diagnosis whereas 'permanent vegetative state' implied a prognosis." His words would eventually be immortalized in the *New England Journal* article.

By suggesting that a permanent vegetative state was a prognostic designation, and not a fixed diagnosis, I believe the task force was sending a cautionary note about diagnostic accuracy. Echoing a caution voiced by Jennett and Plum in 1972, the task force suggested that in the absence of a clearer understanding of mechanisms of injury and recovery it would be difficult to be categorical about the prediction of diagnostic states in some liminal cases. This is a point that Bernat confirms when noting that, "Prognosis was an important issue but should be stated separately for different groups (traumatic vs. non-traumatic etiologies)."

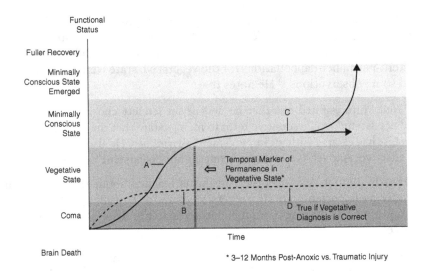

FIGURE 4. Temporal Markers of Recovery.
Image by the author.

Absent such distinctions, and without more etiological and causative refinement, a diagnosis becomes attenuated, much how light dissipates over distance as an inverse square. Put another way, time *delimits* a diagnosis and morphs it into a more uncertain prognosis when attempts are made to achieve an enduring prediction of outcomes.[19]

We can crudely model this if we think of the slope of a curve over time. The more acute the tangential slope at a point in time, the more uncertain the fixity of the diagnosis. Once the slope gets close to zero, the diagnosis becomes more certain. We can understand this if we imagine a patient who is rapidly recovering after an injury. His diagnosis is changing significantly over a time course and he will have an acute slope (see Figure 4, A). Contrast that to a patient who is in the permanent vegetative state, such as Terri Schiavo, whose condition remained unchanged for a decade and a half after sustaining a cardiac arrest and whose slope was zero (see Figure 4, B).

The slope of these curves is positive in the direction of a recovery, negative in the setting of decline, as in an intercurrent illness, or flat in the setting of an injury that does not portend recovery.

These slopes can lead to time-delimited prognosis for patients who are comatose or vegetative, and can help clinicians provide guidance about prognosis without resorting to overextended predictions about outcome.[19] Linking functional status to the rate of recovery and the reaching of certain temporal milestones sets parameters within which outcomes are likely to occur. For example, it would not be appropriate to offer a definitive prognosis to the family of a comatose patient with traumatic brain injury who has regained brainstem function and is moving into the vegetative state as this might portend a more favorable outcome.[20]

EXPLAINING "LATE" RECOVERIES

The years since the "Multi-Society Task Force Report" have confirmed the wisdom of those scholars who published the guidelines in 1994, when they urged caution with the classification of permanence. We now know that *their* categorization of "late recoveries" from what was described as a permanent vegetative state were in fact patients like Terry Wallis, who was actually minimally conscious and misdiagnosed. This unfortunately represents an unacceptable standard of clinical assessment and constitutes what the late Bryan Jennett presciently characterized as "late discoveries of earlier recovery."[21]

The possibility of such errors was reason enough for the drafters of the "Multi-Society Task Force Report" to urge caution. But it was not the only one. Prudence was also warranted because there is a profound discontinuity between when we contrast the question of prognosis in the vegetative state before the three-month or one-year cutoff points for anoxic and traumatic injury with that of the minimally conscious state. Lest we oversimplify something that is quite complicated – and overdraw too heavily upon the calculus analogy – once a patient reaches the minimally conscious state, there appears to be *no fixed time variable* linked to the question of recovery and emergence. There are a mix of temporal patterns, of possibilities, linked to discrete trajectories – yet to be charted – that reflect different mechanisms of injury and regenerative processes.

Paradoxically, it is the *absence of temporal determinism* that informs our growing scientific understanding about these brain states. When we turn to the status of patients who are in the minimally conscious state we find ourselves in the discomfiting place of noting that once one achieves that designation what happens thereafter is *not* time sensitive in any predictable way. So although reaching the functional level of MCS before the three- or twelve-month interval after injury is an important time stamp, once the patient is minimally conscious the more conventional correlation of time and injury seem not to apply, as Lammi has shown. That is, recoveries to emergence and the restoration of reliable functional communication can occur after long periods of dormancy ... *or not.*

DON HERBERT

One of the most poignant of such recoveries was that of Don Herbert, a Buffalo firefighter who was injured in a house fire in 1995.[22,23] He sustained both traumatic and hypoxic injuries. In the months following his injury, he appeared to meet criteria for MCS, responding to sounds in his room and tracking those who entered. He even began to make halting efforts at speech. Without a clear precipitant, he stopped talking by the fall of 1996, appearing to all the world as if he had become vegetative. That is until 2005 when he was given a mix of medications – including ones used for depression, Parkinsonism, and attention deficit disorder – by an earnest physiatrist new to his care.

With this mix of medication, Herbert suddenly and fluently began to talk. His functional status and level of awareness far exceeded his most functional early months following his injury. Though cortically blind, he could identify his old firehouse mates by their voice and recall past events. Poignantly, he too had a temporal dislocation reminiscent of both Terry Wallis's eternal present and the psychologist cited by Professor Winslade. Herbert was incredulous that his youngest son, Nicky, but a toddler when Don was injured, was now a teenager. In disbelief he spoke to his son on the phone, "This isn't Nicholas – he's a baby, he can't talk!" Nick responds, "I can talk. ... Do you know how old I am? ... I'm thirteen." Don laments his protracted absence with a father's guilt, "I've been gone a long time. ...."[22,23]

Cases like Herbert's – whose recovery and survival were regrettably short-lived – raise the question of whether or not he was really "gone a long time." Where exactly was he when he was unreachable? And more importantly, what was the state of his brain such that it was capable of returning to a high functional status from such a seemingly quiescent state?

Diagnostically, he was in MCS, a state latent with the possibility of an *atemporal* recovery. It has this capability, in contrast to the time-delimited possibilities of the vegetative state, precisely because the *biology of the two states is different*. Despite their behavioral resemblance, patients who are MCS are fundamentally different than those who are vegetative. In contrast to the disintegrated vegetative patient, MCS patients' brains may be functionally integrated.

The reader will recall that Schiff and colleagues first demonstrated in 2005 that spoken narratives can activate large-scale language networks in some MCS patients.[24] In contrast, vegetative patients who are exposed to auditory stimuli only have first order activation without secondary somatosensory areas and higher-level associative areas.[25] In this way, the vegetative brain is disconnected functionally and without the capability of achieving functional integration as seen in MCS.

DEGREES OF COMPLEXITY

This contrast between the architecture of the vegetative and minimally conscious brain reflects the hierarchical structure of each. The former with isolated modular networks is contrasted with preserved large-scale networks capable of activation in MCS.[26] This differing degree of neurological complexity might help explain why time is such a salient variable for vegetative patients, but not one in the MCS. Indeed, the difference between the vegetative state and MCS is nothing short of consciousness, what the Nobelist Gerald Edelman might describe as the emergent or evolutionarily distinct systems biology and combinational complexity of the conscious human brain.[27]

The differing spatial organization of these two brain states, and their contrasting impact on the capability for consciousness, cognitive complexity, and time, suggests an analogy to the discontinuities between Newtonian and relativistic physics. In the former, time is a constant. In the latter, space and time are melded into *space-time*, a composite in which time is no longer a constant but rather a variable whose value can be influenced by gravitational fields as well as an object's velocity relative to the perch of the observer. At least through a relativistic frame, time becomes a fourth dimension contextualized against the other spatial dimensions and forces that might distort or alter its "usual" pace.[28]

It is useful to think of time as a *fourth dimension* in MCS, reminding us that how we view the temporality of an MCS patient's recovery depends upon the rapidity of that process *relative to the observer*. To make the analogy clear, let us illustrate this with a quotidian example. Anyone who has sat on a train and observed the swish of a train passing in the opposite direction appreciates that the speed of that second train relative to the observer is the composite speed of both trains, not the speed of the single train going in the opposite direction. Because velocity = distance/time, time has a relative value informed by the context of the observation.

The passage of time can also look different within the health care system depending upon where the observer is situated. When considering an MCS patient in the acute care setting, an admission for more than a few weeks after injury is considered too long or too slow.[29] Utilization reviewers will assert, at least in the United States, that the patient who is lying dormant in bed is not making overt improvements and hence not meeting the reimbursement criteria for medical necessity. In that regulatory sphere, which is blind to underlying brain mechanisms that undergird recovery, time passes quite quickly. Contrast that, with the expectations of practitioners working at a brain-rehabilitation center who expect the time course for recovery to take months, if not years.

This perspectival difference reflects more than a regulatory stance. It also implicitly indicates that a different value is being attached to time in the acute care and chronic venues. In the acute care context, the temporal constant that is invoked is reflective of what I have termed a *somatic time frame*. Time constraints relate to relatively simple systems and problems like recovery from an infection or wound healing after surgery. It is linear, and in our analogy, Newtonian in scope. As such, it is ill-suited to the actual biology of the recovering brain.

The neurologist or physiatrist working in chronic care, whether informed by habit and experience, or through emerging scientific knowledge of mechanisms of recovery, views time differently, influenced by the biological complexity that is the recovering human brain. The time stamps associated with the recovery of ambulation following hip surgery or the resolution of pyelonephritis are not the temporal frameworks applicable to a brain regaining its capacity for consciousness.

More fundamentally, the differing time constants in the vegetative and minimally conscious states bring us back to their differing biologies and the importance of understanding underlying mechanisms of recovery to explain the "aberrant" recoveries of some patients who seem to have violated the expectations for permanence noted from the "Multi-Society Task Force Report."[15,16]

This is a phenomenon that we will likely see reported with more frequency as recent papers from *Neurology* indicate.[30,31] These papers show marginal predictive aberrations centered around the task force's prior three/twelve month demarcation point for distinguishing between the persistent and permanent vegetative states.

TOWARD MECHANISMS OF RECOVERY

The issue is that our descriptions of these brain states remain *descriptive and are not yet mechanistic.* If we look at mechanisms reflective of underlying biology then those who make late recoveries to MCS beyond the heretofore marker for "permanence" are those patients who are *biologically different.* James Bernat hints at this point by noting that predictors of late recovery are a patient's relative youth and traumatic versus anoxic injury;[32] demographic characteristics that I would assert are more likely to track with mechanisms of *recovery* that correlate with the emergent characteristics associated with the transition from VS to MCS as well as the transition from an unconscious to a conscious state.

There is preliminary evidence to suggest that patients who are capable of becoming MCS, but who still appear vegetative on clinical exam, *are biologically different* while they are behaviorally VS. That is, they have the biological substrate that has the potentiality for the emergent phenomenon of consciousness, whether or not they have demonstrated that capability vis-à-vis overt clinical manifestations seen on behavioral assessment. This can be seen if we return to Owen and colleagues' report of the twenty-five-year-old woman who was clinically vegetative five months after injury and showed network activation patterns consistent with MCS, a behavioral state that the patient subsequently reached, as evidenced by behavioral criteria.[33] Notwithstanding behavioral progress out of VS into MCS on a subsequent examination at eleven months,[34] the discordance between behavioral exam suggested the novel diagnosis of "nonbehavioral MCS."[35]

Di and colleagues similarly reported on two vegetative patients who showed both primary auditory cortex activation and associative temporal activation comparable to those who subsequently improved to MCS.[36] Conversely, the bilateral absence of the cortical components of the middle-latency auditory evoked potentials has been taken by some investigators to correlate with a lack of potential for functional integrative recovery into MCS.[30]

To be sure, this line of work – to borrow another temporal marker – remains *preliminary*. It remains important to acknowledge that these neuroimaging tools are investigational and are not vetted for clinical practice.[37] But they all help substantiate my larger point about the biological discontinuities between VS and MCS, a point made epidemiologically by Estraneo and colleagues from their longitudinal follow-up studies.[31]

The most suggestive of a biological difference between VS and MCS is the nosological question posed by studies that demonstrate that a patient's diagnosis is changed when a therapeutic intervention is received. Consider the diagnostic challenge, grounded in actual experimental work, of the patient who is behaviorally vegetative for a period of time that qualifies for "permanence" under Multi-Society Task Force criteria and then receives a drug that moves their brain state to MCS.

Whyte and Myers report on the case of a patient who had been vegetative for four years following TBI.[38] After receipt of the hypnotic Zolpidem – more commonly known as Ambien – in a small trial of fifteen patients with disorders of consciousness, this single patient transiently demonstrated behaviors reflective of MCS, making the fixity of the "permanent" vegetative state problematic.

As encouraging as this is, nosologically such cases present a labeling problem. If a patient is behaviorally vegetative, and "permanently" so based on Multi-Society criteria, and then moves into MCS with treatment, what is their diagnosis? To make it more complex, suppose the patient reverts back – as he is most likely to do – to the vegetative state once the drug's effect has dissipated? Behaviorally, at *a moment in time*, he may be vegetative or minimally conscious if we want to temporize our nosological thinking.

Has the patient's diagnosis changed? Has their prognosis been altered by the intervention? Or did the drug tap into the potential for biological integration that existed in this solitary patient? These cases suggest that even within the syndromic "permanent" vegetative state, some patients have the biological heterogeneity indicative of a latent capability for recovery to MCS and beyond. Indeed, these patients should be considered to be MCS or diagnosed at their highest functional status. For these select patients, progress is no longer represented by the time-bound constant of the vegetative frame, but rather that of a potentially more favorable MCS space-time continuum.

Given the emphasis that the Multi-Society Task Force placed on temporal markers and their import in the polemics over the diagnosis of Terri Schiavo,[39] it is tempting to view outliers as violating our rules. Otherwise dormant patients who show responsiveness on neuroimaging, ones that have "late" recoveries, or those who respond pharmacologically from a state of "permanence," seem to challenge well-worn norms. These (still) exceptional cases seem to threaten what has become familiar, undermining categories that have served us well. They have helpfully influenced how we think about end-of-life care and justified the right to die since *Quinlan*.[40,41]

But as comforting as it might be to marginalize these exceptions and hold fast to our temporal conventions, it is far better – and scientifically more honest – to reexamine our temporal expectations about recovery. As I have demonstrated, time has been an imperfect proxy for the biology of disorders of consciousness. It has been descriptive but not explicative and led us astray from a hidden complexity that awaits a more thorough explication of neural circuitry and mechanisms of recovery, which Schiff and Posner have advanced as their mesocircuit hypothesis.[42]

In lieu of a descriptive approach to these disorders, we should reset our clocks – and priorities – and turn to a mechanistic one grounded in biology. This will make a profound difference for scientific advancement, diagnostic and prognostic accuracy, therapeutics, and decisions about the adequacy and timing of rehabilitation.

14 Heads and Hearts, Toil and Tears

WHERE'S MAGGIE?

Maggie did not get better in time, and like so many others was dispatched to a skilled nursing facility. For her mother, Nancy, it was as much a strategic decision to accept the transfer as a practical one. She was still new to brain injury and being her daughter's advocate. She did not know she could have appealed the denial for more time on the grounds of equity, "... there were lots of people that were there longer and I could have fought for insurance." But she did not pursue an appeal because she was frustrated by the quality of communication with families, or more specifically profoundly upset by one event. In the context of the Worthen's narrative what upset her seems almost trivial. But in the psyche of Nancy as a mother, it loomed large.

When Maggie was found to be colonized with Methicillin-resistant Staphylococcus Aureus (MRSA), a virulent bacteria that is resistant to most antibiotics, she needed to be isolated from other patients until cleared of the infection. Consequently, Maggie was moved out of her room to another floor where she could have a private room. This is common medical practice.

The only problem was that Nancy did not know about the transfer. When she called up to Maggie's old floor to check in, she was gone and the staff on the next shift did not know where she had been sent. For a brief time, Nancy lost track of her daughter.

It was a little thing in the scope of all that had happened and Maggie was soon found. But this degree of insensitivity was especially upsetting to Nancy. Her daughter had been moved as if her connection to her family did not matter, either to Maggie or to Nancy. But it did.

She had been transported without advance warning: "they didn't tell me so I'd come in and one time I called on one floor and they didn't know who she was, the floor she'd been on. And I'd been in that day and they didn't tell me she was moving." It was incredibly frustrating, "I'd just had it with the sort of organizational structure of the hospital."

The critique, though directed at the hospital – perhaps the finest rehab program in the nation – spoke to something deeper: the connection between mother and daughter, seemingly severed by injury, no longer mattered. Maggie had been depersonalized, turned into someone – or something – who seemingly had no interests and in whom others would have no interest. Even

at a world-class rehabilitation hospital, a patient with a disorder of consciousness had been stripped of the remnants of personhood, or so it seemed to her
mother. She could be moved and that move could occur anonymously without consequence because sentience was lost.

Even if others thought the relationship between mother and daughter must have been attenuated by injury, Nancy was still connected to her
child. And she had hope that her daughter might still be aware and have a
connection with her. Indeed, in many ways the asymmetry of the relationship deepened it when seen from Nancy's perspective. Because Maggie could
not participate and respond, Nancy had to do so much more to maintain the
bond. In that sense the relationship she had with her daughter was intensified
even if not reciprocated. She became her surrogate both legally and ethically,
entrusted with making choices on her behalf and preserving the relationship
which had become one-sided.

And in her decision making for Maggie, her surrogacy had evolved
from bringing her daughter's wishes to the fore, and being a vessel for her
self-determination. Simply fostering her autonomy no longer made sense and
wasn't particularly useful in Maggie's state of dependency. Nancy would have
to take the next steps and make decisions on something deeper and draw
upon the relationship she had with her daughter. That was the font of her
authority and source of moral guidance.

So when it came time to leave rehab, Nancy went with her gut. She
made a Faustian bargain that she thought was in Maggie's best interest. She
traded their world-class high-end rehab for Middleboro Skilled Nursing,
which provided good nursing care and seemed to have a heart. The amount
of rehab was less than she would have liked, but their "nursing care was so
good." It was what Nancy thought would be best and it was her choice, at
the moment.

When pressed on giving up better rehabilitation, Nancy was frank about
her thinking, "For Margaret, at that time, it was the right choice, I think.
Well, I made the choice. You have to make the choice and then you have
to say 'I made the best choice I could at that time' and then live with it and
go on."

And then there were ever-present practical concerns about paying for
care. Middleboro was also something Nancy and her family could afford. Her
husband's insurance had run out and Nancy secured Medicaid for Maggie. It
was both good and bad, "it does pay for everything ... but you only get a very
limited amount of physical therapy."

And then the now common refrain about medical necessity: benefits are
limited "because in order to get physical therapy you have to progress. And
if you're in MCS or PVS or in a coma, well, duh! You wouldn't be progressing
but you might still benefit from PT [physical therapy] or OT [occupational

therapy] but you can't get it after a certain number of weeks because you don't progress."

Nancy was frustrated asking, "What do you mean she can't get physical therapy?" and resigning herself to the answer that, "you can't fight Medicaid; you have to change the bureaucracy." But she had neither time nor energy for that. Her advocacy would not be toward policy but directed toward her daughter. Nancy would tend to her daughter. Her advocacy would not be for a cause, but for Maggie.

THEY TALK WITH HER

Nancy's most important choice was deciding where Maggie would live after leaving Spaulding. And sending her to Middleboro was a good choice. Nancy felt that it was the first place that seemed to show Maggie genuine affection. Not one for hyperbole, Nancy actually felt that the staff at Middleboro "were loving." And Maggie responded to the love, a sign perhaps, that she was in fact in there.

Finding a welcoming facility becomes a respite for fatigued caregivers. Shirley Green had similar sentiments when she found Inglemoor for her son Josh. It was unlike the first facility where "they constantly called about maintaining him ... it would be frustrating just to hear that, it was like, 'shut up already.' It was maintenance, maintenance, maintenance." The word annoyed and even offended her, because maintenance was not seeing if a patient could be helped to improve. It was just maintaining the status quo, like maintaining a home appliance.

She recalls that "the first nursing home was like that. They had a couple of people who had been in comas for a long time, just sleeping, laying there sleeping. And mothers would come and sit with them and everything. And they had a man in the same room with Josh who was angry and bitter, had got in a car accident or something and they weren't doing anything for him. And he was just angry, constantly angry, he would throw things, he could move his arms and things like that." Shirley offered to be of help and was told "that's not something, we don't do that."

And when Shirley sought outside consultants for Josh, one administrator at "the nursing home would yell at me that it wasn't my place and I shouldn't have said that I wanted to bring this person in to see him. Things like that would happen ... I guess it was that word maintenance that just bugged me."

The alternative, another facility nearby, was far more welcoming to Josh. It was a faith-based place. Shirley felt that the church affiliation made a difference, the "head nurse was a strong believer in, was a strong faith kind of person ... after I'd gotten there I found out that that was a lot of how she ran the nursing home. ... And it sort of transmitted to the people that worked there, because when I was going to transfer him, they were, 'oh we're so happy, we'll have a young person, we'll have somebody we can work with and do things with, because it's hard always just having old people that we know are going to die.' "

Like Josh at Inglemoor, staff at Middleboro paid attention to Maggie. It was the little things that seemed to make a difference. Nancy told us, "... they dress her; they get her up every day. She got a really good wheelchair that fits her. They *talk with her*, you know. ..." And all the attention, "... it actually turned out, I had felt that she had a moment where she was more responsive there ... she could open her eyes a little more, and kind of just being more present in small ways, so that seemed positive."

NOT ALL SANGUINE

As receptive as Nancy was to Middleboro, all was not sanguine. One of the first barriers she confronted, like Shirley Green, were rules that limited efforts of families to supplement rehabilitation services. Even though physical therapy time was pretty limited, families could not supplement care and bring in a private physical therapist: Medicaid did not allow it and the facility was wary of the liability.

So Nancy improvised and set up a Supplemental Needs Trust with funds provided by her father, Maggie's grandfather. It was a strategy recommended by the counseling staff at Spaulding to provide Maggie with extra services. The trust provides both current and future resources for Maggie's care. Importantly, although the trust is in Nancy's name, it is not part of her estate, ensuring that all funds remain for the discretionary use of Maggie's guardian. It does not devolve back to the nursing home or the state Medicaid authority.

Nancy has creatively deployed these funds so that Maggie could get extra physical therapy. Although Middleboro does not allow outside physical therapists, they do allow massage therapists. So Nancy found a massage therapist who was also an occupational therapist. Although she was not a physical therapist, she could provide the range of motion exercises that would prevent Maggie from stiffening up and developing contractures.

It wasn't perfect, but was good enough because "she does the closest I can come to PT in Margaret's bed. But it's called massage therapy because I can pay for that, and that's allowed in the nursing home. So I'm paying out of pocket maybe $500 a week of additional daily treatment for her that gives her stimulation and circulation."

Other families have acted in a similar vein. And in many cases, they step up to the plate and try to provide some semblance of care themselves. When the Quigley's encountered curtailment of services and rapid staff turnover, they took it upon themselves to provide their version of physical therapy to Kenny. Elinor, Kenny's mother, told us that the "turnover for the therapists is astronomical, and every time they would turnover they'd start doing the same things again." Care became disorganized and each new therapist would take it from the top, leaving Kenny without the maneuvers that would prevent contractures. Elinor lamented, ". . . his arms were bent, one of his arms was bent up, he had no range of motion whatsoever." Their solution was to have family members take on the task, "I'll tell you honestly, my sister quit her job and went up there every day and she did range of motion and she's the one who got his arm to work."

IT'S LIKE A DORM

Despite the challenge of inadequate therapy, Nancy was pleased with the overall feel of Middleboro because it was not the typical nursing home with the usual geriatric cohort. Instead, it was a residence filled with young people. It was at once a tragic and uplifting setting where the story behind each curtained bed was sadder than the next. Each held a young life that had been inalterably changed by an accident or an illness. And though there was sadness all about, it was also a forward-looking place. It had to be, because the residents were young people.

As Nancy told us, "Most of the patients are young. . . ." And then in a phrase which stays with you, she notes that, "*It's like a dorm of young people, they just happen to all be brain injured.*" For the first time, Nancy sees, and we see with her, that Maggie is part of a group. There is a community of young people who are similarly affected and whose needs are not going to be met by being placed in a nursing home filled with elderly patients with degenerative disease. No, Maggie and her mates needed something else.

She needed to be with her peers. Nancy made a point to pay attention to context and sought this place out: "It's the only place I found, I mean I looked, but so the average age of people is forty, so there are some elderly because it used to be a nursing home for elderly so they're still there. So there's like the ninety year old, ten or fifteen of them."

In this way Middleboro was different than other venues, "I went to visit lots of nursing homes. So there's all these seventy, eighty-five year olds and they have a community together, playing bingo and watching whatever movies. But this place, the people playing bingo are twenty to forty year olds."

Instead of the nostalgia of Glenn Miller for a musical backdrop, Maggie is "in a place where they at least play appropriate music for her age group." The music fit her generational cohort: "They have this radio that's always playing like sixties and seventies; I don't even know what it is exactly, whether it's tapes, but it's kind of hip music, you know, it's just different music than you would play if you were in a senior citizen's home." At Middleboro, Nancy told us, they seemed to favor The Grateful Dead and The Beatles. Not bad choices.

Maggie's roommate is a twenty-five year old with Huntington's chorea, the inherited degenerative disease of the nervous system, which afflicted Woody Guthrie. Hers is a tragic story but also uplifting, "She's deteriorating before our eyes. But she is loving Margaret. I mean it is incredible the gift that she is giving to Margaret. Because she has this person to love, this person with Huntington's chorea, who's worse off than she is, but she can give something to her."

She also looks out for Maggie. She "reads to Margaret, calls out when Margaret has a problem." She "is her voice." Her presence comforts Nancy, who worries about Maggie's inability to speak. When she is not there, her roommate is "her advocate in a particular way that I can't be every day. I mean it's incredible."

I MEAN SHE'S TWENTY-FOUR

Although they play karaoke, as maybe the seniors do, at Middleboro it seems "kind of like a young person's thing." But the ethos of the place transcends the music, "I don't know, I think that the conversation, the treatment, I think it's more that the nurses and the staff are all dealing with young people so they're, they're thinking of them differently because it isn't about it being the end of their lives."

Nancy's insight is a profound one. Like Josh's experience as a young person at Inglemoor, Maggie benefitted at Middleboro from staff differentiating the young MCS patient from the elderly one with advanced Alzheimer's disease, a too common conflation that stems from a frequent, but flawed analogy. Although two such patients may share many common needs and be functionally equivalent in their dependency at the moment, as we have seen, care happens over time and over a trajectory. Over a longitudinal span, the two patients may split company and go their separate ways, one with a progressive debilitating condition, and the other with an acquired injury with the potential for recovery to a higher functional level.

It is important to make this rather obvious point because the loss of consciousness in routine medical care takes on so much prognostic and ethical meaning.[1] In the context of routine end-of-life care in the general hospital, most decisions about withholding or withdrawing life-sustaining therapy hinge on the presence or absence of consciousness. When consciousness (and resulting decision-making capacity) is lost, surrogate decision makers take it as an important prognostic sign and use this loss as a prompt to make end-of-life decisions.[1] As we have already seen, in the acute care setting DNR orders get written and ventilators are removed.

This link between consciousness lost and end-of-life decision making can prove problematic for brain-injured patients in chronic care as well. Perhaps this was the change on ethos that Nancy sensed amongst the Middleboro staff working, as they were, with the younger brain-injured cohort. Taken away from their usual proximity to nursing home patients with the dementing illnesses of older age, Middleboro patients were seen differently than the older patients closer to life's end.

Beyond the historical links between the evolution of a right to die and the vegetative state discussed in earlier chapters, the association between loss of consciousness and end-of-life decisions has a bearing on how physicians classify patients. Just recently, I served as vice-chair of the Ethics, Professionalism and Human Rights Committee of the American College of Physicians. Every five to ten years, this committee rewrites the American College's ethics manual. One of my goals for the new edition was to move the discussion about patients with disorders of consciousness out of the end-of-life care section,[2] where it was located in prior editions.[3]

My rationale for this was encapsulated in an exchange with Nancy. When we asked her if she thought it was reasonable for others to think of Maggie as someone who is near the end of life, she paused and responded, "But why? Why would you say that? I mean she's twenty-four. Because I think there's a possibility of some recovery for her."

As a mother, the stakes of her child's recovery for the rest of her life is more consequential than the rehabilitation or recovery made by others in their old age. It is more than an arithmetic calculus about the longevity of the subject or the durability of the rehabilitation. It is also about children and young people in the prime of their lives being struck down with a severe injury and having some sort of opportunity to reclaim a part of what was expected of a normal life.

Nancy told us, "Putting Margaret aside, the people around her that are in their twenties, they're learning to walk again. So if they're in rehab at twenty-two learning to walk again, they have another sixty years of walking. But if an eighty year old is in rehab learning to walk again because of a hip replacement, if they're not really, really successful. ... I'm not saying it doesn't make a difference for the quality of their life, but it's not the same."

Perhaps the greatest benefit of the generational grouping of patients was for their parents who had struggled in their own isolation, alone amidst a wave of chronic care that saw their loved ones as invariably close to death; clinical and rehabilitation failures who were just biding their time waiting for an inevitable death to take them. At Middleboro, this was neither the expectation nor the sentiments of the parents attending their children. Nancy found this support from other parents at Middleboro helpful and a way to pierce the isolation she had felt since Maggie's injury.

Nancy confessed that she did not know if it was better for "Margaret to be around people who are progressing in their lives ..." but that "It's better for me."

GERIATRIC GROUPTHINK

And even if the benefit is limited, the alternative formulation of admixing young people with brain injury with older patients is a recipe for neglect and marginalization. This is what Jamila Baucom encountered when caring for her middle-aged mother, Melva, while she was in a nursing home. There, care became routinized as if she was an elderly nursing home patient. Melva had one doctor who was her primary care provider and other specialists as needed, who are all on "pretty much the same page."

Jamila was worried about their formulaic approach to care and how they seemed to characterize her mother. She questioned their actual expertise to take care of patients with disorders of consciousness and worried that "there's a low quality, or low standard of continuous learning that happens, and I think that ... the doctors in a nursing home could still have some burden put on them to understand the latest in what's happening in brain injury."

Short of that, she looked for a way to get an outside consultation to break up the geriatric groupthink that seemed to have evolved around her mother's care. She hoped to alter rather reified expectations, which Jamila characterizes as, "I'm the doctor, I know what's set." Such views are reinforced by interdisciplinary team meetings that only include department heads and not the clinicians who know the patients best. Absent the participation of those most familiar with the patients, the process becomes scripted: "it's just the heads, which is in and of itself very odd, so it's like the head nurse, the dietician, perhaps someone from rehab, and so they just go into her chart. It's not an opportunity to like think forward in terms of what's been observed or things you can do differently."

Although Melva had improved during her nursing home stay, her local team of doctors had not budged in their prognostication. Echoing Nancy's observations about seeing MCS patients as invariably at life's end, Jamila observed that, "The biggest barrier with the nursing home facility as opposed to a rehab facility, is I think their view of patients overall. I mean people enter a nursing home and it's likely that they're never leaving because they're usually much older. Whereas if they're there for rehab it's ... the need to know what they think is going to happen, if the person is going to get better." There is a need for greater clarity about the future, about a prognosis when patients have the prospect of leaving and getting on with their lives.

Absent this future frame, staff can limit their efforts to medical details and lose the bigger rehabilitative picture. The approach fundamentally constricts their patients' prognostic horizons and prospects for recovery. Jamila felt that such views adversely affected her mother. It "lends itself to ... the staff not spending a lot of time with her, especially the staff that has influence on her care." A doctor's assessment is often limited to a visit a few times a week for five or ten minutes to do a brief exam and inspect her feeding tube, "her PEG site and her trach [to] make sure it's functioning properly," echoing Shirley Green's remarks about "maintenance."

These visits are not occasions to articulate goals of care or ask probing questions about the patient's quality of life. Care is all in the present tense and the prospects for a future are limited because everyone else is old and at the end of *their* lives. And because this is so, the consequences of a missed future are limited and those who determine it of less consequence. But not so for patients who are still at the start or the middle of life's journey.

Jamila worried that the practitioners who attended her mother were more in touch with the elderly patient's needs than those with complex brain injuries. As she put it, "... the reality is this physician, I don't think, is well versed or even qualified to even know anything about brain injury. ... I don't think he's qualified to even know how to assess someone with a brain injury. ... I think he's doing what *he's used to doing with old people*, and making sure that they don't have pneumonia and aren't getting bed sores."

Jamila and her family attend all family meetings at Melva's facility to help the clinicians see the differences between the patients under their care. They "go at almost every opportunity," seemingly at the annoyance of staff, who they simply want to educate. It is frustrating for Jamila because she has good intentions. She just wishes to alter their tone and broaden their gaze to the distinct experiences of patients with brain injury. Instead of a defensive posture, she wishes that staff would "take more of an opportunity to listen to families, especially those that are active in a patient's care and often there with the patient." It is a balanced request as she acknowledges too that "there are families that are I think overly optimistic and sometimes see things that they want to see." But nonetheless, Jamila concludes that "physicians should take the opportunity to at least investigate further instead of shrugging their shoulders." Indeed, they might learn something.

RESPECT FOR PERSONS ... ON THE SECOND FLOOR

It would seem to be the least that staff could do. Families are under extraordinary pressures seeking to safeguard those they love from real and perceived indignities. Much of their stress comes from their loved ones being treated as if they were not there, victims of a lost personhood.

This is neither a semantic concern nor a trivial matter. In the realm of bioethics, respect for persons has been enshrined as a central principle for ethical conduct since the National Commission for the Protection of Human Subjects of Biomedical and Behavioral Research authored the historic "Belmont Report" in 1979.[4] "Respect for persons" was one of three aggregate ethical principles that reflected what was described as the "common morality," universally held values and norms shared within society.[5] The articulation of that principle was to set minimum standards for how we treated each other and was tied to the worth and dignity of individuals. It was an ethical mandate after the abuses of the Holocaust and the Tuskegee syphilis study,[6] whose public disclosure in 1973 led to Congress to establish the National Commission the following year.[7,8]

In the context of patients with disorders of consciousness, the "Belmont Report" presents a curious twist. Paradoxically, these patients historically have not been under the Belmont Report's protective shelter, or so it seems to this observer. To state the obvious, Belmont's articulation of respect for persons requires that personhood exist. But in the clinic, patients with disorders of consciousness have been prone to depersonalizations, almost relegated to the status of nonpersons and hence deprived of the respect that has been linked to personhood. It is an irony and a tragic one, because the very principle articulated to guarantee respect for the most vulnerable of persons has been unable to protect individuals most in need of it. These patients have been denied this principled protection, so central to respect and standing in the human community.

This often takes the form of indifference, a lack of professionalism, poor care and even negligence. Staffing problems are legion in the nursing home space according to the families we interviewed.

Burt Brody told us how interest in the patient fades when progress stalls and how his wife, Jean, was segregated from other patients whose pace of recovery was faster. As he told us, "They lost interest ... this was a rehab facility where people who had surgery would go to and they get rehab and were there for three or four weeks and then go home. They'd have knee surgery or hip replacement or something like that. They were used to more of a patient like that."

Those patients whose recovery followed a different path were placed aside. Burt "found out that there was a second floor where they just put everybody who just had no opportunity, or no prospect of ever being very alive. Alzheimer's patients, people who were in a PVS. So they had this horrible second floor. If you went up there it was filthy, the staff was bad."

He describes a particularly disturbing scene of unprofessional behavior when he made an early morning visit to check in on Jean and found the nursing aides dancing in her room. He had just purchased a nice little stereo because Jean enjoyed listening to music. When he arrived "at about two in the morning and two of the CNAs [certified nursing assistants] were jumping up and down and dancing and doing foolish things and I said 'what in the hell are you doing?' And they said, 'well we know you have a nanny cam in your stereo and we wanted you to be able to see something, so we're putting on a show for you.'"

After that, Burt decided to take Jean home, "I took her out on her birthday, which was December the tenth, and realized I could give her medications, and change her, I could keep her comfortable. And I was much more happy with her in my house, in our house, than a nursing home." The aides' response to Burt's late night visit is disturbing in and of itself and also evidence that his heightened vigilance was entirely necessary.

CLOCK WATCHERS AND DISLOCATIONS

Other families have been equally guarded about the safety and well-being of their loved ones when in a nursing home. To them it was not even ensuring "respect for persons," it was making sure they were safe.

John Harmon moved John Jr. around a great deal from one nursing home to another citing quality concerns: "... some of them were worse than the other ones. And that's why he's not in them now." He worried about the adequacy of staffing, "... especially on the weekends [when] they don't have full staff ... and that's why I went and saw John twice every single day unless I didn't feel good or the wife didn't feel good. . . ."

Mr. Harmon had seen poor care up close and what he felt were breaches of integrity that were then, in his view, covered up when his son developed a serious bedsore. Saddened still by the experience, he told us, "I don't like to look back when John had a bedsore that you could put your whole hand in it. And the ladies, they lie and they say, 'no that's not a stage four bedsore, it's only a stage three.' And I said, 'don't tell me,' because the next day I went back after I read stuff on it and I said, 'that's almost a five!' and she said, 'Yes.' Well she lied to me. And I just don't like that kind of stuff. ... I've noticed in these places that they've got clock watchers and they've got professionals ... they watch that clock and if she is in John's room changing him, she does not care if John's completely changed or not, if she looks at that clock and her eight hours is done, she's walking out of that room. That's a clock watcher, a professional won't do that. That's a lot of things I've seen in the past."

A no-nonsense mid-Westerner, Mr. Harmon is blunt in his counsel to others, "Unless you're there all the time and they know you're coming, then they're going to do what they're supposed to do. But I've seen where patients, nobody doesn't come to visit them and the staff, they don't give a damn about them. That's why I saw my son, to make sure he was taken care of."

He made his views clear to a nursing home administrator that "... if I didn't come here twice every day I believe my son would be dead by now.

And that's exactly what I told them and I've had no problem with them after that. They knew I was coming *but they didn't know what time.*"

Other families are more cautious about voicing their concerns for fear of some sort of retribution. The mother of one patient told us, "I didn't like the nursing home at all. I always had complaints. And then his father would tell me, 'stop complaining, stop complaining 'cause they might not take care of him and do what they're supposed to do.'"

Heidi Hansen, Kathy's daughter, tells us that she felt that her mother had been neglected because she developed painful contractures. A speech therapist, Heidi was astute in her criticisms of the chronic care her mother has received. Unlike many other families who are new to this clinical space, Heidi has told us about the antecedent care omissions that lead to more obvious sequelae. The contractures were a case in point. As she explains, "She's in the nursing home. She has a lot of pain, so she is developing contractures. She was getting physical therapy for range of motion and everything else but I guess her physical therapist was not in tune enough or in tune to her body. ..." As a result, "my mother has dislocated her own knee. So now the only way to fix that is surgically. . . ."

The tragedy was that this was a complication of neglect, a failure to prevent the contractures that stressed her knee to the point of dislocation. In hindsight, Heidi thinks that "this really could have been prevented because our orthopedic surgeon yelled at the physical therapist, 'how can you have let this happen, because this is unacceptable.' So that's just another kind of thing that we are ... all upset about."

The chain of events is much like that cascade of medical errors that the Institute of Medicine's *To Err Is Human* made famous.[9] One small omission, or oversight, leads to a minor complication, which is then compounded by another failure or dereliction until something really significant happens. That is the pathway, but sometimes such a root cause analysis is obscured by the fact that the problem is brewing in chronic care where medical errors can be misattributed to the natural history of disease progression and *not* human error.

Without requisite rigor, one could look at these immobile patients and say that complications like contractures or blood clots or bed sores are all the norms. And yes, they are the sequelae of immobility from brain injury, but they are hardly inevitable with proper nursing care. So, it becomes a convenient misattribution of cause and effect, when the complication that occurs is blamed on the patient's condition and not the conditions of care. In Kathy's case, the dislocation of her knee was the consequence of a number of smaller adverse outcomes, each of which could have been prevented. Without a requisite level of nursing care, they snowballed into a significant complication, a true dislocation of care.

Her mother had become contorted into a fetal position because of untreated contractures and this in turn put stress on her knee. Heidi did not parse words when reflecting on the quality of Kathy's care, "But it's just the negligence of, I think, the whole team, whether it's the physical therapist or whomever, because if they just go in and see day after day she's in this position that it can't be good, she's just getting contracted and contorted, you know, 'okay let's put her in an immobilizer at night, or let's do more range of motion.'"

Echoing Mr. Harmon, Heidi has pursued vigilance through presence. She points to the importance of showing up and visiting, "I think she gets more attention now but if we weren't there she wouldn't get the attention. Sometimes I'll go up there ... [and] there was only one person taking care of the wing. One person. So [her] food would have sat on her table for, you know, who knows, 'til 10:00 in the morning before she got fed. And the woman next to her didn't eat."

RAGDOLL

Even those who are locked-in, and fully or nearly fully conscious, suffer from these indignities. And most concerning, they experience the outright subjection to pain, that is neither promptly nor adequately addressed. Take Angelo Donato, who we have already met in the locked-in state. He told his wife and his sister that he had been treated like a "*ragdoll,*" a word he spelled out with his spelling board. He was evidently very upset with a nursing assistant who had callously transported him in and out of bed. According to Glenie, his wife, his day is full of such affronts.

And like those patients on the second floor, where Jean Brody once resided, Angelo is wholly ignored, even though he is completely aware of his surroundings and the neglect and insensitivity with which he is treated. And to add insult to these real physical injuries, his medication orders for analgesics are written with the designation of PRN, an abbreviation of the Latin, *pro re nata,* for the thing born or in the medical context as the need arises or as needed. The problem is that the only way a nurse would know that Angelo was in pain would be for Angelo to say so, which of course he cannot do. He needs to be asked, and with the help of a spelling board, have the direction of his eyes decoded into meaningful content. If he is neither asked nor assisted with communication he will remain functionally mute, but sentient and in untreated pain.

Like so many others, Angelo has also been the victim of less than attentive care because he can't communicate independently, or at least without a willing interlocutor. The only difference is that he can bear witness and tell us about it; locked-in as he is, he is still open to communication. So he was able to tell Glenie when his leg was caught in the railing of his bed for six hours and he could not complain. When Glenie arrived, he told her what had happened, "And you could see the mark. This is why I never want to leave him at night. This is why I get very upset. This is part of his dignity. He should never be forced to have his knee ... stuck there. He should not be slumped over for eight hours at a time. And that's his dignity. ... He knows he's slumped over, and he knows that he looks ridiculous, and he knows he can't reach anybody and they just walk by. And not just for Angelo, for anybody. I watched a caregiver, a nurse, pacing down the hall with a patient's arm hanging out of the wheelchair, burned his arm on the wheel. And I said, 'look, his arm is hanging out of the chair.' And she picked it up, it fell off [again], and she just continued. I don't want this to happen to my husband. This is not fair to that patient and it's not fair to my husband."

It is of little solace that things like this are occurring at a good place with a national reputation for excellence. Glenie acknowledges it as such: "And this is at the best place. So I have to go home going, 'calm down, it's still better than other places.' But this is why I'm there, this is why I complain, this is why I go to the head nurse everyday ... because Angelo is my concern. I feel bad for everybody else around me, but Angelo is my concern."

But Glenie's major worry is that his inability to communicate causes him to be in pain. Because he can only communicate when assisted, she knows that Angelo's pain goes untreated and he remains uncomfortable. On one occasion he was asked if he was in pain. When he answered yes, it was assumed the pain was in his head because he had chronic migraines. The staff didn't wait for him to elaborate because they don't have time. Glenie voiced her concern, "None of the nurses even try to let him say something. It's just a yes and no question. So if they ask him if he's in pain – he's had a migraine headache since February – and all they do and say, 'do you have a headache?' and [wait for a] nod. They don't ask if there's other pain, 'does anything else hurt you?' They just assume it's the head."

She continued, "I went in one day and he said he had a chest pain at seven in the morning, and I said, 'well did you tell the nurses?' And he said no, because they're not going to ask him if there's any other pain. And I just don't think they're aware of how aware he is. And he needs someone who is going to talk to him and ask him if there's anything that he needs."

This is her job. As she sees it, "I only have his dignity to look after; the medical part is up to the doctors." Glenie's attentions though, come with a price. It has imperiled her ability to work and she is frank about this, "You shouldn't have to be made poor to help somebody ... I'm at the hospital every day."

Glenie is admittedly frustrated that she can't get her husband's caregivers to pay more attention to him, a man she still clearly loves, "I can't get through to them. You know, he's so aware, he knows when he's been sitting in a wet diaper for three hours. And when you ask to change him or put him back in the bed, I said to them one day, 'Angelo's been sitting in his chair for three hours, he's soaking wet.' You have to wait for shift change. There's no reason he should have to wait for shift change. This is a man that's fully aware of what's going on. And this is his dignity. You have him sitting in urine and feces for three hours." As she begins to cry she tells us, "This mortifies him" and petrifies her.

She is afraid that Angelo's inability to communicate will have dire consequences for his well-being, "I'm so afraid something is going to happen because of the lack of communication and understanding of these patients with this condition. I don't want to come in and find out that Angelo had a heart attack because he couldn't communicate and get help. He needs a computer in his room; they need things to be able to communicate with the staff in order to continue."

I WANT TO HEAR THE WORDS

But then Glenie engages in a bit of self-confession. It is not just about Angelo, it is about them as a couple, and the relationship with a husband she so sorely misses. Again crying, she tells us, "But again, a lot of it is woe is me. I want to hold my husband. I want to give him a kiss and have that feeling. We're married thirty-three years. And it's like an empty shell ... it's just like a shell."

It feels empty because everything is mediated by something that comes between them. Although knowing that they can communicate at some level "eases it a little," communication without the corporeality or timbre of his voice is just not enough. It seems false and hollow like an echoing sea shell. Glenie desperately wants to hear Angelo's voice, "Not writing it down, not spelling it out on a board." She explains why verbal communication is so important to her, "I think a verbal communication, I mean, we've been married thirty-three years. I want to hear the words 'I love you.' I don't want to write them down. His new thing now is if I say 'do you love me?' he has to give me a smile, and then he'll give me a smile." But she concludes, "I want to hear it."

Almost waxing philosophical, she tells us that while there is no person without the brain, the brain does not constitute a full person: "sometimes I think we're just keeping the brain alive, but I really think that without speech, he needs to communicate, he needs to talk." From her perspective, "There's no person without the verbal, hearing the words 'I love you,' or getting mad at you and yelling at you. That is the person ... his voice, to tell someone you love, what makes you feel. ... Not the holding of the hand or the actual kissing, it's having the person talk to you."

Short of those exchanges, her marriage is in a netherland between what she once knew and the loss she fears is drawing nigh. With an eloquence borne of experience, tearfully expressed, she puts it frankly, "As I said, I'm stuck and I'm lonely. I'm stuck between being married and being a widow. I don't have the person to share my problems with; he's who I told everything. I'll never kiss him with feeling."

And turning to a topic that may be taboo to some, she speaks of her continued desire for intimacy, "Corny as it sounds, I'll never make love again. And these are important things, not just to me, but to him. And I know he feels the same way. I can give him a kiss and be excited that he puckers and kisses, but I'll never hold him again. You want that part of that person, that intimate part of that person."

IN MEMORIAM

Sadly, Glenie would lose Angelo. She applied for hospice a couple of years after we first spoke because Angelo was losing his sight and hearing. Without these two senses he would be totally isolated from others, completely locked-in without even a spelling board to step out of his own head. He would neither be able to hear, read, nor communicate. The future was complete solitary confinement, total and unspeakable aloneness.

It was an impossible fate that prompted a wrenching decision for the Donatos. Angelo did not want to live that way and Glenie respected his preferences, his wishes as much as she hated to let him go. But she would allow for the removal of his feeding tube.

We spoke after he passed. Heroically, she told us, "I gave him ... this is what he wanted and I gave him what he wanted." It was a painful and difficult ten days precisely because he remained conscious and aware. Unlike most decisions to let nature take its course, Angelo's end was different; he had not lapsed into unconsciousness but was, at the outset, awake and alert. The balm of sleep, with one's eyes closed, did not lessen the sting of loss for Glenie. That flicker of life, and even hope, lingered as long as he was awake, until the lack of food and water eventually caused him to lapse into a stupor and then a terminal coma.

Glenie was courageous and loving until the end. Once he did drift into sleep, she made sure he remained medicated so he would not awake in pain or in terror. She took care of him and protected him. But the experience took its toll on her. Her vigil was, "Worse than the three years I've spent feeding him. ... Because there was nothing worse than watching your loved one die slowly." With tears in her eyes, she told us how she protected Angelo, "I didn't let them wake him up; I kept him sedated."

But she felt terrible that she had held on to him for so long, "I feel guilty that I want him, not that I gave him what he wanted. That I was selfish enough to want him to be around. I needed him, I still need him." Crying, she told us how important he was to her own well-being, as impaired as he had become. Even though he had become invisible to others, a ragdoll to be tossed about, he was ever present in Glenie's life. "He's what kept me going, he was my comfort. He was my friend. I couldn't let him go blind and deaf and not know what was going on, who was touching him, what they were doing to him."

When we tried to console her, assure her that she had been faithful and had protected him, it was to no avail. In fact she rejected the comfort, blaming herself for prolonging his agony. With a broken heart, that will never – it seems – be healed, she confessed her felt guilt and her enduring love, "But I was also selfish because I wanted him ... I love him, I still love him."

15 What Do Families Want?

Many look at patients with disorders of consciousness and think that it is a fate worse than death. If we had a choice, we would never choose a life like theirs, devoid of mobility, independence, and the ability to communicate a preference. From a distance, we look at these unfortunate ones confident that we could avoid their fate.

It is almost an act of denial, not to imagine the unimaginable because the unforeseen is an outcome that none of these families desired. Instead, the reality they confront is one that emerged, *almost accidentally*, because of a series of therapeutic goals that were only partially met.

Let me explain. As patients are brought into the emergency wards of hospitals, loved ones are thinking moment to moment and hoping only for survival. Gripped by the suddenness of the tragedy they cannot think ahead to the deeper questions we are confronting now: Is my wife still there? How much of herself does she need to lose before she is no longer herself? And even if she had lost a part of herself, how would I know if she was unable to communicate, blocked as it were, by a lack of motor output from her injured brain?

These later questions are overshadowed by wondering simply about survival. These deeper issues are subsumed by the heroics of acute care: the emergent neurosurgery that prevents or mitigates herniation and the moment to moment vigil hearing the hum of ventilators and watching ICU nurses hanging IV medications. During those early days, patient surrogates are hoping for the best, a full and outright recovery and restoration of the person whose brain injury has fractured a life. And if that is not anticipated, then decisions are made to withhold or withdraw life-sustaining therapies. It is as if there is no middle ground.

But like all things in biology, recovery and therapeutics happen on a spectrum. Though the hopeful and dire extremes exist, most survivors end up between cure and catastrophe. They represent *form fruste*, or incomplete, efforts to heal, presenting ethical challenges of what the bioethicist Daniel Callahan called the "troubled middle."

No one is protected from this middle ground, these lost horizons, if their families initiate therapies meant to salvage a life and restore function.

Many, of course, will choose to withhold or withdraw life-sustaining therapies and sidestep these dilemmas. That much is true, but so too is the truth that families who ended up grappling with these liminal states never chose to be in this intermediate state. Their intent was something better, or better yet, something ethically less complex.

It is too easy to sit on the sidelines confident that you might have avoided their fate. That was then, but this is now, and the operative question is what are the goals of care that should motivate treatment decisions once the patient is medically stable and in – or approaching – a minimally conscious state?

PERCHANCE TO SPEAK

Families we interviewed are quite consistent about their goals of care and how their objectives changed and evolved over time. Burt Brody, like most surrogates, notes that, "First of all I wanted her alive and I wanted her to recover, but I didn't know what I wanted her to recover the most. And it's the ability to speak and communicate, and we have 30 percent of that back."

For Sandy, like Glenie, the restoration of functional communication was "... The world. To be able to communicate with her, to hear that she loves me, to know that she knows that I love her, to be able to ask her, 'are you thirsty, are you hungry, do you need to be changed?' It's a whole new world."

The Wexlers felt the same way about their daughter, Sarah, and fostering communication is their primary goal: "I am hopeful that ... we will know what part of her brain is functioning. It is obvious that she receives information, there's no question about it." But the challenge was verbal output: "She cannot project any information. So our hope is that when we find out what is working, that maybe something can be done either through drugs that she is not presently taking or through stimulation in some form that perhaps, we can hopefully stimulate the communication center."

Without some form of communication, the Wexlers worry about what Sarah is experiencing and wonder what she might be able to achieve. Communication is most important "... because I think once we get that, her ability to follow commands will get better." Ultimately, communication also helps families know if their loved one is conscious.

Although the only consciousness that we can truly know is our own, in practice we know the consciousness of others through communication, which is a proxy for the cognitive experience within. Without communication, others cannot know a patient's level of awareness, thoughts, and desires. Families routinely worry about what they cannot know without some semblance of expressive communication. It limits knowledge of the patient's current state and their future capabilities.

The Wexlers spoke for many families when they confessed that, "I think the hardest part is that we don't know anything. We don't know what she's potentially capable of. I know she's not going to be that same person she was but we're hopeful that she can have a better quality of life than she has. . . ." And their goals are modest, the most rudimentary communication scheme would be valued: ". . . that Sarah at some point might be able to give us a 'yes' or 'no' . . . that would be important."

Sarah's mother, Betty, also reminds us of communication's importance in restoring relationality and the familial connections that have been tested by Sarah's silence. She tells us, "That [communication] to me is the key to all of this . . . because she has a son." It is hard to admit, but a sad reality that, "we have no clue as to whether or not she knows that Max is her son, or the word 'mother' or 'father.' We don't know." It is a mystery upon which the reciprocity of their relationships hinges, even as their parental obligations continue.

Betty hopes that she and her husband, Immanuel, could know if Sarah's "cognitive skills are good enough" to simply "answer 'yes' or 'no' " so they could know, "That I'm her mother he's her father, [the boy] is her son, etc." Betty concludes by reiterating the importance of knowing whether Sarah is capable of having a relationship with others – that ". . . relationship with people is so vital . . . ."

To Rich Hansen, Kathy's husband, speech is important because it recreates the normalcy of family life. So, "instead of just going to the nursing home every day and just saying 'hi,' instead of staring at the TV, this way she can tell you, 'I was cold last night' or 'a bird flew into the window.' I don't know, stupid little things she used to come out with. To be able to say, 'do you want something?' "

And that simple question represents the practical side of communication. Many families told us that they were worried sick about what happens when they are gone and no one understands, or cares to understand what happens to their loved ones. The ability to communicate mitigates these fears to some extent.

Family members worry about the ability of their loved one to express a desire or complain of pain. Anita Myers, the mother of Thomas Perdue, a young man who was in a car accident, told us about the importance of communication. She elaborated, "We can take better care of him because of what his needs are and what his wants are. Whether it's food, or TV, or he has an eyelash in his eye. It's like an infant; you have no idea what they're thinking. Communication is the key."

And beyond that, for Thomas, communication was also central to knowing something about his abilities and quality of life. Thomas had been an inveterate reader. It had been central to his existence and happiness. His mother recalled that, "the thing that was important for Thomas was reading, he loved to read and that's all he does. Read and read and read ... he could read three books a week, it was living. So that was his quality of life. ...." But now Anita does not know what he can and cannot do. She concedes her ignorance: "I don't know if he can read."

It is an old philosophical impossibility of knowing the mind of the other: we can only attest to our own sentience. Each of us can only speak to our own consciousness. But practically, in the pragmatics of brain injury, an expression of knowing would be a good proxy for consciousness and would ease the doubt of the surrogates who watch their loved ones *not* knowing if understanding remains possible. Anita spoke of how crucial it would be to know "... if he can comprehend, if he still has comprehension or cognition, or see if he understands, to see if he has any intelligence there, to see if he has any comprehension or understanding and communication. ...."

It was perhaps Heidi Hansen who said it best when she told us why restoring her mother's ability to communicate was most important to her. "I think," she said, "it's because speech and language are a clear sign that she's in there."

A RIGHT TO RESULTS?

Nancy Worthen also had views on this topic. We spoke about them during her first visit to New York in February 2008. She came to Weill Cornell with two distinct goals, which were linked. What was Maggie's diagnosis and did that diagnosis suggest that she might be able to communicate with others?

To begin with the first question, Nancy wanted to know if Maggie was in the vegetative state, the diagnosis she carried up until then? Or was it something else as suspected by Dr. Doug Katz, her Boston neurologist who had suggested she come to New York? Nancy was hopeful that neuroimaging studies at Cornell would help address this quandary, even though we were careful to caution her that we were doing research and not engaging in clinical practice. Neuroimaging work was still speculative and not an established way to make a diagnosis in isolation, and certainly not apart from formal neurological and neuropsychological assessment which would be part of the studies done in New York.

The place of neuroimaging in the assessment of these patients when Maggie first came to New York was complicated and it remains an area of debate. Just a year earlier, in 2007, I had cochaired a conference at Stanford on the uses of neuroimaging in disorders of consciousness with the Canadian neuroethicist, Judy Illes.[1] Though we had no doubts that this was an important emerging technology, we felt it was premature to disseminate these methods outside of a research context, especially before we had learned to reconcile how to make sense of patients whose classical neurological exams were widely discordant with their scans.[2] That is, for patients whose bedside exams did not show evidence of consciousness but whose neuroimaging studies showed widely preserved neural networks indicative of more function than was behaviorally manifest.[1] Now eight months after the Stanford conference, it was possible that Maggie might be such a patient.

I tried to be cautious with Nancy. I told her about the limits of our methods that were still *speculative*. I explained, "We're doing research. There's a difference between something that's research and something that's a vetted diagnostic or therapeutic intervention that's real and we know what it means. We can diagnose images for pneumonia because we know exactly what it is and how it relates to a phenomenon. Here we're still at the very early stages, and it's at the stage of discovery, and so you know, it's prone to be misunderstood." This is the reason tests are often not shared with subjects.

But Nancy pushed back, challenging the clear-cut distinction we ethicists like to make between research and therapy. It is a distinction that fades at the margins, especially when patients and families have nowhere else to turn and there are only a few research centers that explore these questions and provide credible advice. Asserting her rights as her daughter's surrogate, Nancy told me that she was willing to take the risk of evolving knowledge to answer a fundamental question about the state of her daughter's mind.

And that struck me as quite reasonable. To withhold information of such importance seemed to be a paternalistic judgment designed to protect institutions and investigators and not empower families and caregivers. Of course, the information would need to be properly cast as contingent data and shared through an intermediary like the patient's treating physician, but share it, it seemed we must, albeit with all those provisos.

When I first came to this conclusion I felt that I was alone in my judgment, but, increasingly, research ethicists are beginning to have a more expansive view on data sharing of research results, even drawing the attention of international consortia.[3] The scholarship of Susan Wolf on incidental findings and the return of research results are particularly useful in this regard. Wolf suggests that investigators share information that is of "potential health or reproductive significance" and outlines an approach that discriminates the risks and benefits of disclosure, taking account the validity of the test.[4]

Most critically, for patients with disorders of consciousness, Wolf breaks down the rather dichotomous distinction between research and clinical responsibilities asserting that sharing results is "consistent with an emerging view that researchers bear some clinical responsibility toward research subjects."[4] This is an important statement for investigators who study individuals who have disorders of consciousness and find themselves providing needed clinical guidance to surrogates who often have nowhere else to turn for important medical information. There are many reasons for this evolving stance, including the reciprocity owed to research subjects who participate in clinical studies.[5]

More recently the philosopher, Henry S. Richardson has written of anciallary care obligations to individuals who are subjects of clinical research, further eroding the false dichotomy dividing the research and clinical context, a space united in the realization that individuals are both patient and subject.[6] These obligations, which Richardson describes as "moral entanglements" become more pronounced if subjects otherwise are unable to receive informed and competent medical care, a state that sadly exists for the majority of patients with disorders of consciousness.[7]

But what and how to share the information? Wolf, echoing the earlier work of Reilly,[8] writes of a research participant-based notion of "utility," what a subject (or in the case of studies of individuals with disorders of consciousness, a surrogate) would find of importance. She suggests three levels of net benefit with corresponding obligations of offered disclosure. When there is no likely benefit, disclosure is not indicated. It may be disclosed when there is possible benefit and should be shared when there is strong net benefit, unless the subject opts not to know.[4]

To my mind, there is nothing more important than knowing that a patient may be conscious, especially when there is a paucity of motor output and the possibility that neuroimaging data, obtained through research or not, might suggest that an individual thought to be vegetative might actually be aware. Nancy agreed.

And when I asked Nancy what her thoughts were about the receipt of research data that was still contingent, she asserted that she must be informed. She maintained that even research data was valuable, "But I think it still has implications for treatment. It should. It would be important if you had information." In Wolf and colleagues' framework, the information gained from neuroimaging would seem to offer a "strong benefit" to Nancy, and others concerned about Maggie's state and well-being.

Nancy appreciated the subtlety. Our solution for the tentative nature of the knowledge was to funnel it through the patient's doctor. And Nancy understood that "... At least don't share it with me but share it with Dr. Katz so he knows everything, so that he could decide treatment and he and I could use that speculative information how we want to treat Margaret, because we need it in order to decide on treatment and plans."

I HAVE TO CONVINCE PEOPLE

But there was an even more compelling reason why the information had to be conveyed. Nancy faced skeptical friends and family who thought that Maggie could not possibly understand or ever be understood. Any effort to intervene on her behalf, and her mother's continued ministrations were considered quixotic. But if she could prove the skeptics wrong and have some evidence that Maggie *was there* then Nancy could carry on and possibly gain some needed support and encouragement. Nancy put it this way, "I want to be as aggressive as I can to help her communicate." "But how can I?," she asked capturing the isolation she felt in her efforts. Her solution, "So I have to convince people that she could communicate ... if I could convince people that she would be able to." Then it would be simpler, "... if we could just find a pathway" or "... a speculative idea" and say, "let's try it."

And here we have the importance of science, and perhaps the image in particular, as a way of convincing people that Maggie still had the capability of communicating. The odds were so against it, the biases so fixed in her nursing home culture, that Nancy needed *proof* attesting to Maggie's potential. It was as much about the neuroscience of her mind as the sociology of her injury. She had to convince her peer group about Maggie's viability, her potential. Here one picture might be worth a thousand words.

But it all hinged on whether Maggie could think and if there were a way of knowing that she was processing information. If we could come to that conclusion, then the rest of the goals would at least be theoretically possible. If she was not thinking, as evidenced by some form of communication, then the scope of the problem would be beyond repair.

Nancy reiterated her key point with an apology, "I'm sorry to go back, but if she couldn't think then I might say, 'well could she walk?'" But that would only be a distant consolation. "It wouldn't be that that's a secondary goal ..." because walking is "... not as important as if she can think, because then she has a life of the mind. But if she can't communicate, then there is no way for her to share the life of the mind with everyone else."

THAT IS WHAT DOCTORS DO

Fundamentally, it was a scientific question of whether Maggie had the requisite brain mass and structures necessary to enable communication. And herein lay the promise and the peril. Suppose she had the structures that suggested a retained capability to communicate but was unable to generate voice? Would that not be the most tragic paradox, the most terrible of outcomes? A case in which the promise was not realized, or only to the point of holding the specter of a silent awareness of one's unmitigated loneliness?

With both a touch of stoicism and pragmatism, Nancy responded, "Like you were saying ... is it awful to know that she has brain function but can't communicate? Well it is awful, but then," she said regrouping with the implications of this knowledge, at least her daughter would seem to be thinking. And if she "... can be thinking ... how can we help her to communicate?"

Her final rejoinder was a reminder of our obligation to help achieve that lofty goal: *"That is what doctors do."*

Indeed, it was precisely what we did the year before for a young man named Greg Pearson. That story begins both a literal and figurative next chapter, for this volume and for the field, in the move from observing and charting disorders of consciousness to their actual manipulation in the service of health. We'll now turn to Greg's story and the first use of deep brain stimulation in the minimally conscious state, a project designed to foster, or restore, functional communication for patients who have been silenced by severe brain injury.

16 Deep Brain Stimulation in MCS

According to his mother, Corinth Pecco, Greg was a sharp dresser who liked nice things and always had a good job. He had a number of girlfriends and was a sweet guy. He never got into trouble and did not like to fight. But that, unfortunately, made him "an easy catch" for local hoodlums who viciously attacked him. Greg, whose nickname was Freedom, was thirty-eight, unmarried, and with a young daughter when he was assaulted.

As his mother told us, his attackers "got high and they went out and riding around and they saw Freedom and they know what type of person he is." And she continues with resignation, "They knew he wasn't going to fight."

When Corinth arrived at the hospital, Greg's father told her how badly their son was beaten. "His brain was smashed in" and he was not expected to live. The situation was so bad that it was initially thought he was brain dead when he arrived in the emergency room of a local hospital. According to Corinth, "... they said, 'DOA.' That he was like dead ... brain dead."

It took her aback because she hadn't imagined Greg's injury was serious. She remembers that when she first got the call from the hospital, everything "was going well, I mean nothing like this happened before this happened, so I paid it no mind. Believe it or not ... I got my nails done. I went to the hairdresser and got my hair done. Then [I thought] I'll stop by the hospital 'cause Greg has never been in any problem, never had any problems with him, so you wouldn't think of anything."

The medical record confirms his dire condition. The assault had resulted in a closed head injury to the right frontal lobe, which caused bilateral subdural hematomas, or blood collections. These collections, in turn, caused increased pressure within the brain and significant degrees of herniation, the actual expulsion of the brain out of the skull through its large opening at its base where the spinal cord connects to the brain. He had lost his light reflex in his right pupil, a sign that he had herniated and his status was grim, just above brain death. His initial Glasgow Coma Scale (GCS), a marker of severity of injury and prognosis, was "three," the lowest score one can receive and not be dead. It was an unequivocally grave situation. Greg was in critical condition.

A doctor spoke to the family, " 'I want you to go in, you look concerned,' he says that, 'I want to tell you right now that we've done all we can for him and there's nothing else we can do. He's on a respirator and you have to make up your mind today what you want to do. If you want to take him off or let him stay because right now, doing the surgery and all he's going to be a vegetable the rest of his life and you have to decide if that's what you want to live with.' "

Corinth went in with Greg's father to see their son and "...then I lost it, you know, he's laying there with tubes and everything is coming out and I couldn't take it and then we went out the room and I asked his father, I said 'well what do you want to do?' "

He thought that it was for Corinth to decide but she placed the responsibility firmly on both their shoulders, "... we have to make a decision together whether we want him to stay on it or take it off." In the end, they "decided we'd just take it as one day at a time and see what happens." But while they did not withdraw life-sustaining therapy and agreed to a craniectomy to relieve pressure on his brain, Corinth decided she should agree to a DNR order. She told us, "... they did ask me if I wanted him to be resuscitated. But after looking at him and seeing him the way he was I made that decision ... Do Not Resuscitate ... And I kept that and I still have that."

She made that choice "because of the condition that he was in. Why would you want somebody to try to save somebody when you've already been told he's a vegetable and wouldn't do anything on his own?"

She was realistic about how things were and resigned to a dismal fate. The DNR decision was a reflection of practical and more philosophical considerations. She did not have the resources to ever imagine taking him home. And she brought an almost aesthetic consideration to her deliberations, one that also reflects a mother's ethical sensibility. There was a visceral revulsion to his injured self, both in body and state of mind, "Like again ... I just didn't want to see him in the condition that he was in. I mean you would have to see him, to see how he was to say that you would not want him to be resuscitated." And perhaps most importantly, she did not want him to suffer, especially in his diminished state of mind: "Why try to keep him alive and he's still suffering, he's not the complete person that he was before?"

UNDER DR. MCCAGG'S CARE

Greg had not fought back against his attackers, but he did fight for his life. He was vegetative for about three months after his injury when he first began to show signs of conscious awareness, such as visual pursuit and simple command following. After leaving the hospital, he spent two years at the JFK-Johnson Rehabilitation Center in Edison, New Jersey. There, he had made minimal progress, was able to eat regular food and – according to his mother – move the wheels on his wheelchair, but then the pressure in his brain increased and he deteriorated, a not uncommon complication. A ventriculo-peritoneal shunt was placed draining cerebrospinal fluid into the peritoneal cavity. He was never the same after the pressure surge. He was left unresponsive and mute save for inconsistent command following using eye movements. He was then transferred to a nursing home. More than six years after his injury, Greg was stuck at a low-level MCS state without incremental change.

That was when Dr. Carrie McCagg, Greg's former doctor at JFK-Johnson came calling. Dr. McCagg asked Corinth if she might be interested in enrolling Greg in a trial of deep brain stimulation (DBS) in the minimally conscious state, a study in which electrodes would be inserted into the thalamus – a central structure deep in the brain – with the hope of improving cognitive function.

The work was originated by my colleague, Dr. Nicholas (Niko) Schiff at Weill Cornell Medical College. Schiff had been a sometime visitor to JFK-Johnson in Edison because it was one of the few places in the world with so many patients with disorders of consciousness, and a mission targeted to their diagnosis and treatment. Amidst a generic sea of neglect, JFK-Johnson was an island of interest with a devoted and talented staff of clinicians and investigators, including Joseph Giacino, who McCagg later introduced to Schiff.

It was a welcoming environment and evidence of that was the hospitality that Dr. McCagg showed Schiff when he visited her center. She had invited him to visit to meet families and examine patients. Schiff recalls his first meeting with Greg around 2000, "I had seen Greg on a trip to JFK where Carrie McCagg had taken me not just to JFK, but to nursing facilities all over the area that they sent people to. And we saw a bunch of patients there, and one of the patients who was still at JFK was Greg."

KEEP TRACK OF HIM

Years before enrolling in the DBS study, Greg had participated in the neuroimaging studies looking at forward-backward language processing discussed in Chapter 11. Schiff remembered Greg's normal activation to forward language and his lack of response to backward language. At the time, the finding was an utter surprise, not because there was no response to backward language but because there *was* a response to forward language.

At the time, even before the official designation of MCS as a brain state in 2002, patients like Greg were thought to be more like their vegetative patients than the rest of us who were conscious. That imaging study began to change things about our understanding of MCS, indicating to us that they retained brain activity suggestive of consciousness, albeit showing few consistent signs of it by standard behavioral criteria.

So Schiff, being the good scientist that he is, took his surprise about Greg's response and filed it away for another day of inquiry. He asked McCagg to keep track of him, thinking that this young man's brain injury had more to teach us. Carrie did just that and remained close to Corinth. She even went to the trial of Greg's assailants and comforted Corinth when they only got three-year sentences for the lifelong wounds they had inflicted on her son.

One can sense the gratitude that Niko has for Carrie, "Carrie has an incredible, personal connection to all of her patients. An incredible warmth. And Greg, of all of her patients was one of the ones that she had this very special place for. She'd brought me to see Greg. . . ."

McCagg was a pioneer in the field of brain injury, even before it became an area of broader interest. She toiled in that lonely vineyard with a keen clinical eye and a level of compassion to which all physicians should aspire. As Niko tells it, "Dr. McCagg graduated one of the first, I think maybe the first, graduating class from Yale Medical School when women were admitted. She's an internist. She was a longtime medical internist and ran the brain injury unit at JFK. She was the principal doctor taking care of all of these patients. And she told me that Greg was one of her favorites, that he was really, you could tell he was a very sweet person."

But there was more, there was this critical observation that distinguished him from other patients who were in the vegetative state. Schiff explains, ". . . when she brought me to his bedside he was able to follow a few commands with eye movements and then within about a minute and a half he just kind of faded out, and he'd stop responding."

"He was a perfect patient for the fMRI studies . . . because he clearly was not VS. And what we were interested in at that point was to look at some patients who were just above VS, who weren't so far into MCS that they spoke a little bit or that they did complex things intermittently."

So when they got Greg to Manhattan in 2001 for scanning at Memorial Sloan Kettering in Joy Hirsch's lab, they were stunned with the results. Niko vividly recalls the moment, "I remember we, Joy and I, were sitting in her lab, which was in the basement of Memorial, and it was the first day the data had come out of the processor and was all laid out on her table and we just stood there and looked at it. And I said, 'this looks like the normal subjects. It does look like the normal subjects.' And it slowly kind of crept up on everybody that, wait, this is a finding because our expectation even though it is so obvious in retrospect, [is] that MCS is totally different from VS. And we were looking at this because we thought that they would be different and we found all this variation in VS. It was still the case at that point, these were new measurements. . . ."

It was what Thomas Kuhn, the philosopher of science, might call the emergence of a paradigm shift, that overused designation for a change in a scientific worldview.[1] But this was the real deal; something was different. Propelled by contrarian data that did not cohere with a preexisting theory and his clinical intuitions, it was gradually dawning on Schiff that these patients were fundamentally different than vegetative patients.

The data he was seeing from Greg and a few other patients was a game-changer, though an uncomfortable one with profound implications. He recalls his emerging understanding, "There's a certain gut level, intuition you have about things. Whether you are admitting to it or not. And that was the reality check that our gut level, intuition ... that these patients wouldn't be that different than the VS patients with little bits and pieces of brain. We just thought we'd have a little bit more connectivity but not the complete network."

This was more than "vegetative-plus." Patients like Greg, who we now know to call minimally conscious, would represent a new category: "we were looking for a little, but more than what we'd seen in these residual cerebral fragment studies. But instead what we saw was what looked like a normal network response at a very high level with bi-hemispheric language, and occipital stuff. And it was, it was a mismatch on our expectation. It was a violation of expectation. It just, no one ever had shown a bona fide study of a patient like this."

It took four years for this work to come out, as revolutionary as it was, because the data would have such a radical effect on how brain states would be understood and classified. But when it did, it garnered front-page *New York Times* coverage.[2] And during that long delay, Schiff never forgot Greg Pearson.

PER CHANCE TO SLEEP

And there was another reason Schiff remembered Greg. It was a more subtle observation but one that was equally important. Working with Erik Kobylarz, then a neurology fellow at Cornell, and earlier with Matthew Davey,[3] an Australian medical student who would later die valiantly as a medical officer in the Australian Navy on a humanitarian mission,[4] Schiff realized that there might be recruitable cognitive reserve in Greg's brain and others with similar injuries. Greg had down-regulation of his cerebral cortex on the side of his brain where his thalamus was severely damaged. But this down-regulation *went away* during sleep. This was a critical observation and "... was a clue that there was a dynamical aspect to this that was reversible."

In other words, Greg had cognitive reserve that was unleashed during the differing circuitry that produced sleep. For Schiff, this "was a full background intuition into what was going on" and suggestive of the possibility of harnessing the same potential through another means.

His brain was *dynamical* or changeable, as "he had a recruitable system, and that maybe, if you increased that level of activation, you might get a bi-hemispheric change."

This state change with sleep and its metabolic implications for brain activity put Greg at the top of Schiff's list for DBS. "So he was, from that moment on in my mind, was the patient out of every patient I had seen to date in studies or outside of studies, the one if I had my choice ... to be the first DBS candidate if we got the protocol in line." Perhaps DBS could also induce a dynamical change in brain state and function.

TUTORS AND BOOKSTORES

What Niko proposed had its origins in his undergraduate work as a history and philosophy of science major at Stanford. Under the tutelage of physicist and historian Peter Galison, Niko was looking for a thesis project. He was influenced by Galison's path into sciences through the humanities and his experience earning a PhD after getting his first doctorate studying the *history* of particle physics. In his work, Galison sought to revive a promising line of inquiry "that died out but didn't answer important questions it had originally set out to answer. ..." In response to this unfinished business, Galison "designed and carried out experiments to answer them for his physics PhD."

Schiff wondered if there was a comparable good, old idea in the history of biology that needed to be resurrected and studied. He had always been interested in consciousness and was primed by his chance encounter with *The Mystery of the Mind*[5] by the neurosurgeon Wilder Penfield, founder of the Montreal Neurological Institute (MNI).[6] A slim volume, it would have a huge influence on Niko's life and the life of this work.

Schiff was in a San Francisco used bookstore with Ray Ravaglia, a Stanford classmate, when he "saw this one book and it had this weird kind of candy striping blue and black on it and it caught my eye and it was called *The Mystery of the Mind*. I pulled it off the bookshelf and I was looking at it and I thought, this is interesting. I quickly looked through it and said I'm definitely buying this."

It was the perfect volume for a senior thesis seeking to demonstrate how the history of science might yield clues still relevant for scientific inquiry and how discourse between the humanities and the sciences was important. *The Mystery of the Mind* was the ideal text for the young scholar seeking to bridge what C. P. Snow had famously called the "two cultures" problem,[7] that divide that too often isolates the sciences and humanities from each other.[8,9]

But Penfield's book was different. His premise was interdisciplinary engagement with the humanities, overcoming the sequestration of the disciplines. Like Snow. Penfield was both a scientist and a novelist and the literary quality and narrative of *The Mystery of the Mind* reflects that predilection. Remarkably, the volume is his decades-long dialogue with philosopher Charles William Hendel about the mind-brain problem. Their colloquy was informed by the writings of the American pragmatist and psychologist, William James. According to Schiff, those exchanges helped develop from Penfield's "thinking about the mind-body problem and what neuroscience had to do with it." For the young scholar, "... that was like absolutely perfect for the narrative I was looking to write."

MONTREAL

Schiff learned that there was untapped archival material at the MNI and obtained a grant to go there for two weeks during the summer of 1986 to get materials for his senior thesis. Along the way he met famed neurosurgeon and medical historian William Feindel, who had written the introduction to *The Mystery of the Mind*, and Theodore Rasmussen, both Penfield's former colleagues and directors of the MNI.

Beyond Rasmussen's syndrome, a neurological condition affecting children, Rasmussen's legacy to neuroscience was the cortical mapping of the motor homunculus that he did with Penfield. That diagram of the motor strip and the localization of function is in Schiff's words, "classical, canonical."

But what Rasmussen told Schiff during one of their meetings was not accepted dogma. The sagacious Rasmussen told him a scientific secret, a "truth" known to few but still in need of proof. When Schiff told him his thoughts about his thesis, Rasmussen started off politely but then told him what really mattered, "... yeah that's interesting, the mystery of the mind, consciousness. The important thing is centrencephalic integration."

Centrencephalic was a word that Penfield coined at a conference in New York in 1950 to describe the central part of the brain, below the cerebral cortex, which he felt had an integrative function essential to consciousness.[10] Penfield came to this realization by studying seizures deep in the brain, in the centrencephalic region, which had the curious ability to produce what Penfield described as *automatisms* – seemingly unconscious behaviors – in which motor and mental functions become discordant.

Another former MNI investigator, Herbert Jasper, explained Penfield's observations in a tribute written after his colleague's death in 1976. In this scientific eulogy, he explained Penfield's view that petit mal automatisms and generalized convulsions were "expressions of two separate divisions of the hypothetical centrencephalic system that might be called mental and motor. In automatism they become dissociated, so that preprogrammed behavior that is coordinated and semipurposeful may continue during petit mal seizure *even though conscious mental activity is arrested. . . .*"[11]

Integration was the other key legacy from Penfield that Rasmussen shared with Schiff. And it was important that he stressed the concept. It was a fine old idea that needed to be dusted off in the wake of countercurrents in neuroscience that prized the study of the single neuron and discarded the study of large-scale neural networks and consciousness. Rasmussen told Schiff, "... how upset he and everybody else who worked in integrative physiology was when basically people stopped funding research to do consciousness ... it just sort of lost its cache."

What Rasmussen meant was that the real scientific issue was the role that nuclei within the central thalamus played in organizing brain dynamics during conscious behaviors. Such integrative neurophysiology, however, was hard to do. The trend within the scientific community was to study the receptive fields of single neurons in the visual cortex, emulating the seminal work of David Hubel and Torsten Wiesel who won the 1981 Nobel Prize in Physiology or Medicine "for their discoveries concerning information processing in the visual system."[12] And Penfield's theory also suffered from attacks asserting the evolutionary primacy of the cerebral cortex over central "old" brain structures described by one vitriolic critic as but a "Procrustean bed."[13]

No matter. Niko had found his historic relic, a shibboleth from Penfield and coaching from Rasmussen. And emulating his Stanford mentor, Peter Galison, he had discovered important – and promising – work that had seemingly come to an end before its full potential importance had been mined. His time in Montreal – and meeting with Rasmussen – informed his senior thesis at Stanford[14] and was destined to direct the course of his career.

Twenty-five years later, Schiff is still exuberant about his meeting with Rasmussen and his early work on Penfield. Niko explains, "And that's how I first found out about the linkage there and then the science worked its way into my thesis in various ways. And I'd always wanted to study the central thalamus and consciousness from that point on. And then it was a matter of how to do it."

DR. PLUM

From there all roads led to New York and Fred Plum, where he would learn how to do the sort of science he had until then only been able to write about. William Feindel, Rasmussen's successor as MNI director from 1972 to 1984,[15] told him, "there's only one neurologist left in the country who is seriously interested in consciousness and that's Dr. Fred Plum at Cornell Medical School." Beyond this parting advice he gave Niko an inscribed copy of *No Man Alone*, Penfield's wonderful autobiography, and the suggestion that his destiny was as a neurologist, predicting that "one of these days maybe we'll get a reflex hammer in your hand."

Getting an appointment with Fred Plum as a Cornell medical student was not easy. Early on after the welcoming white coat ceremony, Schiff approached Dr. Plum and "... he was completely gracious and he said, 'I love to talk to students about research, set up an appointment, come talk to me.' ... Then it took like months because I had to get through his wall of people, they were all like, 'forget it, why do you want to talk to Dr. Plum? You're not a third year medical student? You don't have a dean's letter? Why do you want to talk to Dr. Plum?' Finally I wore them down and I finally got an audience with him maybe four or five months later."

The start of their meeting was not auspicious. The conversation at the white coat ceremony was long forgotten and Niko worried that his perseverance could have been mistaken for being "this impetuous medical student who was trying to harass them to get an appointment." When he entered the office, Dr. Plum is "turned around with his back to me with a rolled up magazine and I hear this thwack, and there's this bug on the window ... and he got it too."

Then he fixed his gaze on the first-year medical student, "... it was just totally as classic as they get. ...'So why are you here and how can I help you?' or something like that."

In typical Plum fashion, known to all Cornell medical students, it was a difficult start. As Niko recalls the meeting, "... it's like, 'I'm an important guy, I was just testifying down at the House Committee, or the Senate Committee' on such and such, he was kind of razzing me at first and then it was fine. Once we got to why I was there, he was amazing. He totally changed demeanor, he was just into it."

Plum appreciated that "this is the time for research" and went on to recommend that Schiff work with Dr. Jonathan Victor, a brilliant mathematician-neurologist who could teach Niko the skills he would need. Plum, "... really emphasized how smart Jon was and that I should look into what he was doing."

Niko was a bit disappointed because he had his hopes on applying for a joint MD-PhD degree but was dissuaded by Plum. He remembers, "... talking to Fred about it and he said, 'you know, apply, go through this, but let me tell you something, science is a young man's game. Think about doing this instead. Think about taking a year off from medical school and doing research and then going back, do your residency and figure out what your problem is and what techniques you're going to need because if you're an MD-PhD you'll learn your techniques, you go and you do your residency and you need to relearn everything over again.'" It was sound advice and of course an implicit invitation to the young medical student to join a very exclusive team of investigators.

Niko joined forces with Plum and his colleagues and sought to study absence seizures that involved the intralaminar nuclei of the thalamus,

because it had been central to Penfield's focus on consciousness and automatisms. But this time, in lieu of methods in the history of science, Schiff was
exploring the same terrain using mathematical modeling under the tutelage
of Jon Victor. It was a difference that would make a difference.

EARLY TREMORS

At the same time, the modern era of neuromodulation using DBS had begun.[16]
The technique called for the placement of small electrical leads into structures deep in the brain using three-dimensional positioning called stereotactic localization. Electrodes are then connected to a pacemaker that resides
in the chest. This device is much like a conventional cardiac pacemaker and
is battery powered. The voltage, frequency, and shape of stimulation can be
modified by programming the stimulator in the patient's chest.

Although electrical stimulation of the brain dates back to the nineteenth century,[17] its current phase began in 1987 when the French neurosurgeon, Alim Benabid, discovered that the stimulation of the thalamus could
reduce Parkinsonian tremor.[18] He had been operating upon a patient with
Parkinson's disease and engaged in brain mapping to optimize where he would
place an ablative or lesioning procedure. As he stimulated the proposed site,
he observed that the current used to map the precise locale of the electrode
and its distal effect had actually *decreased* the tremor. It was an unexpected
finding, but it prompted Benabid to wonder whether stimulation alone might
treat the tremor without having to destroy brain tissue.[19] This would be less
invasive, have decreased risk, and potentially could also be reversible, unlike
a destructive lesion in the brain.

Benabid's observations – and the possibilities of this alternate approach
to Parkinson's disease – inspired him to develop the modern deep brain stimulator in use today.[20] By 1997, the Food and Drug Administration approved
the use of the deep brain stimulator as a *treatment* for refractory Parkinson's
disease and essential tremor.[21] Subsequent research has shown it to be effective in prospective, double-blind studies of Parkinson's disease.[22,23]

Contemporaneously, in the early 1990s, multinational investigators
applied this nascent technology to a group of some fifty vegetative patients,
including Terri Schiavo who was a part of this trial.[24-26] These papers caused a
sensation because two of the investigative teams showed functional improvement in some patients,[24,25] a result that was methodologically problematic for
two reasons. Firstly, DBS was applied three to six months after injury, which
is within the time frame for *spontaneous* recovery from a vegetative state
caused by traumatic injury. Secondly, some of the patients who did improve
did not meet the criteria for being vegetative at the time of enrollment and
were more likely in the, *as yet to be described*, MCS. The reader will recall

that MCS would be described using the Aspen criteria in 2002[27] and that it carried a more favorable prognosis for recovery.[28]

Even as this work was coming out, and a decade before these efforts would come under closer scrutiny and critique, Schiff was puzzled. Although "they were a huge sensation ... I remember looking at these papers ... and I was thinking, these people are like dead, I mean, what is the point here? Why would you put electrodes in these patients? They're not going to do anything, it doesn't make any sense."

The aforementioned investigators were putting the electrodes in the same nuclei involved in the absence seizure. Penfield had shown that you "could functionally disable conscious awareness and behavior" in an intact brain "by changing the pattern of stimulation in this area." In an uninjured brain, this area of the thalamus was important to changing the brain's functional state and moving it into a state of unconsciousness. But it did not follow logically that you could do the same in a severely damaged brain because the ability to alter one's brain state required that the responsible circuitry be intact. The expansive networks were just not there in the permanent vegetative state.

Schiff recalls thinking, "... there is no point in doing this in this very structurally brain injured people who are permanently unconscious. In fact there's probably only a point in doing this in patients who you absolutely know are conscious and have fluctuations and have wide behavioral fluctuations." In other words, those patients who had the circuitry that could sustain consciousness, even if that circuitry was understimulated.

INSIGHTS

And that was the key insight. What if the circuitry, that expansive neural system, was structurally intact but offline, like an interstate highway system just waiting for traffic? The roadways were intact and could host the cars, but were – for some reason – underutilized in contrast to highways that were destroyed and impassable. So the question was identifying those patients whose pathways remained intact but that were seemingly, or rarely untraveled. How could these patients be distinguished from those whose circuits were physically disturbed and interrupted?

The answer was that occasionally the patients with the intact pathways would sometimes show flickers of activity of their intact circuits. Not all the time, and rarely so, requiring careful observation. But these would be the patients who might be jump-started with stimulation in the thalamus.

That observation of self-generated activity was the key to Schiff's thinking: the patients most likely to respond would be those who showed wide behavioral variation on their own. They would not be vegetative patients who simply remained in that state because their injuries were so much more pervasive. The more likely candidates would be ones who were conscious, who Schiff and others would come to call *minimally conscious*.

The point was that it took a more *intact* brain to move in and out of an unconscious brain state. Vegetative brains did not have this in their repertoire. They were, in Schiff's words, "structurally wiped out, the cells are dead and like, it didn't make, it made sense to me that you could get different patterns of activity." More intact brains "produce altered consciousness just like when Penfield would push on the area of [healthy] brain with his finger and cause a loss of consciousness."

With these thoughts in mind, Schiff began his residency in neurology at Cornell. He had learned that DBS of the thalamus was being studied by Robert Fisher to suppress seizures[29] and wondered whether he could use DBS to study the loss of consciousness that occurred during the absence seizure. To do this, he sought to understand whether sensory signals could be disrupted by the seizures during low frequency stimulation of the intralaminar nuclei within the thalamus. He would record the effects of the thalamic stimulation in the primary visual cortex, thus marrying the "integrative physiology models" with the more *au courant* work utilizing receptive fields, emanating from the legacy of Hubel and Wiesel. As Schiff told me, getting these two approaches to work together to understand consciousness "was the grand idea of this experiment."

It was 1994 and Schiff told Dr. Plum, "If we can figure this out we might be able to change the stimulation and turn it into a way to help people with cognitive impairments." Plum agreed and Schiff set off to write a patent. The patent had three key criteria that would need to be met for patient eligibility and the physiologic tenability of the hypothesis to work.[30] First, the subject had be a conscious patient who had behavioral fluctuations that suggested the presence of an intact wide spread neural network that would be amenable to stimulation. Second, the intralaminar system of the thalamus, the sweet spot where electrodes would be placed, would need to be mappable and intact to the level of its subdivisions. Finally, there were intact projections from these thalamic nuclei out into the areas of the brain that could be correlated with behavior.

Schiff had a powerful hypothesis that would take ten years to come to fruition, surmounting a number of challenges, most notably ethical ones. And in the process we would come to Greg Pearson's aid.

17 Mending Our Brains, Minding Our Ethics

I first met Niko after he submitted his patent. He was a few years behind me at Cornell and I knew him by reputation as someone who was deeply interested in consciousness and had a close relationship with Fred Plum. As a former student of Dr. Plum's, I was really impressed by his proximity to a professor who had a reputation for both toughness and excellence. If Niko had been taken into that club, he had to be both tough and excellent.

At the time, I had just founded the first hospital-wide ethics committee at The New York Hospital and was busy doing ethics consults, most of which related to questions at life's end. On a national level, I was working to develop the field of palliative care, building scholarly bridges between clinical ethics and that nascent area of medical practice.

To that end, I was editor of a section in the *Journal of Pain and Symptom Management* called "Ethics Rounds." Its purpose was to address ethical dilemmas in end-of-life care.[1] Typically, I would line up a case with two commentators with opposing or supplementing points of view. I had received a case from Bezalel Dantz who was doing a joint residency in medicine and psychiatry at the New York–Presbyterian Weill Cornell Medical Center, in which the question arose whether or not comatose patients should receive opioid analgesia for pain control.

The patient in the case was a fifty-nine-year-old woman with metastatic breast cancer to the brain.[2] On a political level it was a question about the right-to-die, double-effect, and whether a morphine drip was providing relief or hastening death.[3] That was the conventional read at the time.

But there was something more profound about the case, and that was whether or not unconscious patients perceive pain and experience distress? I wanted someone to comment intelligently on the question of consciousness and pain. By chance, I ran into Niko at the coffee shop at The New York Hospital. I asked him to remark on the case and he did, presciently noting the possibility that "patients who exhibit minimal interaction with their environment do register painful stimuli."[4]

That chance encounter, in 1997, started our collaboration and quickly led to in-depth discussions about these altered brain states and ways in which they might be treated. The DBS project intrigued me, and I began to think about the ethical challenges that would need to be addressed, and overcome, for the work to go forward.

ETHICS AND STUDY DESIGN

From the get-go, Niko appreciated that he needed to do this work in the most ethical fashion. He intuitively understood that the only way the science could proceed would be through an ethical argument that underscored its importance and articulated an appropriate structure for its conduct. Schiff's appreciation of the centrality of ethics to the science led to our partnership and still sustains our ongoing collaborations.

The place of ethics began at the level of study design. There was the issue of which patients were the appropriate ones in whom to conduct the study.[5] It was clear that, unlike the Japanese studies,[6,7] ours would require at a minimum, subjects who were conscious. In contrast to the vegetative patients studied by the Japanese, our patients would need to have dynamic range as evidenced by some variance in their behavioral repertoire.

To satisfy this requirement, Schiff initially thought of enrolling subjects who had already emerged from MCS and who were fluctuating at much higher levels of behavior, for example patients who were already reliably communicating. The effects of stimulation would be assessed more easily and perhaps more robustly in these patients than those who were still vegetative.

Although I appreciated the scientific rationale for selecting these patients, I objected and felt that the functional status of the patients was too high. It seemed to me that patients who were already at this level of communication were at an incremental risk from the placement of electrodes, especially because any value associated with the study was still hypothetical. Given this, the risk-benefit ratio would be disproportionate.

Instead, I argued that we needed to find subjects at the lowest functional level at which the operative hypothesis about activating brain networks might work. Clearly, the bright line distinction was in patients who were *not* vegetative with their nonintegrative brain function, but at a minimum, low-level minimally conscious patients who had preserved or recovered integrative brain function. That is, brains that had retained widely distributed neural networks that could be activated.

Niko recalls our conversation about study design and how ethics at the inception altered the course of the work: "... that takes me to a very clear remembrance of a pivotal moment in how things changed direction in your office on the first floor of the hospital. The first thing I remember about the ethics of this study changing the study was that in its first iteration, in the first grant that was proposed to go to the Veterans Administration, it was not primarily MCS, it was mixed MCS, emerged from MCS, and in my mind the patients who this really was focused on were above MCS. And I remember we sat down and what was not in my canon, my experience, was this incredible valence of the negative right and how much that weighed on the intervention, as you would say, in this population."

Schiff continues, "And you said, 'look, this is an unproven thing and you've got to start just above these VS patients where you think you can make a difference.' So that's when the ethics came into this. We were writing the protocol that became the main FDA protocol ... when it became focused entirely on the range of MCS patients where there was a potential benefit. And it was the ethics that brought that in. It was your influence saying, 'look you really have to go just above what's been done where you think it might make a difference.' "

SURROGATE CONSENT IN RESEARCH

Even more challenging than the question of who the subjects might be was that of who would provide consent for such an invasive study? That is, how could we obtain consent from patients who were unable to provide it and do such a study under the guise of surrogate decision making, where others provide authorization in lieu of a competent patient?

This has long been a fraught question in research ethics. Subjects who cannot provide autonomous consent constitute a vulnerable population, open to exploitation, unable as they are to protect their interests or defend themselves against unwanted and unconsented to interventions. This inability to provide consent for research participation may either displace authorization to surrogates or lead to a protectionist ethic that excludes this population from research of more than minimal risk without the prospect of direct benefit. Or it can lead to distortions, or confusion, in what is meant by the prospect of direct benefit and confusion about early phase research, which is primarily concerned about safety and not efficacy.

Going back to the history of bioethics, there has been a large lacuna in our regulations – both at the state and federal level – because of the competing challenge of protecting a vulnerable class of patients from exploitation and giving that same group access to scientific progress. But there was a protectionist slant to the deliberations because of the egregious history of abuse. Just mention Tuskegee or the abuse that occurred at Willowbrook, a state hospital on Staten Island in New York, and the deliberate inoculation of the hepatitis virus into retarded (to use the then current nomenclature) children.[8] These children were institutionalized and convenient research fodder for zealous investigators who exploited them to do their "science."

In response to the Tuskegee studies, which involved syphilis experiments in more than four hundred African American men[9] and revelations of other research ethics abuses disclosed in 1966 by Henry K. Beecher in the *New England Journal of Medicine*[10] – earlier of the Harvard Committee that sought to define brain death – Congress passed the National Research Act of 1974.[11] The act established the National Commission for the Protection of Human Subjects of Biomedical and Behavioral Research, which was constituted and staffed by prominent bioethicists who would write reports that would alter the landscape of research ethics for a generation.[12]

Given its historic moment, the National Commission made human subjects protections its primary focus. The commission articulated three overarching ethical principles in its seminal product, *The Belmont Report*[13] which reflected a broader "common morality."[14] These three principles stressed the centrality of respect for persons, beneficence, and justice and the associated applications of these principles in the process of informed consent, risk-benefit assessment, and selection of subjects.

But given the shocking revelations of Tuskegee, the National Commission appropriately focused on human subjects' protections and not the promotion of access to research. When it came time to consider the question of distributive justice, the emphasis was that the *burden* of research be properly and fairly distributed across society. Vulnerable populations should not shoulder a disproportionate share of the load simply because they were available for research. But neither should they be excluded from participating in research because they cannot provide consent. That too would be a violation of a justice principle.

But given the legacy of cases like Willowbrook and the Jewish Chronic Disease Hospital – where Chester Southam, an immunologist at Memorial Sloan-Kettering Cancer Center, injected cancer cells into patients who could not provide consent to observe variability in immune response[15] – the National Commission recommended the modern institutional review board (IRB) process to assess the ethics of any proposed study. Their emphasis was on the importance of informed consent, as a marker of respect for persons, one of the key Belmont principles.

But what I think became confused over the years was the linkage of informed consent and respect for persons. The two had become synonymous with research done without a patient's informed consent becoming an indicator of a lack of respect of persons, a clear violation of the Belmont principles. But this was only half correct. Clearly the conduct of research without consent or over the objections of a patient who could provided consent and was competent would be an ethical lapse without justification.

But what of the situation when a patient cannot give consent because of decisional incapacity, as occurs with severe brain injury? It would be erroneous to put that kind of research into the first category because it is impossible to obtain consent from an individual who cannot provide it. In those circumstances one would logically need to turn to a surrogate decision maker for guidance.

But logic seemed to have little to do with surrogate consent for research with more than minimal risk that was experimental and could not honestly promise direct medical benefit. Such authorization was suspect because the permission did not come from the patient and, absent that, such research could be exploitative and disrespectful of persons and thus morally proscribed, making research on those who are decisionally incapacitated off-limits.

While research over the objection, or without the consent, of an autonomous individual is an ethical breach, this does not translate into making research authorized by surrogates suspect, or research on those who are decisionally incapacitated off-limits. Such a stance is paternalistic and robs the surrogate of an important decision-making role. Through my interviews with families of loved ones with disorders of consciousness, I came to appreciate the burdens they have assumed and strongly believe that with this assumption of responsibility should come additional authority to consent to research with appropriate IRB oversight.

Nor should research without autonomous consent be problematic when the object of the intervention – as in the case with our work with DBS in MCS – was the restoration of functional communication and some degree of personal agency.

MAROONED IN MIDDLECOURT

In the winter of 1999–2000, I was at work on a first paper outlining some of the ethical requirements for the DBS trial. I vividly recall completing the paper while I was a Woodrow Wilson Foundation Visiting Fellow at Hampden-Sydney College, a venerable old school dating back to 1775. As a Woodrow Wilson Fellow, I was on campus to talk about the importance of the humanities in my work as a physician and as a bioethicist. Each year I made week-long pilgrimages to small liberal arts colleges and enjoyed the chance to teach and talk across many disciplines.

But this trip was different. I was immersed in the paper on the ethics of DBS and in a space that was quite conducive to the writer's muse. I was put up in old slave quarters, a nineteenth-century wooden frame house adjacent to *Middlecourt*, the President's home at Hamden-Sydney. Now called a "carriage house," it served as a guest house for the college's visitors. I noted with a sense of irony that one of my predecessors in the guest book was Douglas Wilder, the African American former Governor of Virginia. It was a charming space with a large kitchen and a stone fireplace.

During that week I took every free moment to work on the manuscript. And by mid-week, meteorological magic struck. A winter nor'easter had landed precisely over the Virginia tidewater. I was marooned in my quarters by the "Blizzard of 2000," which dumped more than two feet of snow in front of my wooden plank front door. Even if I wanted to leave, I couldn't open the door; I was a prisoner of the past without electricity, so I started a fire in the fireplace and lit a candle. The apple on the lid of my Mac lit up its environs as I wrote and hoped for prolonged battery life. I had a spare in my bag and wrote 'til the mid-afternoon when the maintenance guys drove up in their snowplows to rescue me and clear the walkway to the cottage.

The results? I soon published "A Proposed Ethical Framework for Interventional Cognitive Neuroscience: A Consideration of Deep Brain Stimulation in Impaired Consciousness."[16] The paper had a bold and confident title, especially because the trial was still but a figment of our imagination. But with the enthusiasm of relative youth, I was confident of the scientific and ethical merit of our mission.

HISTORICAL LEGACIES

The historic backdrop of the antebellum South was somehow fitting for this ethical framework, which I hoped might liberate patients from disorders of consciousness, bound up, as they were, in broken brain circuitry. I had yet to learn that these patients were also trapped in a health care system that isolates, or even, dare I use the word, *segregates* patients once they are in chronic care. I did not understand all this yet but had a visceral premonition that the scientific work and its societal implications would be consequential and tightly linked.

I argued that to justify this study in human subjects, certain prerequisites would need to be fulfilled. The first criterion was that the work was hypothesis driven and that the hypothesis, thalamic stimulation for disorders of consciousness, was robust enough – justified by preliminary studies and natural observation – to allow studies in human subjects. I maintained that the study of human consciousness could only be done in humans and that the studies were not "done on these individuals because they are an available and 'captive' population. Studies would be conducted on this population precisely because they have the cognitive dysfunction under investigation."[16]

But this was not enough to move the work forward. After making the assertion that there was the probability of a hypothetical benefit, I turned to the question of burden and risk. This proved to be an interesting question because it became clear that how we understood proportionality – that is risks versus benefits – had become rather distorted.

To most observers, what we proposed remained incredibly disproportionate and something that should not be done. I recall riding in a Manhattan taxi with a prominent bioethicist describing our plans to use DBS to hopefully treat patients with disorders of consciousness. We were riding north on Park Avenue above Grand Central when he turned to me and asked, "Why would you want to do that?"

His question was an important one and it prompted me to ask why he and I could so disagree on the ethical propriety of the work. We had similar values and usually would be expected to see moral and ethical questions in the same light. An explanation, therefore, was that he and I were operating on a different factual base and reaching differing conclusions because our predicates were different. That was a lesson I learned from doing ethics consults. Disagreements were seldom over fundamental differences but usually related to misconstruals of the facts.[17]

It seemed to me that the conventional view of DBS in MCS suffered under the burden of two conflicted legacies, which taken together led to a moral prohibition. Putting aside logistical questions like consent, the work appeared unimpeachably disproportionate because of perceived *therapeutic adventurism* and *therapeutic nihilism*. Let me explain.

When DBS first entered the public space as a new form of treatment, journalists were eager to link the promise of DBS with the perilous era of psychosurgery[18] with *The Economist* even going so far as to suggest that these developments pose a "greater threat to human dignity" than cloning.[19] At a personal level, excesses of psychosurgery were linked with the egregious ablative lesioning of the lobotomist, Washington neurologist Walter Freeman.[20,21] The tone was cautionary and prudential[22] so as to avoid a repeat of the sort of therapeutic adventurism that Freeman represented.

If this connection to psychosurgery were not enough, the population on whom the intervention was to be performed were patients whose resemblance to, and proximity with, the vegetative state called for therapeutic nihilism. That is, even if an intervention could be done, it should not be done in patients who were beyond hope and remediation. This population called for a strategy of less is more and a nihilistic, not an aggressive, clinical stance.

Starting with that paper from the Tidewater, I sought to untangle the suppositions that informed my colleague's views. I came to understand it implicitly carried an aversion to therapeutic adventurism and a respect for therapeutic nihilism when it was indicated.

The adventurism had its roots in what is proverbially described as the "yuck" factor, that squeamishness that ensues when, in this case, something is placed into the living brain. Add electricity and the overtones of Mary Shelly and her monster and one begins to see the experiment as frightening and dangerous. But as the philosopher Mary Midgley wrote in *The Hastings Center Report*, in an essay aptly entitled "Biotechnology and Monstrosity: Why We Should Pay Attention to the 'Yuk Factor,'"[23] philosophical reflection requires more than an emotional response. There is much more to it, as we shall see.

Admittedly the brain is a fragile organ and operators should trespass within it with prudence and caution. A 1972 *Lancet* article said as much when it spoke of the "peculiar penumbra of sacrilege" when surgically interfering with the brain.[24] But on closer examination, by the time we began to plan our study of DBS in MCS the risks of DBS for disorders of consciousness were neither excessive nor without precedent. At that time, DBS for Parkinson's disease was already widely accepted as proportionate and eventually as a vetted therapy. It had ceased to be experimental and was viewed as safe and effective.

PSYCHOSURGERY

So why the aversion to DBS for disorders of consciousness? I began to study the history of psychosurgery to understand why electrical stimulation of the brain for a motor disorder – the tremor of Parkinson's disease – was viewed favorably and why its use for psychiatric or cognitive purpose evoked a more visceral response.[25]

I began to publish on the topic in light of more recent science that caused us to examine the past with a bit more nuance and care.[26] It was a complicated story replete with a Nobel Prize in Medicine to the Portuguese neurologist Egas Moniz for the development of the prefrontal leucotomy.[27,28] Done before the advent of major tranquilizers, or neuroleptics, the technique was a solitary treatment for severe and refractory psychosis.[29] The inscription of the 1949 Nobel medal said it simply enough, "For his discovery of the therapeutic value of prefrontal leucotomy in certain psychoses."[30] And in contrast to later media portrayals of DBS, the American media viewed the therapy positively, at least at the outset.[31]

In light of new science, it was no longer sufficient to condemn the clear excesses of the past[32] and falsely analogize what Freeman had done with modern neuromodulation using DBS. DBS was different in a number of salient ways. Targets in the brain could now be precisely localized with neuroimaging and electrophysiology and, unlike psychosurgery, DBS's effects could be reversed, either by turning off the stimulator or removing the electrode.[33]

But while one might be able to turn off the stimulator to eliminate any adverse effects on a patient, it was far more difficult to undo the sociology of psychosurgery; especially true in its more modern iteration dating from the 1960s and 1970s, which began to focus on electrical stimulation of the brain.[34] The focus during that period transcended damage to the individual. It now resided on the impact psychosurgery might have on society as a means of behavior control to address the civic unrest, crime, and tumult of that era.

It is hard to grasp the state of society at that time but it was a period of social dislocation for many. The middle class who fled the cities amidst upheaval and shed the more liberal politics of the decade for a wave of conservatism, which as Rick Perlstein depicts in *Nixonland*, persisted through the second Bush administration.[35] Amidst the chaos, people were searching for order and a way to return to prior norms. Jose Manuel R. Delgado, a Spanish physiologist at Yale, sought to answer the call by advancing the notion of *psychocivilizing society* using an implantable brain implant – he named the "Stimociever" – that could be operated by radio remote control.[36] He hoped that a better understanding of the neural substrates of violent behavior would lead to a greater ability for individuals to direct their own behavior.[37] His work was funded by the U.S. Public Health Service, the Office of Naval Research, and the Department of the Air Force.[38,39]

Delgado gained international notoriety in 1965 when he demonstrated that he could make a fighting bull stop mid-charge by activating the "stimociever" he had placed in its brain. The feat made the front page of *The New York Times*.[40]

Amidst concerns of civil liberties and mind control, Delgado's work and other cultural depictions – such as Michael Crichton's *Terminal Man*[41] – led to concerns about abuse and the violation of civil liberties. Crichton's book was based on the work of UCLA's Vernon Mark who studied the relationship between organic brain diseases like temporal lobe epilepsy (or absence seizures) and violence.[42] Mark, like Delgado, sought to liberate patients from the organic conditions that compelled antisocial or destructive behaviors. He asserted that, "correction of that organic condition gives the patient more rather than less control over his own behavior. It enhances, and does not diminish, his dignity. It adds to, and does not detract from, his human qualities."[43]

Although it seems hard to seriously consider solving society's problems through the use of this technology, back in the day, the idea was not as far-fetched as it might seem now. A "Medical News" column in the *Journal of the American Medical Association* attests to contemporaneous sensibility when it noted in a 1973 piece that, "Logistically, psychosurgery for social control is highly unlikely, simply because there are not enough neurosurgeons."[44]

The fears of psychosurgery were strong enough to bring together a coalition of civil rights, antipsychiatry, and minority groups opposed to psychosurgery, aided by critics within the professions such as Willard Gaylin,[12] a psychiatrist and first president of The Hastings Center. Their advocacy led to hearings convened by the National Commission for the Protection of Human Subjects of Biomedical and Behavioral Research to issue a report on psychosurgery in 1977,[45] a sister report to *Belmont*.

Perhaps explaining why DBS for Parkinson's disease has been less contentious than neuromodulation for psychiatric disorders or disorders of consciousness, is that the National Commission did *not* define psychosurgery as including electrical stimulation or surgery of the brain for the treatment of somatic disorders, such as Parkinson's disease, epilepsy, or pain management. In a classic nod to Cartesian dualism it asserted that "psychosurgery includes the implantation of electrodes, destruction or direct stimulation of the brain by any means . . ." when its primary purpose was to "control, change, or affect any behavioral or emotional disturbance."[46]

The Psychosurgery Report had all been lost to the archives until I studied it as I was preparing a 2003 essay.[26] Their findings remain a surprise given theory cultural and historical context. Against expectations, the commission did not recommend a ban on psychosurgery. The commission found enough evidence of therapeutic efficacy to allow experimental work to go forward, so long as there were strict regulatory guidelines in place concerning patient selection, physician competence, and informed consent. Neither the National Commission nor other leading panels[47,48] found good evidence that psychosurgery had been used for political purposes, social control, or as a means to foster racist repression as had been charged. Contrary to expectations of the day, the commission did not ban psychosurgical procedures. Harvard professor of obstetrics and gynecology Kenneth J. Ryan, who headed the commission, had a more favorable view, surprising himself and countering his preconception. Ryan recounted his experiences in an interview with *Science*:

> We looked at the data and saw they did not support our prejudices. I, for one, did not expect to come out in favor of psychosurgery. But we saw that some very sick people had been helped by it, and that it did not destroy their intelligence or rob them of their feelings. Their marriages were intact. They were able to work. The operation shouldn't be banned.[49]

Although allegations of mind control were never substantiated, contemporary media reports about modern DBS still invoked these earlier fears,[19] distorting our ability to accurately assess this new technology.[50] They were exacerbated when those considered for the intervention were so closely associated, as we have seen, by the relationship of patients with disorders of consciousness and the establishment of the right to die.

NEGLECT SYNDROME

In a *Nature Reviews Neuroscience* paper I sought to draw this link between the right to die and the marginalization of this population.[51] I advanced the metaphor of a *societal neglect syndrome*, invoking the neurological analogy of patients with parietal lobe lesions who neglect part of their visual field. That is, if a speaker is so afflicted addressing an audience, he will neglect everything that is stage right all the while thinking that he is speaking to all assembled. Similarly, I argued that patients with disorders of consciousness have been out of our gaze amidst polemics and notions of futility, which lead to the mistaken belief that nothing can or should be done to ameliorate their condition. Hence the nihilism . . . .

When a risk of therapeutic adventurism is admixed with a rather profane violation of an edict for therapeutic nihilism, the result is stasis or fundamental neglect of a population. And the result of that are the staggering diagnostic errors and errors of omission and commission that the previous chapters catalogue. Mary Midgley was right, the question is far more complex than simply a yuck factor.

And the reason for the ethical complexity is that patients who are minimally conscious make a justice claim upon our health care system. Being falsely labeled as permanently unconscious and left to linger in a nursing home bed becomes ethically unacceptable when the person in the bed is conscious. They make a justice claim on neuroscience research to be able to partake in the benefits of new technologies, which might restore or augment their abilities. A similar claim could be made upon medical ethicists to foster beneficial research in light of the ongoing challenge of surrogate consent.[52,53]

18 It's Still Freedom

"Indulge me," I remember asking the research team. It was winter 2003 and we were at a round table in the corner of Weill Cornell's Griffis Faculty Club. Niko, Joe Giacino, the surgeon, and I were finalizing the research protocol that would eventually be approved by the institutional review boards at JFK-Johnson, the Cleveland Clinic, and Weill Cornell.[1-8] It would also inform the basis for an application for investigational device exemption (IDE) from the Food and Drug Administration. IDEs are required when a new device is tested or when an established device is proposed for a novel purpose. Our plan was to use a DBS device routinely used to treat Parkinson's disease in our study to address the impairments seen in the minimally conscious state.[9-11]

By this time, the details of the protocol were being finalized. We decided to restrict the study to individuals who were MCS secondary to TBI. We agreed that going into patients with a higher level of function put them at risk of incremental harm when exposed to an intervention that was experimental and of unclear benefit. We specified traumatic brain injury over other etiologies because of their more favorable prognosis, as compared to anoxic injury. Inclusion was limited to patients from eighteen to fifty-five years, so as not to have data complicated by either the developmental processes of a younger brain or the degenerative ones of an older one. All subjects had to be past the one-year postinjury mark for study inclusion so as to not confuse the *natural* process of recovery, which can occur up to a year in TBI, with the *facilitated* recovery we were trying to prompt using DBS.

I next turned to the remaining ethical issues and explained that we had made a good argument for the use of a surrogate decision maker, the legally authorized representative, to consent to the surgery. But, I asked, what happens if a subject got better and could give his or her own consent? The response was, "we should be so lucky," but I insisted that for ethical symmetry we needed to put a reconsent provision into the protocol, asking the subject if he or she wanted to continue with the intervention if he or she regained the capacity to make autonomous choices. As far-fetched as that codicil amending the original provisions for informed consent seemed at the time, if our purported goal was the reestablishment of functional communication, then it seemed only logical – and ethically correct – to revise the consent process for an outcome that was possible, although improbable. My colleagues indulged me and we modified the draft, moving ever closer to our first surgery.

WHENEVER YOU'RE READY

On November 5, 2003, Niko was at the JFK-Johnson Rehabilitation Institute. He was giving a talk at the 15th Annual Conference on "Rebuilding Shattered Lives," and saw Carrie McCagg there and asked her if she knew Greg Pearson's whereabouts. He recalls that, "Carrie had kept track of Greg from the moment he left. And when I was at a conference ... when it was getting clear that we had things in place to get the IDE approved ... I said to Carrie, 'do you know where Greg is, and do you know how he's doing?' She said, 'I know exactly where he is and he's had some problems with bedsores, but he's fine. I have contact with him. Whenever you're ready. . . .' "

The team met Greg in October 2004 at JFK when he was readmitted to Dr. McCagg's service. Carrie was a co-investigator but we had designed her role so that her fundamental responsibility was to protect Greg's welfare as his physician.

When Greg arrived back at JFK his well-being was in doubt. He had large and deep bedsores that concerned all of us. Corinth, his mother, remembers, "... his bedsores were horrible I mean they showed, it was like all the way down to the bone."

It had been a really hard time for her and Greg. With the Schiavo drama playing in the background, she struggled to feed her son only to have any gains reversed by hospital stays for bouts of pneumonia, most likely from aspiration of the food he could not swallow.

Corinth said she felt for Mrs. Schindler, Terri Schiavo's mother, "... well I felt like the mother, you know, the child's trying to eat." She felt the maternal urge to feed her child and the desire to eat as a life force geared toward improvement. Sharing sentiments any parent can appreciate, she confessed, "Every time you see any little gesture, any little movement, you think that they're getting better and I thought if I keep feeding Greg, he's trying to eat." No matter the biological distinctions between Schindler's daughter and Corinth's son, which I thought were meaningful, her words made me appreciate that there was something rather universal about a mother's desire to nurture a child. It was something that fundamentally transcended politics and science.

But this urge was frustrated because she could not feed Greg. "At the nursing home it never happened." His course was fraught with episodes of aspiration and pulmonary complication: "... every time he turns, it's been pneumonia, pneumonia, pneumonia." Her desire to help, to do *something so normal like feeding a child* was thwarted and she was at her "wit's end ... I just couldn't take it anymore."

So she went to a brain injury support group to recalibrate her hopes. It was a reality check and acceptance of diminished expectations. She had to learn "what to expect and what not to expect and it was good. I enjoyed going to it, it did help me, accept his brain injury ... that this is how it is and I'm going to have to accept this, nothing's going to change. He's not going to be back the way he was from day one." Fundamentally, "he'll never be that way again so I just have to ... deal with that and work with it."

So when she was approached by Carrie McCagg about enrolling in the clinical trial, she was taken unawares. She had felt that the end was near and that when Greg was going to die, he would take his earthly leave from his nursing home bed, "That was my dead-end right there. I didn't look any further just then. I knew when he left, he's going to leave me from that nursing home."

But that wasn't to be his fate. Instead he came back to JFK and into Dr. McCagg's care. She would tend to his wounds and get his weight up so he would be ready for the surgery.

SURGERY

We went through a multistaged approach to get Corinth's authorization for study enrollment. We made no promises of efficacy as it was a phase I study, an early trial designed to assess safety. Although we had more lofty goals, questions of therapeutic effect typically come later in a study's evolution. On reflection, Corinth recalls that "nobody knew how it was going turn out. But at least they wanted to try on him because he met the criteria and I was willing to go with that, even if he had been paralyzed or something or whatever afterward."

Niko and I flew to Cleveland on the night of February 14, 2005 for the surgery the next day. Corinth and a friend drove out to Cleveland. I found out later during a subsequent interview that she went by car because she did not have the money to lay out for a plane ticket, even though she would have been reimbursed by the study's funding. I wish we had known and prepaid for the ticket to have made it easier for her. All the more so because it was not an easy trip: her car broke down and needed repairs. Greg came out in an ambulance.

The night before the surgery we huddled in a conference room in the department of restorative neurosurgery at the Cleveland Clinic looking at three-dimensional images of Greg's brain. All eyes were envisioning the various surgical approaches that would get the electrodes into the intralaminar nuclei without doing damage to surrounding blood vessels and tissue. The electrode had to come in at angle that would pass under an arching artery and above a tissue plane landing in the target in the thalamus. It was a complicated approach. At the time, I remember thinking that the surgical skill in placing the electrode on target without hitting the blood vessel lingering above the site would be akin to a golfer getting to a small green with one shot across a long fairway. It would require a fair amount of skill.

The next morning the operating room was cold. Greg was on the table getting prepped with a stereotactic titanium frame circumnavigating his head. This device allowed for three-dimensional localization within the brain and precise placement of the electrodes. After extensive prep work, the operation began in earnest at 12:45 p.m. A Beethoven *adagio* was playing on a CD player as burr holes were drilled into his skull. They would provide a portal into the brain.

Like all stereotactic functional neurosurgery in which electrodes are implanted for DBS, the patient is awake. Remarkably, all the anesthesia that is needed is for the skin and the skull. The brain is insensate. Paradoxically, the organ through which we process stimuli from the outside world is without feeling. This allows the patient to participate in the surgery when different areas of the brain are stimulated.

The pace was excruciatingly slow with careful efforts at mapping the locale of the electrodes as they progressed slowly into the brain, one side at a time. At each cellular juncture the electrodes would pick up a different tune sung by the local chorus of neurons through which the thin filament passed. Like a microphone the electrode captured the signature melody of each crop of neurons, distinctive signals made up by various cell types in the brain. Ken Baker and Jerry Vitek, both master neurophysiologists, manned a tall frame of electronic gear alongside the patient reminiscent of NASA and Mission Control during the moon shot.

At their post, Vitek and Baker used all their senses – aesthetic and scientific – to discern where the electrodes were headed. They knew the angle of the insertion, the anatomy of Greg's injured brain, and the melody of the different neurons down into the thalamus. The oscilloscope on their console provided pictures of the wave form as the electrode moved deeper, millimeter by millimeter. Niko and others frequently consulted large plexiglass salami-slice maps of the thalamus that could be stacked one upon another to approximate three dimensions. Even with the computer simulations, the team seemed to prefer these translucent maps. Dressed in surgical garb, they bent over them as if they were ancient scrolls that contained some distant truths.

Niko's first recollection of the day was when it seemed that an early shot of stimulation might have had an effect, "One thing that leaps into my visual memory was something in retrospect that was highly significant but at the time just struck me as important. It was the ... apparent change in the rapidity of his command following when he was being stimulated for the first time in the left hemisphere. And one thing that I had thought I'd never seen him do . . . when they asked him to stick out his tongue, his tongue came right out and into the midline and I was like, 'whoa!' "

It was as if the processing speed of a computer had been increased with the insertion of a new chip. But whatever the analogy, the important thing was that something *changed*. The delayed latency of response so characteristic of MCS patients had been sped up. Greg now followed a command at normal speed, which was an indication that his brain was acting more normally.

A few minutes later, Joe Giacino asked Greg a question as part of his testing for the Coma Recovery Scale-Revised (CRS-R). To our surprise, Giacino's question elicited Greg's first verbalization *in years*. I recall seeing him pursing his lips as if to say something and then barely hearing his weak whispery voice. In response to Joe's question, Greg simply said, "Yup."

Niko had actually forgotten this important detail because Greg's speech became even more impressive during the trial. But at that moment, in the OR, it was really something to hear. Our astonishment was met with a desire to be sure it was not wishful thinking. We looked around at each other and asked, did you hear that? But there was no doubt he had done it and at 4:31 p.m. Niko turned to us and said, "Pretty cool gentleman."

My notes from the operating room confirm his recollection and also report the following, "eyes are open, conjugate, keeps eyes open longer, more alert." All of that was an indication of Greg's state change and a higher level of awareness and consciousness. When he was not being stimulated his eyes had been droopier and would go askew. With the stimulation, the eyes came back to midline, opened up and he became visibly more responsive. Something was indeed happening here.

Although we were all delighted and surprised, I confess that I expected a good outcome. I had seen the diligence in Niko's hypothesis generation and its rationale. When I later told Niko, he suggested, "you had good faith and you figured that if all of your friends and people you knew who invested so much thought and energy, and you had put all this together, there should have been at least some weight of a higher probability of success than failure."

But Niko had not been so sure. "The fact is I didn't feel that way. I felt like, I don't know what I thought. I have to say, there was another moment, you know what the other moment was? When I looked up at the board that has the notations that you wrote down and I saw 'diagnosis: MCS,' and I saw 'target B' with a circle around it, which meant bilateral, and 'CL,' central-lateral thalamus. And I'm like, that is unbelievable . . . whatever happens . . . getting here to see that, this medical history, because that has never happened before. Ever."

And it was quite the achievement to simply have persevered and gotten so far, against the skeptics and naysayers, against the inertia that meets innovation and new thinking. So even getting through the surgery safely was an accomplishment, "even that was history because just to get everything in place to do it right and the way we did it, to be in an operating theater at a major medical center and have a new diagnosis on the board and a new surgical location on the board was gigantic. That was cool, that was really cool."

HIS FATHER'S VOICE

Corinth remembers waiting for news as we were in the operating room. "I was worried, I was outside the hall, I was on pins and needles, I was like twitching and I was like, 'what he's going to be like? What he's going to do? What is his reaction?'"

She had been taken in by the clinical team's guarded optimism but wanted to be tempered in her expectations, "I mean, here everybody had all these good hopes and vibes and they just felt so good with me, I don't know, I just, I didn't know how to expect it."

When she was told that Greg had said a single word she told us, "I didn't know what to think or how he's going to be and when they came out and said to me, 'he just said a word, he said yup!'"

It was a familiar word. Where had she heard it? Immediately, she tried to place the verbal fragment into the context of Greg's broken life. She asked herself, "Where did that come from?" Then she realized that the expression came from his Dad, "that's his father, that's what him and his father always said to one another, 'yup, yup.'"

It was joyful, "And then it was just like, just like something just overcame me, I was just so happy." But then a dose of realism set in. This would not restore fluent speech but would be something. She "thought maybe, you know, when they said, 'he's going to be speaking,' that he would just start speaking like you and I. But then, it wasn't that way, but it was still hopeful and happy because he still, he could communicate. He couldn't communicate before. He couldn't say anything before."

CAMP DISAPPOINTMENT

Over the years leading up to that trip to Cleveland, Niko and I had analogized our voyage to the transcontinental explorations of Lewis and Clark. We had both read Stephen Ambrose's *Undaunted Courage* and were drawn to the adventure and scientific objectives laid out by their patron, Thomas Jefferson. But we were also inspired by their partnership and the collegiality and hard work needed to reach shared objectives.[12,13] I still have a map of their passage in my office wall as a reminder of the journey that got us to Cleveland.

When we heard Greg speak that first time in the OR, it was as if we had seen the first vistas of the Pacific, as if through the eyes of those great explorers two hundred years earlier. But we had to be sure of our observations, recalling that Lewis and Clark had misread their position and mistook the estuary of the Columbia River for the Pacific.[14] Their response to their miscalculation during the dreary approach of winter in November 1805 was to name their resting place *Camp Disappointment*. And we were more than prepared for the same, knowing that the trek back East would be arduous.

All we knew was that if there was a discovery to be made, it would be demonstrated by the rigors of science and method, and a great deal more effort. Like the Pacific, getting to Cleveland was but part of the journey. The trial would continue back in New Jersey over the next eleven months at JFK where massive amounts of data would be collected using the CRS-R that Joe Giacino had devised to track behavioral changes in MCS patients.[15] It was a measure that had been validated and used in this range of brain injury worldwide and its utility was key to the team's efforts.

The data was collected by Giacino and Kathy Kalmar who oversaw the work of teams of colleagues who assessed the subject three times a day, four days a week for six months. After a period of titration, or gradual increase in the frequency and amount of stimulation, parameters were locked in for a double-blind crossover study in which stimulation was randomly turned on one month and turned off the next. All the investigators, except Dr. McCagg as Greg's physician, were blinded to whether the stimulator was on or off.

We used the CRS-R to collect objective evidence of any behavioral changes. In the study the CRS-R was divided into three domains. Schiff notes, "The CRS was essential because you needed to have operational, quantitative, behavioral assessments so that you could have data collection done by multiple people, be calibrated across them, be reliable ... [and have] inter-observer reliability."

The instrument was an essential ingredient in our design. Simply stated, the project could not have been done without its superior metrics. Schiff agreed. It was "the core of the study because in the end it's the primary outcome measure. Our primary outcome measures were subscales of the CRS-R. That carried the day because they were measures that we could understand, that had numerical values that could be computed once the data were collected and we knew what they meant. They told the story. They told the story in a way that was much less evocative and sensational than the real story."

Schiff continues, "The real story was amazing. The real story was we had a man whose family didn't even think was conscious [who] could now speak and eat. ..." But as compelling as all that was, it was not the scientific proof necessary to convince skeptics. Nor could it be. Our goal was scientific proof; that was the threshold. Lest we forget, "the numbers told this unequivocal, unambiguous story."

Niko is quick to emphasize that Giacino and Kalmar gave us the means to empirically track the recovery process in these complicated patients, "Joe Giacino gets all the credit, plus Kathy Kalmar for developing the scale, but Joe Giacino gets the credit for the structured assessment and the setting up of the teams and essentially putting in place the data collection mechanism that made it possible to have a database that could be analyzed to demonstrate this."

With hundreds of examinations, the data was meant to be massive in order to give us the statistical power to identify and validate changes in a subject's behaviors. It was necessary, in Niko's view, "because we'd had at that point seven years, or six years of very negative peer review about the project, so we knew what kind of reception the work would have. So when the trial was structured, it was structured to have huge amounts of data collection and validation and all the rest of it."

Our preliminary data showed behavioral improvements in attention, limb control and spoken language, and what seemed to be a causal relationship between DBS and the outcomes. Or so we thought. Niko recalls, "And then despite having very strong and very clear ... cut and sort of unambiguous data, the first review came back with effectively, 'we don't really believe this.'"

It was our *Camp Disappointment.*

PROOF OF PRINCIPLE

In years past, this setback would have been the time for a huddle with Dr. Plum to figure out the data and plot one's next steps. Unfortunately, by this time his health had deteriorated and he was unable to provide the guidance we needed.

And so Niko went back to his other key mentor, Jonathan Victor, the mathematician turned neurologist to whom Fred Plum had first sent him twenty years ago. The only difference was that now, Jon had just been named the first Fred Plum Professor of Neurology at Weill Cornell, a fitting tribute to both of them.

When Niko speaks of Jon Victor, his words convey deep respect for his intellect and his mathematical genius, "So when we got the records back from the review process I went to Jon and it's, 'look, we know what went on here, we can see it in the data.'" Victor helped the data convey the biological transformation that was evident. It was a subtle task and elegantly done. The data was complicated.

It turned out that Niko and Joe Giacino had undersold the data by comparing maximal scores before and after stimulation. Before DBS the maximal score in the arousal domain was two. After stimulation it rose to three and was strongly and causally linked to DBS. Schiff and Giacino minimized the effect because they compared frequency of the maximal two scores with maximal three scores.

The other problem was that the study was divided into three distinct periods. During all three periods his CRS-R was recorded three times daily. The first period was a six-month warm-up, when Greg only got conventional rehabilitation. The idea was to establish a stable baseline and/or to see if there was any effect from rehabilitation. In essence there was none. Then the next period was what we called the titration phase, when stimulation parameters were increased gradually to higher settings determined to be most efficacious just after surgery. Following five months of titration was a six-month period during which stimulation was turned on and off at monthly intervals.

The second problem Schiff and Giacino made in the first submission of the paper was that they had only compared the on and off effects with what Greg was doing after the completion of the titration phase. But *the stimulation during the titration had had a large effect.* It would be akin to comparing the reading scores of first graders who had gone to preschool and kindergarten with those who had not.

So it was with Greg. Measuring his progress after titration failed to account for his improved functionality after those first five months of "titration" before the cross-over stage of the trial started. Again, it undersold his progress from his pretitration baseline. The ascent had already started. We needed to make a comparison from the pretitration baseline.

All of that was the simple stuff. Then came Jon's singular insight. He asked Niko, "Okay, have you ever put together a logistic regression model?" Schiff responded that he had not and Jon told him that was needed to capture the study's complexity in all its many facets. And then with his typical modesty, he added, "Let me think about this because I've done a lot of these and it's complicated."

A week later Jon had worked his magic and was able to provide Niko a mathematical framework that was able to "analyze every aspect of the trial ... making a sort of time history of when this stimulator was on and when the stimulator was off. ... For the five months of data when we're titrating it was very complicated. But the model would also have terms that would allow us to deal with whether Greg was slowly getting better, whether he was getting slowly worse, whether there was no change at all . . . ."

It was a breakthrough. Niko is appreciative when he notes that "Jon's models allowed us to rigorously investigate the data for how robust it was. ... And in the end, what we were able to show in all of the data was an absolutely clear, unambiguous story of what was strongly modulated on and off DBS, which our primary statistics already said was there. But [there was] also a way of helping the reviewers and us ultimately show very clearly what had happened in the run-up to the crossover trial in the five months where Greg started getting exposure to brain stimulation. We had so much data that we could actually see that he was totally flat for six months and then everything started to move as he started to get DBS."

Our paper was eventually published in *Nature* in August 2007.[16] The six-month double-blind crossover study showed an increased level of arousal and function in multiple domains. Before DBS, Greg could only eat using a feeding tube placed in his stomach. But with stimulation he was alert and coordinated enough to eat by mouth, for the first time in years. He also began to speak again, having regained the ability to communicate up to six- to seven-word sentences. And as the press coverage emphasized, he could say the first sixteen words of the Pledge of Allegiance and *tell his mother that he loved her*.

It was heady stuff. We ended up appearing on *Charlie Rose*[17] the night the paper came out and the story was covered by all the major media outlets. We sought to temper our achievement by putting the focus back on the patients and their unmet needs and the residual cognitive capacity that might exist in patients who were in MCS. Appreciating that this was not yet a therapy but a proof of principle we echoed our comments at the end of the paper. We hoped "that confirmation of these findings in other patients might influence the current practice of excluding individuals with inconsistent behavioral responses from structured rehabilitation programs."[16]

Most critically, we sought to redirect attention to the long haul and the work that remained suggesting that "our findings should motivate research to elucidate the mechanisms of recovery and to facilitate the identification of patients who might benefit from neuromodulatory interventions."[17] We did not want our accomplishment to be like NASA's fabled Apollo program, which made its last moon shot in 1972, but to be the first step toward additional discovery.

Niko said it best when he told me that the *Nature* paper was "the end of the beginning. That's how I see it. It was the end of the beginning. We got proof of concept, it took ten years or more, it was nearly ten years exactly, plus or minus a few months from when I submitted the final version of the patent on this to when the *Nature* paper was actually published."

MOTHER AND SON

For us the work had just begun. But for Greg and Corinth, the surgery meant the end of their exile from one another. DBS had breached the isolation that separated them and allowed communication for the first time in years. An electrical current had reconnected mother and son.

Corinth was satisfied with the results, "... like I tell everybody, if he doesn't do anything else, as long as he can open his mouth and say, 'I love you Mommy.' He can call my name. I can call my son. I can say, 'what do you want to watch?' He can say whatever he wants, but if you ask him, 'do you want to watch this on a TV?' He'll tell you, 'no.' "

To be sure he understands what she is saying, after all the many years of silence, Corinth has tested his reasoning. She knows he does not like sports. So she tests him. With an element of pride she recounts her method, "... so if you put sports on and ask, 'Greg do you want to watch this?' and he responds, 'no.' "

She continues, "Then you know he knows." It is an indication that Greg's old preferences and personality have returned intact from his years of hibernation.

The improvements have been a balm to Corinth who had been "angry from the day when it [the attack] happened." She has asked herself why it had to happen to Greg and why it had left him in his condition. But with the surgery and his improvement, she is able to tell us, "... I'm starting to overcome that, because each day I come in and I see him it makes me feel a little bit better and I'm a little happier."

But Greg's father was upset that his body was now unable to keep up with his brain. Because he did not receive range of motion therapy, he has contractures and joints that have petrified. Corinth explained Greg's father's concern that the focus has been on the brain at the expense of the body. She explains, "... this is where his father is upset ... you all are most focused on the brain image than all the other parts. But he wants to see all of them working in connection – brain, the hand movement, and the legs." Now that there is new potential for some degree of functional recovery, Corinth tells us that "his father doesn't think he's getting enough physical therapy."

And it isn't just Greg's father who had an opinion. For the first time in years, Greg had one too. Corinth tries to explain it, almost embarrassed by suggesting it, that her son, mute and distanced from her, might in fact *now* have a point of view or an interest in something.

And for Greg, the ability to respond to questions and voice a preference is to gain a part of himself that had been lost when he was beaten, that part of the self that is volitional and directive, which assumes control over one's destiny. All of that had been lost, either substantively – he had not recovered enough to have preference – or procedurally – he had preferences but could not express them. Either way, the result, absent the intervention, is the same: isolation and sequestration from others, families and friends, one's past and future.

But now it was different. Corinth prefaces her comments, as if to apologize, "And, you're not going to believe this either. ... Greg is a sharp dresser

... I keep buying him nice clothes." And to her amazement, Greg enjoys going shopping and has strong preferences. So Corinth took him to Old Navy.

Her plan was, "To get some clothes, just to buy him some shorts, and I picked up a pair of, I think, I don't know if it was these green khaki shorts, and I said to him, 'You like these shorts, Greg? Do you want me to buy you a pair of shorts like this?'".

She continued, "He looked at me," and said, "'No.'" Laughing with delight that her son could talk back and question her taste, she recalls telling him, "Well guess what? Mommy's buying them anyway!"

Such an exchange may seem trivial, a mother and her son buying clothes at the store, but it represents the reemergence of Greg's ability to make a choice, to voice an opinion, to express his wishes as an individual, something that had been taken from him by his injury. But now he is able to participate in choices that matter to him. No matter that his mother initially vetoed his decision – she did it with a laugh that recognized that Greg was back in the room *interacting*.

Now they were able to share in a dynamic of parental authority versus a child's defiance they undoubtedly rehearsed many times when Greg was a teenager. It was a healthy interplay, a return to normalcy that brought a smile to Corinth because it represented a reconnection.

And it is still Greg, her son. After all that has happened, after the long silence, the Greg that has returned is still familiar to Corinth. Although philosophers might struggle with questions of personal identity and discontinuity after such an injury,[18] for Corinth, the young man with the deep brain stimulator was her son and no one else. The essential elements remained, despite the disabilities, both cognitive and physical.

When asked if the old Greg remains within, Corinth is unequivocal about it, yes, she replies, he is the "same kid." His identity is preserved, his interests are constant, and his relationships with his family still important to him.

How does Corinth know? She responds with concrete answers, "Because he smiles at certain things and he still likes to watch the cartoons on TV. He knows the *Simpsons*, he likes that. If he was up and about he would have been in that line for *The Dark Knight*. I mean, those things I can tell. Reading a comic book. You can bring a comic book and he can usually look at it and he'll smile."

Then comes the most telling comment, "So inside *it's still Freedom*."

Note the use of his nickname, Freedom. Corinth did more than say it is still the same Greg. Instead, she said to me it is "still Freedom," the nickname he has carried since a teen. Her use of a nickname, known only to those who knew Greg the best, is more than a term of endearment. It signifies – and preserves – an essential aspect of his past, of who he was and who he remains.

It is a symbolic marker of continuity, if not a philosophical proof of Greg's return through a technological intervention.

And beyond theories of the self, in the real, in the relationship that has been restored, or better yet, amplified, between mother and son, Greg remains. There is a new degree of reciprocity between them. The relationship between them had been unilateral. Now that Greg can communicate it is now mutual and shared. Moreover, their relationship has grown over time, like it always does between a mother and a child.

Corinth has become more respectful of Greg – or deferential to his new-found ability to express a preference and emerging sense of autonomy. In this, his recovery seems to recapitulate a developmental process that occurs during the period of latency as a child becomes a teen and takes tentative first steps toward independence under the surveillance of wary parents.

She appreciates that Greg is less dependent and that he has views that warrant deference. With time it is different. Now when they go shopping, she explains, "... if I take him and buy things and bring them to him and ask him if he likes it, he can let me know what he likes and what he don't like, and *I'll take it back.*"

Asked if she returns the merchandise with "great joy," she responds, "Yes. He decided that this is what he wants and what ... he didn't want." It is all the more meaningful because, "He couldn't do that before." She explains, before Greg was passive to his environment. "Now there's moments where you can put a movie on and Greg will stay there and watch the whole movie without falling asleep. Now that to me, I'm happy and I'm thrilled and I enjoy that moment."

NO MEANS NO

Months after completing the formal seventeen-month study, we went to check in on Greg and be sure that the settings on his two stimulators were optimized. It was time to see if he needed to be recalibrated because his brain had likely changed during the stimulation. He had likely outgrown the original settings dialed at the start of the protocol back in Cleveland. As important as hitting the right target in the brain is the way in which the target is stimulated, the size and shape of the charge as well as the frequency of the current. All of these elements are critical variables that could yield a range of effects both good and bad. The wrong stimulation parameters at a proper target could be ineffective at best and dangerous at worst. They could set up malignant circuits that could undermine cognitive functions and even result in seizures, a complication to which patients with brain injury are already prone. Alternately, the optimization of parameters could have significant impact on Greg's level of arousal and his cognitive abilities.

We set out to New Jersey to pay a visit, where we were in for a significant surprise. It was June 16, 2006 late in the afternoon, after a full day of
revising the settings for each of the four leads on each electrode planted on
either side of the brain. It was hot and all of us were exhausted, including it
seemed, Greg. Brian Fritz, a physical therapist colleague, had noticed that
Greg looked fatigued. He was crouched in front of Greg's chair and assessing
his responses. Greg was rather stoically going along with the process, dapper
in a black shirt but looking tired.

But Brian sensed that his longtime patient was getting a bit too tired.
He felt that we had asked him to do too much. So Brian paused and asked
Greg if he wanted to continue with the stimulation tests.

Greg looked him straight in the eye and said, "No." It was 2:50 p.m.

Of course everyone stopped. It was the ethical thing to do. No means no
when a patient refuses an intervention. It is a basic tenet of informed consent
and informed refusal that a clinician needs the moral warrant – or permission – of the patient to invade one's space or to treat.

No news there, but there was big news here. I stopped the proceedings
to make a point of telling the group what we had just witnessed. Greg was
asked a question, he responded, voiced a preference, and his clinical team listened and respected his wishes.

I was immediately brought back to that lunch three years earlier at the
Griffis Faculty Club at Cornell when we were finalizing the protocol and
I asked that we insert the reconsent provision into the protocol if the intervention restored decision-making capacity, or the legal competence, allowing
the patient to make choices for him- or herself. That authority would no
longer reside in the surrogate but return to the subject once he or she regained
capacity.

And here we were: an assertion of wishes by Greg Pearson in response to
a question by a clinical professional who heretofore was operating on the moral
authority of his mother, his surrogate and legally authorized representative. In
that instant, all that changed, Greg was no longer represented by his mother;
he was representing himself. Or at least he was partially representing himself,
asserting his self-determination and expressing his autonomy, as best he could.

What he asserted did not rise to the level of a formal consent or refusal.
And it was not a comment on whether he wanted the stimulation to continue
or not. It was only that he was tired and wanted a break for the day. But it
was a huge step forward. Greg had reached the lower level of assent or dissent
in which a preference is voiced, but in a situation in which the patient can
neither explain the rationale for a preference nor independently seek information that might make for a more informed choice.[19]

It may have only been voiced at the lower level of dissent, but no matter. Greg's "No" constituted an historic moment. It was the first time ever

that personal agency – *agency ex machina* if you will – had been restored by a neuroprosthetic device. He could now participate in medical decisions alongside his mother and soon he would share decision-making authority with her over sartorial preferences.

BUT IS HE DEPRESSED?

The literary critic Frank Kemode observed in his elegant book, *The Sense of an Ending*, that we can understand life by imposing the structures of fiction upon it.[20,21] And looking at Greg's life, it takes little to see it as if it were a fictional, indeed, science fiction account. And though it is all true, indeed all the accounts herein are true, it is helpful to ask: How has it ended for Greg? What is the sense of his ending, after all that he has been through?

For his mother, this has been more a continuation than an ending. The careful reader will recall that when Greg left JFK for the nursing home, Corinth viewed it as "my dead-end right there ... he's going to leave me from that nursing home." So, one lesson of fiction – and this true story – is that of contingency. An ending is only known in retrospect, and while there are probabilities that can guide prognostication and judgment, at the margins of scientific advance, there is often more doubt than certainty. Sometimes an ending becomes a beginning.

And in her surprise, Corinth has found new possibilities: happiness and a sense of reconnection. She has regained a son who can engage her at some level and disagree with her on minor issues. And yet, her happiness is tinged with sadness precisely because she knows her son so well. It is a balanced and honest response that distinguishes her needs from his, an instructive distinction relevant to any assessment of outcomes after DBS. A first question then must be, good for whom?

Corinth is honest about making this distinction between his and her needs, "... and I'm still crying because I'm crying because one part of me is happy, one part of me is sad. I mean I'm jumping the gun now. But ... with the surgery, I'm pleased. But on Greg's part with the surgery, I think it made him more aware of his surroundings and it's making him a little depressed."

She observes, "He is aware of what he was ... he's aware of his surrounding now more so than he was before he had the surgery. I think that's what's bothering me because now he's starting to get ... I think he's depressed. . . ."

And Greg's ability to share any sadness raises the deeper, more challenging question, noted earlier, that we can only know one's inner state if it can be communicated. If deprived of an outbound communication channel we would be hard-pressed to know if Greg were depressed or not. Then the question is which is worse, to know his actual state of mind or not? In the former, intercession is impossible, but in the latter it is possible. Of course, without the stimulation, Greg might be unaware and silent, unperturbed by his condition. Alternately, without stimulation, he might be aware of his predicament but unable to communicate with others, isolated without recourse.

As we shall see in the coming chapters, patients who are as minimally interactive as Greg was before stimulation can show evidence of awareness without behavioral manifestations while undergoing neuroimaging. This evidence suggests the worrisome possibility that the minimally conscious state could be one in which there is awareness and isolation, a situation that would seem horrific, if a communication channel such as DBS or neuroimaging were not provided and then only ameliorated for those subjects in whom these experimental methods worked.

So to return to the question of Greg's possible depression, I would view it as the condition that it is and one that is amenable to treatment if diagnosed. Depression can be treated if it is appreciated. And what of the possibility that Greg is *more* depressed with stimulation than before, even as he has regained more functional capacities and with them possibly a deeper understanding of his condition?

Again, analogizing to routine clinical practice, deeply depressed patients often become more depressed – and paradoxically more prone to suicidality – once they are treated. As the apathy and psychomotor retardation of a psychotic depression is ameliorated, the patient gains more energy and interests, which can sometimes coalesce into self-destructive behaviors that were previously beyond contemplation or consummation. This risk, en route to a fuller recovery is managed by medical surveillance and optimization of medical management.

The same can be said for the depression that might accompany patients who, in the future, were to get DBS for the minimally conscious state. First, depression should not be a complication that leads to suspension of the intervention, because like conventional treatment of depression, improvement in some aspects of the condition may be accompanied by negative changes elsewhere. Instead, emergent depression should be managed and the patient carefully observed. I first responded to this then-theoretical objection to DBS in MCS in the paper I wrote at Hamden Sydney College, now more than a decade ago. Commenting on the risk of ego-dystonic self-awareness in the consent process, I suggested that:

> Risks associated with deep brain stimulation should be reviewed including the possibility of iatrogenic injury during stimulator placement and the theoretical risks of reversible ego-dystonic self-awareness. This discussion of risks and benefits should be framed against conventional rehabilitation strategies that ideally would be available to the subject, although it should be noted that in reality many subjects may only be receiving custodial care and not active rehabilitation.[22]

Then as now, the possibility of terminating DBS exists, thus resolving at least the ability to communicate distress but not providing any guarantee that an adverse affective state is eliminated. The worry would be that a patient like Greg could remain depressed, without stimulation, but have no recourse to expressing it. In this context, to maintain functional communication would seem to be an ethical "good," better than the possibility of an isolated depression. By contrast, it is possible that Greg might not experience depression at all. In this formulation, DBS helped resolve a confusional state that precluded an emotional self capable of producing an affective response of happiness or sadness. But that too, is a condition that could be managed with the input of surrogates and the patient who could also decide that the situation was so intolerable as to move toward a withdrawal of the stimulator and life-sustaining therapies. This would also seem to be a justifiable action in the proper circumstances. The point of anyone counseling these families (and subjects/patients) in the future is to be nonjudgmental, neither promoting an intervention nor denigrating its utility. Balance will be necessary to engage surrogates and as able, subjects/patients in these complicated questions. Unilateral judgments will be insufficient for the phronesis, or practical wisdom necessary to achieve a proportionate outcome.

But when critics speak of DBS in MCS they bring biases to the analysis.[23] One commentator creates hypotheticals for its use after erroneously defining MCS:

> The term refers, in fact, to a spectrum where patients at one end may be locked-in-syndrome (LiS) and at the other in a persistent vegetative state.[24]

And after that error-laden definition, he suggests the application of DBS in MCS for which there are no current protocols (for anoxic brain injury) and envisions its application in TBI ten months after injury. The latter, as we have seen, would be a protocol violation given the course of natural recovery. Then, using his two hypothetical cases he seeks to define types of medical futility, including a category he describes as having *"the risk of unacceptable badness* (the RUB)." He concludes with a healthy dose of ambivalence, but not before using this nascent technology as a rhetorical straw man in an article provocatively entitled, "Minimally Conscious States, Deep Brain Stimulation and What Is Worse Than Futility."

TEARS FOR CORY

While we need to be prudent about any intervention that holds both promise and peril, the physician and philosopher of medicine, the late Lewis Thomas, rightly described early innovation as *half-way technologies.*[25] DBS for MCS is no exception. While it represents progress in facilitating consciousness and providing a means for improved motor output in MCS, it is not a cure. It is a step in the right direction but one that comes with burdens and imperfections. These challenges must be borne if progress is to be made. The question is, are these burdens proportionate or not to the hypothetical benefits of the interventions?

We concluded our *Nature* paper tentatively for just that reason, neither endorsing nor rejecting this nascent work in a categorical fashion. Instead we pointed to the need to develop "a neuropalliative ethic of care to establish proportionate goals of care to help families balance the potential for improvement against associated burdens while being guided by the patient's previously articulated wishes."[16]

Having a responsive family does not answer the question of what to do, but it does provide a locus for responsive and responsible decision making. Although there will always be a quest for certainty in these deliberations,[26] it is far wiser to engage a process that will lead to better responses and locate the decision in a proper place. In my view that locale is in the nexus of families, properly informed and assisted.

Families will need to make these judgments with the assistance of their clinicians and investigators. But to pursue these decisions, it is absolutely critical that *a priori* prejudicial preconceptions are abandoned. Residue from the right-to-die debate – which simplifies the ethical choices related to MCS with prosthetically aided communication – can lead to rather unreflective responses. In Greg's case, it could lead to an altogether erroneous reason for his sadness. What exactly is making him sad?

It is a question that needs to be asked given his improved brain state. The reflexive response that equates sadness with a decision to withhold or withdraw therapy or with a desire to die hinders deeper analysis that might indicate that Greg's emotions and feelings are not as primitive as one might think and are more like what you and I might experience.

Consider Corinth's recounting of one episode of Greg's sadness. When asked if this has been a "good chapter," she told me, "Yes, it has." Before the surgery, "... you don't know how he feels, because in six years he didn't say a word. He never opened his mouth to say anything. ... Now to have him say words. ... These are things he couldn't do before."

She continues, "He was crying one day I was visiting him and I said, 'Greg why are you crying?'"

"He says, 'I'm crying for Cory.'"

Innocently, I asked, "Who's Cory?"

"*That's his brother.* That's his brother that does not come to see him, that's in denial."

Corinth's analysis, "And even I started crying because here he is, he's aware, he knows what's going on." To the surprise of his mother, Greg remembered he had a brother and knew that he had not come around to visit. The brief comment that he is crying for Cory suggests memory and implies that he is hurt. And perhaps even that Greg is crying because Cory is grieving for his brother. It is a comment pregnant with meaning and one that begs caution for any commentator who assumes that they know the latent content of this discourse without knowledge of its context and provenance. To engage in precipitous analysis would be to again silence patients like Greg after they had regained voice.

Corinth repeats herself, "So for him to say that day, I said, 'why are you crying?' He says, 'I'm crying for Cory.' "

Greg said it "plain" and softly and "not as loud as I'd like to hear him." Both in tone and substance, there was sadness in Greg's voice and Corinth's recounting. The repetition is to remind herself that Greg's comment suggests a level of understanding that his laconic speech does not fully convey. Here is a person embodied in that soft-spoken voice with a full repertoire of sentiments. Greg is keenly feeling the absence of a brother he still loves.

And his recollection of Cory prompts another admission, the possibility that Greg misses others too. Then, Corinth tells me, "I'm sure he misses [Cory], and he has a daughter that does not come to visit him."

By this point, I had known Corinth for a couple of years and did not know that Greg had a child. But all of a sudden, his ability to communicate had opened the door to the fullness of his relationships. Once again, he has been placed squarely in the room and into the nexus of his family, including his daughter Tamika.

Tamika was eighteen years old when this interview took place in 2008. Corinth thinks she is in denial too. She was ten when Greg was hurt and stayed close to him at the outset. She knows the story but does not talk about her father. The hurt was just too much for the young child.

Corinth admits that Tamika is herself in a great deal of pain, "I think so. Well her grandfather is very angry with her, but I'm not. He thinks that she should come and visit her dad." Corinth wishes she would visit because Tamika would give her pictures to share with Greg. "She would tell me to give them to him. She had a prom picture and I hung it in his room."

Corinth has no doubt that Greg "knows, he knows it's Tamika. He can say Tamika." And she is sure Greg misses his estranged daughter "because if you show him a picture and you say, 'Greg, who is this?' And he'll say, 'Tamika.' "

A painful existence, but not a shallow one. It is a sadness that neither invalidates the feelings, nor the surgery that made those sentiments possible, but rather a sadness that should compel others to act. Corinth agrees, "That's why I feel that he gets depressed now. I bought a van so that I would be able to come and pick him up ... a handicapped van. It worked fine last summer, but this summer it's nothing. I have to have brakes and I got to have shocks, so I have not been able to get the van to come and pick him up and I think that has a lot to do with his depression too because I'm not able to come and get him out and take him on trips like I did ... before he would look forward to coming, they would have him ready, I would come pick him up in the van and take him out."

She also laments her inability to do more for Greg, to provide the companionship he needs, "Most of my main concerns – I can't get up here [to JFK]. I can't do what other mothers are doing that I wish I *could* do ... could be here every day with him. I wish I could bring him home and then bring him to therapy, but I can't. I don't live in that type of housing. . . ."

Given Corinth's comments, it is plausible to think that Greg's "depression" is contextual. It is more the consequence of his felt loss of loved ones than a perspective on his overall circumstances. Although the latter is expected, the former is supported by the facts. So in lieu of condemning Greg's brain state as one "worse than futile," put a brake on the distant commentary. Instead, it might be better to appreciate the depth of his perceptions, *human and complex as they are,* and consider what support might be provided to families like Corinth's so at the very least they could get their "handicapped van" equipped with workable parts.

Perhaps that is all it would take to improve Greg's perspective and have him echo Terry Wallis's sentiments as told to me by his mother, Angilee. There had been a family gathering in their Arkansan town of Mountain View, and Terry was in attendance with all his friends and family, including a bunch of cousins his own age. Spontaneously, Terry turned to his mother and softly declared, "Mama, life is good!"[13]

It was a welcome comment indicative of Terry's state of mind and the happiness he felt being with his family and friends. It also pointed to the importance of context. Would Terry have been as happy if he was socially isolated and his family had been unable to make provisions to bring him home? If they couldn't make the extensive renovations necessary to accommodate his disability? Would he then feel the sadness that Greg feels?

It is an apt comparison and one compelled in part by necessity. Both Terry and Greg (post DBS) have emerged from MCS and now have the ability to express themselves. Both indicate in *their* comments the importance of family to their well-being. Don Herbert, the Buffalo firefighter, also felt the strong pull of family when he briefly emerged from MCS and spoke fluently. His brief awakening did not celebrate the happiness that comes with yearly family celebrations, but rather a sadness that comes from *missing* so many gatherings. His love of family was expressed through a father's guilt, a sad culpability, encapsulated in a remorseful, "I've been gone a long time. . . ."

And the difference in these perspectives also speaks to the caution of painting these patients with a single stroke. Doing so dangerously ignores the unique and reemergent individuality of each of these patients and obscures the human need captured in their personal narratives.[27] Summoned from exile, each of these patients deserve better. Society can ill afford viewing another group through the narrow frame of a stereotype, especially those whose return to a human community has so long been severed.

FREEDOM'S GONE

Gregory Tyrone "Freedom" Pearson died on September 7, 2011. He was forty-three.

Niko and I drove to Patterson to attend the funeral. It was a sunny, indeed beautiful day, against which was cast the inner city decay of a town that the physician-poet William Carlos Williams had written so evocatively.[28] And now another chapter from that storied town. . . .

We found the Hughes Funeral Home, a clapboard building on a tree-lined street with old houses in varying states of decay. We sat in the last row of the chapel so as not to interrupt the ritual. Most of all we wanted to be respectful of the family's grief. But as unobtrusive as was our choice of seats, after the Reverend spoke, we were the first directed to walk past the open casket. So up we went, with his personal physician Dr. McCagg and Jeanne O'Connor, a physician assistant from JFK who was also on the DBS study. All eyes were upon us. The room was full with a few floral decorations toward the front.

It is always sobering for a physician to attend a patient's funeral,[29] but this was different. Greg was not our patient, but a subject in a clinical trial that had shown what might be possible for patients like him who had been cast aside and viewed as irretrievably hopeless. It was work, if it could be sustained, that might make a difference for other patients with disorders of consciousness. But my thought as I walked toward the front was whether we had made a difference in Greg's too short and sad life. We had brought a few moments of joy to Corinth, and she thanked us. But to Greg? That was a question I wish he could have answered. I wish he had had more time, made more progress. Now I hope that this earnest attempt at telling his story is a fitting legacy to a young man who, with his courageous family, made history.

19 Maggie Is in Town

I walked over to the Neuro Unit at New York–Presbyterian Weill Cornell Medical Center on a cold and wet night to see Maggie after speaking with her mother that morning. It was now February 26, 2008, just a few months shy of the second anniversary of her stroke. As I crossed York Avenue, I thought about all that Nancy had shared with me about her daughter and herself. It was an informative interview, but so unbelievably sad. It was the first time I'd heard Maggie's story.

Nancy filled in the gaps of her biography. She was one of those kids who did it all. Academically strong and involved in enough co-curricular activities to keep several students busy. According to *The Providence Journal*, she was an honor roll student, dorm president, freshman captain of the crew team, and an Ultimate Frisbee player.[1] She had studied abroad and did a semester in Granada, Spain. A classmate recalls Maggie as someone who "was rarely ever sitting still."[2] She was a whirlwind.

With no shortage of pride, Nancy told me that Smith College had awarded Maggie her bachelor's degree. Because her stroke occurred at the end of her senior year, she already had enough credits, so she was allowed to graduate. During commencement ceremonies, her classmates wore blue ribbons in solidarity with their friend. Stacey Baird, the president of the Smith class of 2006 and student speaker, dedicated her commencement address to Maggie.[3]

By all accounts Maggie was an exceptional individual. Her friends mourning their early loss wrote essays and poems, all of which indicate the profundity of what a basilar artery stroke can do to injure the brainstem and shatter a promising life. At Middleboro Skilled Care Center, her friends put up one thousand origami paper cranes in her room, which according to Japanese legend promotes the return to health.

Nancy told me Maggie hoped to become a veterinarian. She loved working with animals and their house had been a menagerie with cats, dogs, hermit crabs, and a parakeet. She and her high school boyfriend were going to work at an animal shelter the summer after graduation. But all that had changed.

A few months after Maggie's stroke, she told a local newspaper, "I have to stay strong for her. She'd do it for me. It's definitely not easy. I work 40 hours a week and go to school, but I'd do anything in the world for her." Two lives inalterably changed, "I don't think anyone in the universe has ever felt love like we do."[2] But after several years, he stopped visiting Maggie because he couldn't take it any longer.[2]

That morning we spoke of Maggie's life and Nancy's hopes. At one point after multiple bouts of near fatal cases of pneumonia Nancy told me she had come close to withdrawing life-sustaining care, only to be pulled back from that decision by her ex-husband, who needed more time to adjust to the grim reality of his daughter's fate. He had been less involved with Maggie's daily care and had understandable difficulty coming to grips with the seemingly poor nature of her prognosis. He would need time to come to the decision Nancy was contemplating, so Nancy gave him some time.

Nancy was a realist and pragmatic in her approach about these choices and how far to go. She wanted to give Maggie every chance to improve and felt that she had done more than most would over the twenty-one months since her injury. She had rebuffed early calls to withdraw care by aggressive and opinionated doctors but had agreed to orders not to resuscitate her. She figured that if Maggie had deteriorated to that point, resuscitation would be pointless if not futile. If it got that bad, Maggie would be declaring herself. But in February 2008, when Nancy brought her daughter to visit us at Weill Cornell, Nancy was not ready to give up. The research we were doing was important to her. What we might, or might not, learn would help her think through how to best serve her daughter. It would help set or delay an internal clock about when watchful waiting and keeping the vigil had gone on long enough. Or it could encourage more patience and hope.

Nancy desperately wanted to know if Maggie could somehow be helped and whether there was something neurologically in her brain that might sustain "cognition." She *needed* to know if Maggie was aware, if she knew who she was or who her Mom was. She wanted to know if she was still connected.

We might call that something "consciousness," but no matter, that is what Nancy was looking for and calling it at the time. To clarify that elusive question if there was a "there, there." Might that inner space of her mind be amenable to recovery and allow Maggie to be reintegrated into her family and the outside world? Might she ever communicate? Could she know that people who loved her cared?

This was not a trivial question because Maggie had been diagnosed as being vegetative at her nursing home, a state that would represent permanent unconsciousness, some twenty months after her injury when she came to New York. Dr. Doug Katz had his doubts. He had thought she had occasionally been able to track objects in the environment. That would make her minimally conscious and warranted a closer look.

But to the world, it would be hard to distinguish that she wasn't vegetative. She was nearly always unresponsive, lying inertly in bed, with a feeding tube and tracheostomy tube in place. She was paralyzed. Her face was broken out in acne from bandages still in place and her head still shaven. Her extremities extended themselves involuntarily in a posturing pattern indicative of the severe injury sustained by her brainstem. None of that was under her control. Most of the time, her eye lids were shut, though sometimes her left eye peeked out when she was asleep, skewing off to the side.

DIAGNOSTIC PURSUITS

As I looked at Maggie, after talking with her mother that morning and hearing her story, I reflected upon how far Niko and I had come with our research program. We had made modest progress and still had much to do scientifically and in social policy to help patients like Maggie get the care they need and deserve.

It was beyond tragic that Nancy was still in pursuit of a *diagnosis*, or at least, *a correct one*. I wondered what would have happened to Maggie if Doug Katz had not wondered about her. Like so many others she would have been lost to follow up, anonymous in an uncaring system of chronic care, designed to warehouse people like her, not investigate their brain states or make a credible diagnosis, to figure out if that person who had been labeled as vegetative was actually aware or perhaps conscious.

As I walked over to the hospital, I thought back to a fax I received in 2005, just as the Schiavo case was getting attention in the media. A woman wrote me to help her husband get a proper diagnosis. He was in his seventies and was a nuclear physicist and a professor. He had been lecturing when he had a cardiac arrest and sustained anoxic brain injury. She wanted to bring him down to Cornell to be assessed. Her fax was straightforward and realistic. She was not sentimental about the outcome, she just wanted to know if her husband was awake, alert, or had a chance:

> The focus of my concern is that not-very-stringent diagnostic procedures have been applied to my husband's condition, yet he has been described as Vegetative. He is in a Nursing Home. The consequences are that he is disqualified from any real therapy. I gather from my reading, that this is common practice.[4]

She went on to write that she did not hope for a miracle, just an honest diagnosis so she could make informed choices about his care. She needed to be more confident about his condition and their future. She loved her husband and wanted to do whatever she could and at the same time reflect on the futility of the situation, as he would, if there was no hope of a recovery.

I was touched by her mix of compassion and realism and spoke with Niko to see what we might do. Even bringing him to Cornell was a challenge. If he came to Manhattan, where would we see him? Where could we examine him? He was on a stretcher and the clinics we routinely used for clinical work were too small to accommodate him. We had yet to begin our program of bringing in research subjects and studying them over a three-day period. We weren't prepared to enroll subjects, much less use neuroimaging to peer into his brain and clarify his status.

Yet the fax motivated us to help configure a solution. We were way too familiar with the scenario she painted of a nursing home diagnosis that was potentially out of date, hopelessly wrong or perhaps heartbreakingly correct. Either way, this nice lady needed to know. We could take a good history and do a good neuro exam – the basics – and see what we could learn. We could also talk to her about her ethical choices and options once we knew a bit more.

So we scrambled and figured out a way to bring him down from upstate and have him examined in the newly renovated out-patient rehabilitation medicine clinic. Its director, Dr. Mike O'Dell, had worked with brain injured patients before coming to Weill Cornell. His clinic could accommodate stretchers and he'd lend us the space. I was thrilled by his generosity and our ability to cobble something together.

I think it was a Friday when I called the wife of the patient back. I could hardly contain my own excitement at our small victory in the face of the neglect of patients like her husband. But as soon as I blurted out our plan for him, she interrupted me. "Oh, Dr. Fins," I recall her saying, "My husband, he developed a bedsore and he died last night."

I was so saddened by what she said, and offered my condolences. I sat at my desk and said we could, no, *we must* do better to help these people and their families who are trapped in a state of ignorance that makes life so hard and bereavement impossible. I really pitied her. She obviously cared about her husband and will now be asking herself if he was there all along.

IT IS WHAT IT IS

We could not help him, but at least now – with Maggie and the others – we were at the beginning of a program to learn more about these patients. We had begun to admit patients to the hospital for a three-day stay and multimodal testing. Perhaps it wasn't the inception of our work, but the start of something new, a productive middle geared at the fundamental question of mechanism and why some brains so long dormant recovered that precious thread of consciousness that had been lost.

Maggie's physical exam and her story were a case in point. At the bedside, for example, she sometimes coughed vigorously when her trach tube got clogged. She seemed to experience these obstructions far worse than other patients we had seen. Her discomfort was suggestive of the hyperesthesia seen in a locked-in patient. Was there a clue there about her diagnosis? Was she more locked-in than vegetative, or a case of being both minimally conscious and locked-in, that is, severe motor impairment because of her brainstem injury coupled with some degree of cognitive impairment?

Her face would flush as she coughed violently. Whether it was worse than others, I cannot say, but many of us in the room made that same mental note. It might have been a nod to clinical science, or been prompted by a sense of empathy and projection. Her flushed, acned face and seemingly unconscious self was a stark, almost unbearable, contrast to the photo at her bedside of an absolutely striking college senior on the cusp of a life and accomplishment. And now she was here with all of us, all because of Doug Katz's diligence and curiosity.

Doug thought she was probably minimally conscious, although her nursing home – with far less medical rigor or sophistication – had her labeled as vegetative. So Maggie was here for a number of imaging and electrophysiologic studies administered under an institutional review board and through research protocols – PET scans, functional MRI, diffusion tensor imaging and passive language paradigms with forward/backward narratives, ones like those used by colleagues at Liege and Cambridge. In addition, we hooked her up to a video EEG to look at her brain waves and check for physical and/or electrical evidence of seizures.

So there she was, finally in New York after that long hiatus of recurrent pneumonias that kept her from coming and almost led her Mom to decide to withdraw life-sustaining therapy. We were glad she was at Cornell, but it was curious because it didn't all add up.

Earlier structural brain imaging studies looked better than they should have. Unlike vegetative patients who lose brain mass as the brain ceases to interact with itself, her brain did not show atrophy or shrinkage like those of Quinlan or Schiavo. Their brains weighed progressively less the longer they were in the vegetative state.

In contrast, Maggie's brain hadn't undergone that deterioration. It looked quite "normal" save for the devastating injury in the brainstem and some small, but potentially significant, areas of infarction in the middle brain structures of the thalamus.

The other thing that did not add up was her rare but definitive tracking of objects in her visual field on some prior examinations. By diagnostic criteria that alone would make her MCS. So she was a curiosity worthy of further clinical and scholarly engagement.

As we have seen, patients like Maggie who suggest some sort of diagnostic incongruity are like questions that go unanswered. It is sometimes easier to let the curious pieces be and not open up the prospect that a patient thought to be permanently unconscious, without hope of any incremental recovery, might in fact be conscious with an unclear, and still as yet, unknowable possibility to recover function.

Such questions disturb the status quo and force families and clinicians to address difficult questions about burdens and benefits of these liminal states, the possibility of awareness and reconnection and the specter of consciousness and isolation. It is a moment reminiscent of Jack Nicholson's famous quip in *A Few Good Men*, "You can't handle the truth. ...."[5] But to the credit of Nancy and Doug Katz, they wanted to pursue the truth and address these questions forthrightly. It was a courageous decision, taking whatever reality lay ahead in the search for diagnostic clarity, as best as we can know it.

Dr. Kathy Foley, our teacher and a neurologist and palliative care expert at Memorial Sloan-Kettering Cancer Center always taught Niko and me that, "it is what it is." In her view, once you accepted what you had been dealt you could deal with it and make things, if not good, at least a bit better. Her aphorism became a watchword for us as we sought to deal with the complexity we encountered, not as some might wish them to be but as they were. We were not going to ignore certain findings because they raised difficult questions or challenged convention.

It was a long-held philosophy, and the only one that could possibly work in a field so divided by ideology and partisanship. I had first declared my adherence to this approach in a paper I wrote with Dr. Plum during the Schiavo debate when people were interpreting her clinical exam based on an ideological stance they wanted to satisfy. The title of our paper, said it all: "Neurological Diagnosis Is More Than a State of Mind," and our point was that the diagnostic act should be devoid of value choices.[6] Whatever moral valuation we place on a diagnosis follows upon those facts. Values should not distort the clinical reality. It is what it is ... there was no other way to deal with what we would confront with our patients and their families. We had to be honest because our credibility would be tested as much by what we knew as what we did not know.

To her enduring credit, Nancy was of the same philosophical school and she wanted to know as much about Maggie's condition as she could, whatever the ethical and clinical challenges that might come forth. So she sought us out for that purpose and wanted us to be as honest as possible.

VEGETATIVE ON ARRIVAL

The first day at Cornell was a huge disappointment. Despite Doug Katz's earlier assessment, we found Maggie to be in the vegetative state on multiple clinical examinations across the day. Her eyes remained closed most of the time. There was no evidence of visual tracking. Nonetheless, the first imaging study done was extremely puzzling. It was a high-resolution MRI that showed minimal if any atrophy of her brain above the level of her severely injured brainstem. This was surprising because we had expected shrinkage of her brain, as is found in vegetative patients. With better methods we had confirmed a paradoxical finding *inconsistent* with her being in the vegetative state.

Even our team, known for its optimism and sense of expectancy, had a sense that day of doubt and disappointment that maybe Maggie was in fact vegetative and not minimally conscious as Doug Katz had hoped. We had been surprised before and would have to wait to see her another day.

WITH THE FLICK OF AN EYE

The next night, Niko briefed me on his exam earlier in the day. He was there with our colleagues Jennifer Hersh and Dr. Mary Conte. In contrast to the day before, Niko had confirmed a small degree of responsiveness and had been able to get her to look downward to command with her more functional left eye on four of six occasions. That purposeful action confirmed Doug Katz's suspicion that she was not vegetative but rather minimally conscious. It also raised the possibility that she could be even more aware but unable to *behaviorally* demonstrate engagement with the outside world.

As Niko was telling me about his exams earlier in the day, we were also looking at the bedside EEG monitor. Again, another paradox. The squiggly lines on the screen, reminiscent of my neurologist colleague's handwriting I thought, looked healthier than the patient we saw in the bed. Save for some slowing in the frontal part of the brain and some degree of asymmetry from side to side, the EEG looked pretty good. A suggestive sign that perhaps she was not in fact in the vegetative state, although it was not a conclusive diagnostic test.

And her violent response to suctioning and to noxious stimuli were also something that might suggest a higher degree of awareness and perhaps even the locked-in-state, which again, is a state of normal consciousness without an ability to demonstrate motor activity below the damaged brainstem. As described earlier, such patients, like that depicted in *The Diving Bell and the Butterfly*,[7] can only move their eyes because the cranial nerves that move the eyes are higher up in the brainstem above the injury, much like Maggie.

So confronted by all these paradoxes, we sought to see if we could again reproduce her earlier response of moving her eye down, to signal *yes*. Initially, she was sleeping after her violent coughing spell. Her left eye was askew. Her mother told us that it often went astray when she drifts off to sleep.

We started simply, asking the most basic of questions. Niko asked, "Look down if you want to answer yes. Look down for yes."

Normally, we would hold up a pen and ask, "Is that a pen?" But this time Niko did something different. Without speaking with me about my morning interview with Nancy and knowing the significance of the question, he turned to Maggie and asked, "Is that your mother?"

A long pause, perhaps twenty seconds, and then a clear and controlled look down with her left eye. All of us in the room saw it, including Nancy. It seemed an innocent enough question and was intended as such. We could have easily pointed to a watch and asked, is this a watch? Look down for yes. Or a pen?

But my colleague's simple question and its quiet response was anything but simple. With a silent downward gaze, Maggie spoke volumes. She told us she knew Nancy was her Mom, providing an answer to a mystery that only a parent could fathom.

With the flick of her eye, we all knew that the innocence of the question had vanished. The response was not trivial but consequential. It spoke of promise and peril.

Nancy came over to hug me, sobbing, with what could have been tears of joy or fear. I did not know, but thought at that juncture it was best to just hold on tight. As I looked over her shoulder, I saw that my colleagues all had tears in their eyes.

For now, they were tears of joy.

TO LOOK MORE CLOSELY

Through careful perseverance, we had gotten a glimmer of what might be inside Maggie's head. Later we got her to track to a mirror, firmly establishing MCS as a diagnosis and a functional floor. Her response with her eye, however, raised the question of what her ceiling would be. If she could recognize her mom, what else might be possible? Although she looked down, she might as well have been scanning the heights. It was exciting but equally frightening.

Had this young woman characterized as being vegetative, actually been in a locked-in-state of near normal consciousness without a means of outgoing communication because she had no motor output? Or was she somewhere between MCS and being locked in? Either way, by presenting us with this question, she had embodied the problem space for all of us studying disorders of consciousness and the role that neuroimaging is likely to take in discriminating between such possibilities.

The preliminary data from the neuroimaging studies suggested that she was intermittently following commands and therefore had some awareness, but the results seemed inconsistent and would need more analysis.[8] But the key point was that Maggie's response was *not* nothing – she was responding to external stimuli both by imaging and behavioral metrics. These responses were inconsistent with the vegetative state, raising all sorts of interesting questions but answering the most important one: Maggie was indeed conscious.

WHAT DID THE NEIGHBORS THINK?

The news from New York gave legitimacy to Nancy's decisions and permission to maintain her stance of advocacy. Nancy told her friends, "No, Margaret isn't in a persistent vegetative state. She's totally there, or as much there as we can know."

The information, as preliminary as it was, made a difference to her friends who were skeptical about ongoing care and whether it was motivated by Maggie's *or Nancy's* needs. She told us, "I think it's changed actually. Well I have one friend, a really close friend, who was really vocal in saying 'you're keeping her alive for you. She's really dead, more dead than alive.'" It was a hard thing to hear and even harder to share because Nancy did take it to heart, wondering about her motivations. Now she had an answer to the question she had long sought to understand. Maggie knew enough about herself to know that she was her mother's daughter. And now Nancy knew that Maggie knew she was not alone, isolated inside her head.

Since her return to Massachusetts her friend has apologized to Nancy for questioning her motivations. Nancy adds that it has been an education for her friend who has had "to really rethink her whole, her own attitude" about Maggie, because outwardly she is the same. Nancy explains, "... it isn't that Margaret is dramatically different now then she was; her behavior is not dramatically different. ... So she's [her friend] really had to examine her own attitude about her just comfort with Margaret being the way she was. ..." Her friend has had to reconsider "her own idea that it would be humiliating to have to have someone change your diaper and bathe you, and that wouldn't *for her* be a life."

All that had to change because up to that point her friend could assert that "Margaret wasn't really conscious anyway, she wasn't in there, so she wouldn't want this." But that had changed and to her friend's credit she was open to the results and what they might mean." She has had "a lot of thoughts about it. So she's been doing a lot of reading and she's changed her thinking. I mean, she still visits Margaret the same as she has all along because she was trying to support me, even when she was arguing with me."

The neuroimaging data coupled with the revised MCS diagnosis, has been a game changer in her community. Nancy explained that "people had to really think of their sort of attitudes, or their behavior. I mean even at the nursing home, I wouldn't say that people are treating her differently, but they're thinking about her differently because I think they were careful to always treat her as though she was conscious. . . ."

Nancy thinks that the imaging data, though still unproven and investigational, was the key to the change in attitudes. It both reveals and implores people to look more closely at both Maggie, *and themselves*.

ANOTHER KIND OF MEDICAL NECESSITY

Even Maggie's doctors were affected by the power of the neuroimaging data. For her neurologist, it was a confirmation of a clinical suspicion. For her nursing home doctor, it was information that could prompt a change in her diagnostic status.

Nancy explained, "I would say both Dr. Katz and Dr. Landon needed to have the clinical information in front of them, in addition to seeing the behavior, because they wanted verification of the change. . . ." For Doug Katz the combination of the exams in New York and neuroimaging data helped to confirm his sense that Maggie was conscious. As Nancy put it, "I think he was leaning that way [toward MCS], which is why he wanted to send her [to New York]."

She continued, "Dr. Katz was very familiar with what you had done. So, to him it confirmed his suspicion . . . the possibilities. I mean, when he looked at her MRI [and] what he was saying was similar to what Dr. Schiff was saying. 'It looks to me like she could have consciousness but I don't know.' And so this is why he pushed for her to come, so that there'd be more data that would prove his theoretical idea, because in front of Dr. Katz, Margaret never did it. I mean he tried all the odd testing as well. You're in a dark room with a flashlight moving – she didn't respond to him. It didn't happen. And he had seen her three times . . . it actually didn't happen dramatically since he's seen her, but . . . he sees her one time for twenty minutes."

Dr. Landon, the doctor at the nursing home, was more cautious about changing her diagnosis. He had given Maggie the vegetative diagnosis and "wouldn't change it until he specifically got something from Dr. Katz." I thought that a revealing response given the reports of her visit in New York and wondered whether his hesitancy to change the status quo was a reflection of the forces that led to so many MCS patients being misdiagnosed as vegetative. It *is* difficult to view these brain states as transient and open to change, unlike the fixed diagnoses to which doctors are more accustomed. Patients don't generally go from having diabetes or kidney disease one day and not having it the next, so why should one be vegetative one day and minimally conscious the next? His hesitancy was understandable. He needed some sort of permission to advance her diagnosis.

I suspect it was a different kind of "medical necessity."

YOUR BRAIN IS WORKING

But there was something more profound than the technical aspects of the imaging; it was the receptivity, the openness to the possibility that Maggie might be conscious. Nancy put it this way, "I guess there were two things: there was the fact that Margaret could now show with her eyes and respond. And now that didn't happen because of the imaging, but it did happen because she was here in an atmosphere where people were saying to *her,* 'You are conscious, we know you're conscious. Your brain is working.' So they were supporting her into showing that she could think."

This was a stark contrast to the environment Nancy and Maggie had encountered until then. Even Maggie seemed to have a new image of herself. Nancy contrasted how it was different in New York. Before the trip, "... everyone around you is saying you're in a persistent vegetative state ... and then she is in an environment where people are open to the possibility that she is not."

Nancy admits, "I don't know what she's been doing, nobody knows ..." but she figures that "... even if you're in a weak condition and you're foggy ..." the pessimism of those around her had to have some effect. If Maggie was thinking then was she also "wondering?"

"But then suddenly she's in an environment where there's people, things, for sure, [that show] with certainty" that she might be aware and conscious. Referring to the fMRI studies, she said with a sense of relief and gratitude, "I mean, this image shows that your brain is working." It changes everything. "I don't know, but Margaret was more alert and more present during those three days than she had been for months."

Is this a mother's wishful thinking or a real response by Maggie to her environment? I think it was the latter and that her reaction was quintessentially human. She responded like any of the rest of us would if all of a sudden someone was paying attention. Finally, she was being recognized as if she was there, brought in from the cold. Now that the world was engaging with her, as if she was there, she would make an effort to engage us.

The next morning after she acknowledged her mother, she greeted the team with a flurry of eye moment, looking down for yes, as she had the night before. It was if she was signaling us: don't forget that I am here. This is but a speculation, I admit, but it was the consensus of the team. Maggie had made contact and she did not want to lose the companionship. It was too hard won.

IT CHANGED MARGARET'S LIFE

Back at home, the excitement of New York was met with regret. Maggie's speech therapists were upset that they had missed Maggie's responsiveness.

Despite their earnest efforts, "the speech therapists were mortified, were horrified at themselves that they hadn't found this response, that they hadn't seen it." It was especially difficult for them "because they said, 'We know we tested her. We know we must have done many of the same things.'" Nancy is agnostic on how it happened, "And I'm not saying that their attitude prohibited them from seeing, it could have been just timing – that ... they didn't catch her when she was in."

But it was a time for reflection not recriminations. Leaving New York, Nancy put her feelings in a poem, which she was kind enough to share. Her conclusion captured the ethical ambiguity of Maggie's new found state:

> Not a happy ending, because
> my daughter is still unmoving
>   and silent, but today
>   she can speak "yes"
> by moving her eye.[9]

She was clearly ambivalent about her present condition, but unequivocal about what her visit to Cornell in February 2008 had meant for her daughter. For better or worse, the experience had changed everything.

At our next meeting, in September 2009, Nancy recalls a conversation we'd had, "I remembered that you had asked me that morning a question that really had struck me as important which was, 'what would be the most important thing for you to amplify Margaret's quality of life?' I can't remember exactly how you said it. And I said, 'if she had consciousness, if I knew she had consciousness and she could communicate.'"

She pauses, "So that was at 10:00 [that morning], and at 6:00 that night, she did those two things." It was a piercing mix of elation and desperation almost impossible to reconcile in a moment. She explains, "So, I mean, I was stunned, I was shocked, I was elated, I mean, I was angry, frustrated you know ... I think more happy, but also thinking I can't believe that eighteen months have gone by before this could happen, you know. But I just ... you know, you just put that aside and pray that from now we can do something, and this is what I hoped for."

It was a mix of sadness for what might have interceded and the isolation that might have been better breached, although it is also quite possible that Maggie had only recently entered the MCS and been able to respond with her eyes. Without careful longitudinal tracking of her abilities over time, it would be impossible to know if her recent diagnosis of MCS was timely or late in coming. But whatever its time course, there could be no doubt that things had forever changed for Maggie and Nancy. Their relationship at some level had been reconstituted. What had been one-sided had now become reciprocal and relational. Maggie and Nancy were again communicating. The revelation that this was possible was profound and heartfelt, "And I mean, I think it changed Margaret's life drastically, and it changed my life in terms of my thinking about Margaret. . . ."

IN PURSUIT OF PAIN

One of the things weighing on Nancy's mind was the question regarding if Maggie was in pain. From the interviews we have conducted, it seems that this is a universal concern of families. It seems especially pronounced in parents whose children have a disorder of consciousness, the fear that their child will be in pain and no one will know about it. Unable to communicate, they are isolated and potentially subjected to a torment for which there might be relief, if only someone knew. The ability to communicate, at even the most rudimentary level, allows patients to be asked about their pain and distress.

Nancy shares her relief over Maggie's newfound capability, "I think that at least because she's able to communicate, her speech therapist is able to ask her, for example, if she's in pain, then she can get her pain medication." But communication can also do so much more. It can help distinguish between physical and emotional distress.

Nancy recalls taking Maggie to a meditation class that she thought might be helpful. All went well until the end of the session when "Maggie started posturing and making some movements that I thought looked like that she was frustrated or upset. And so we were asking her questions about that movement, 'are you in pain, are you uncomfortable?' "

At first they asked her if she were frustrated or angry and to their surprise, ". . . she ended up saying that with all those choices of words that we gave her, she chose *happy*." Like Greg Pearson who cried for his absent brother, Maggie confounded expectations when questioned more closely.

Nancy explained that Maggie expressed that she was both happy and in pain. An interesting mix of emotions and sensations not usually ascribed to people like Maggie but which they are *capable*. The explanation was understandable. Nancy told me, ". . . it turned out she was in pain in her leg." It was that simple. Sometimes when she sits in her chair, her legs would stiffen up and she would need them extended. Even Nancy could misinterpret it as sadness or something worse. Her ability to now communicate and differentiate what she was experiencing and feeling was very helpful, "And so to me, her saying her leg was in pain, that's what I saw as frustration or anger, and it helped me to differentiate between a physical problem and an emotional state."

Given the tendency to undertreat pain, or write off distress as emotional when it is physical, Maggie's ability to communicate is critically important.

It preempts the experience of treatable pain and compels caregivers to assure that questions about distress are part of her routine assessment.

TIME PRESENT, TIME PAST

It started off as an innocent enough question about the difficulties of caregivers not having known Maggie before her stroke. How might the absence of a prior relationship influence caregiving when there is neither recourse to shared memory nor knowledge of what Maggie actually remembers?

It was even a challenge for Nancy, who of course shared much of her life with her daughter. But it is a life that is remembered? Does the past influence Maggie's present, much less her future? Nancy reminded me that even when she is with Maggie, *she* does not know what memories Maggie retains of their shared past, if she recalls much at all. After New York, the question became more profound, because if Maggie recognizes her mother, it might suggest that she remembers more than less. If she did not know her mother, the person closest to her, it would be unlikely that she would have access to her past. But now she knows at least something about her family and it prompts the question, how much has she retained?

Nancy cannot presume that the past is known and part of their relationship. And because of that she has resolved to live their new life together in the present. That way they can share the moment and potentially build a new past together as the present recedes into memory.

In the *Four Quartets*, T. S. Elliot wrote

> Time present and time past
> Are both perhaps present in time future,
> And time future contained in time past.
> If all time is eternally present
> All time is unredeemable.[10]

Nancy wasn't so sure about time future being contained in time past. She might have agreed with the poet that time is unredeemable, as ruptured as her family's experience had been. So Nancy decided that she and Maggie would do their best to live in the moment, to allow Maggie to have new experiences, to have a future untethered to the past. Not that the past did not exist, but to allow Maggie the chance to have new experiences and relationships in her current state, independent of the past and memories that may, or may not, still be part of her.

And even if Maggie had full memory of her past, Nancy did not want her to linger there and not have new experiences and enjoyments. That would further impoverish her already constrained existence and seemed unfair, if not cruel. So Nancy decided to make the most of the present with her daughter. She told me forthrightly, "... one of the things that I had thought right along, right from the beginning, was that I didn't want Margaret to only have memories, I wanted her to have experiences, in the present."

So she bought a van and altered her work schedule. She wanted to do things with Maggie, give her a context, "... so she has things that people can reference that they know about ... in her present life. So it isn't only past memories ... that Margaret has access to, which I think is important."

It was also a strategy for *social* engagement. Nancy was creating new memories so that others could meet Maggie in the here and now, the only existence we know she experiences. It was a meeting place for everyone, even for her friends and family who knew her before, "... so that person who had that relationship with Margaret can also have a present experience with her." And for Maggie, it "normalizes her life for those moments."

This normalization is symbolized by their van. It is a vehicle for making their journey in the moment. It allows them to go out together, shop, and have lunch. She asks rhetorically, "what do mothers and daughter do?" Yes, it's time travel in the moment.

The present has also become a refuge because the past is *just too sad.* Nancy is torn between Maggie as she was and who she has become: "I'm sad because I miss my daughter the way she was, and I'd like to let go of that ...not even a hope, it isn't even about hoping she'll be happy again, it's just that I miss her. I miss the way she was. I miss talking to her. So, you know, I guess that it's like a death and at the same time this other thing."

Like so many families touched by severe brain injury, Nancy had to move out of a place of perpetual bereavement where she mourns a daughter who is still alive, though so much hope and promise has died. Unlike conventional bereavement after a death, this phase of mourning is neither temporally limited nor attended by the ritual or communal support that Leon Wieseltier describes so beautifully in his volume *Kaddish* the journey of his year of grief after his father.[11] No, the bereavement of brain injury families can last forever and is generally not met with support, after an initial outpouring of concern. In fact it is chronic and often accompanied by the abandonment of friends and more distant family who just don't know what to do with the pain and sadness of those they once befriended. For her own survival, Nancy needed to start anew and not allow herself to grieve for a past she could never retrieve.

But it wasn't easy to be in the moment. There is guilt in wanting her smart, capable daughter back and knowing that she is gone, as if dead; a discontinuity of selves very different than Corinth's sense that Greg was still the "same kid." But of course Greg could speak and had a bigger repertoire to express and share himself. Perhaps Maggie will achieve that too, if she can communicate more – or be helped to do so. But for now, Nancy and Maggie live in the present. The goal for Nancy is survival and being able to move on from the unbearable torment of unspeakable memories to the present and future.

Her realism allows her to say, "I'm not keen on living a tragedy. ... So from my own personal life, I'm trying to keep Margaret's tragedy," she pauses and regroups: "I'm not saying I'm trying to keep it out of my life, I'm trying to still maintain some normal, some normalcy in my life, *where tragedy isn't the color that my whole life has painted.* That's what I'd like ... that's what I aim for." But she admits, with her usual candor, "It doesn't always go that way. . . ."

It is a realpolitik version of self-care that is protective for herself and for Maggie. Nancy's rather pragmatic and brave response is to try not to think about those really hard questions: "I guess that I really have been trying really hard to stay in the present, and just be with her, in the present." She is amazed by others whose children have been touched by brain injury who have the fortitude to allow time to exist in all its many facets, as if it were redeemable, and the pain of the past could be amplified by the sorrows of a burdensome present and a future that probably will be not much better.

"And I guess my big question is how do other people withstand this hardship, like over time ... and how do people not just collapse with sadness and grief, ... because all the time that I'm in the present with her and I take her to the movies and do things with her, I'm, I'm sad. . . ."

She is frank about the most obvious but still unspeakable fact: "I know that my daughter isn't who she was." It is not about forgetting her daughter, but forgetting *that* she is no longer who she was and keeping their relationship in the present tense.

All she can handle is to take on one dimension of time. It is all very Zenlike. To engage the present, to enjoy its pleasures and experiences, such as they are, limited but real, happy but sad, never as fulfilling as they once were or as a mother-daughter talk. That is enough. For Nancy, to add the past to mix or to contemplate the future would be overwhelming.

Nancy makes every effort "to be in the present with her so that I'm just with her, just 'cause I love her and I want to be with her." There is always "an aftermath," because ". . . then afterwards ... I wish I could talk to her more and have her respond."

WELCOME COMPLICATIONS

Notwithstanding her pledge to remain in the present, now that Maggie could answer yes and no to questions, Nancy is curious about how much her daughter might remember. To test her memory, and retrieve a shared part of herself, she decided to take Maggie to see the movie "The Secret Life of Bees."

She had it all planned out, "... the reason that I wanted to go to that movie is 'cause I had read it, she had read it, her friends at college had read it, it was like a thing that we had read and talked about. And so I wanted to know if she remembered reading it, and she did!"

When I reminded Nancy of her wariness of bringing the past and present together, she now thought that bringing the past to bear was "sort of gratifying." And then she enthusiastically told me about a present-day encounter that suggests that Maggie is much more than just in the moment. She has a past too.

Part of that past took place at their Rhode Island beach house that had been in the family for years. It was a place that Nancy and Maggie would visit during many a New England summer. Nancy had thought of selling it to help make ends meet but it had brought them both so much joy, so she held on to the property. To make it more accessible, she had a handicap ramp built so she and Maggie could go to Rhode Island. The hope was to make new memories and search out some old ones.

Before the trip to the shore her speech therapist asked Maggie if she wanted to go to the beach and what she wanted to do there. Her responses indicated a degree of self-awareness that was startling. When asked, "What would you like to do, would you like to go swimming?" Maggie declined swimming and going to the beach, preferring instead to sit on the deck, which, as Nancy pointed out, "was something she *could* do."

"And she wanted to feel the wind on her face" because it was always windy there. Like Jean-Dominique Bauby in *The Diving Bell and the Butterfly*, who also enjoyed the sensation of a sea breeze against his face at his Normandy hospital, Maggie loved "the physical sensation" of the wind. And that is why she loved sitting on the deck.

Nancy thought it curious and revelatory about Maggie's analytical abilities, "So I've been thinking, from that, I mean it was kind of interesting, because it made me think that she knew, that she remembered the past. ..." And her response also showed a degree of insight "because to answer the way that she did ... she had to be aware of her present situation ... because normally I know she would have said she wanted to go swimming, because she would have gone swimming, because she loved to swim."

Maggie's answer suggested that she knew that swimming was no longer possible and that she was *thinking* about her options and making rational, informed choices, at least at some level. Nancy was clearly pleased, "So those were realistic choices for her, those were things she could experience ... what she chose were things she can [do]. ..."

EAGLE EYES

Nancy was grateful that Maggie's now *overt* progress was making it easier for her to secure benefits. She was now finally satisfying medical necessity and getting, at least part of, what she needs for her speech therapy. Maggie's new found eligibility for help came as a relief to Nancy and caused her to reflect on others who still have not crossed the threshold to behavioral evidence of improvement within the brain. Even her modicum of advancement put Maggie in a different bureaucratic category. For that she was grateful, "... the fact that there's any progress, the fact that she is still getting speech therapy when others in her situation can't continue to get speech therapy because they don't make progress." And then she became reflective about what she and her daughter had been through struggling for the needed services: you need to make "... because that's the only way you can have speech therapy."

Nancy's mix of gratitude for her newfound circumstances and sympathy for other families was bred of experience. She learned the hard way about medical necessity, and it is a tale worthy of Kafka and one worth telling. It all began with *Eagle Eyes*, a system from Boston College that placed electrodes around the eyes looking for directional eye movement that allowed Maggie to use her left eye to point at an alphabet board or to capture simpler yes/no movement.

From the start it was a rush. The speech therapy sessions lasted forty-five minutes and it took twenty of those minutes to set the thing up. It was not very efficient but along the way her therapist, Robyn Dragonetti, discerned that Maggie could actually read. This expanded her choices beyond yes or no on a wipe board. But it was slow and tedious and there was a better technology on the horizon called *My Tobii*.

In her typical manner, Nancy pushed the envelope. "So *then*, I guess I pressed ... she had actually had a trial on the *My Tobii* system, which is an infrared sensor for eye gaze."

But then the problem was again medical necessity. Nancy explains, "... in order for Margaret to get her own there had to be a, what they call, a trial, a month, four week trial that cost $2,000." And in the ultimate of inanities, Nancy explains, "Medicaid doesn't pay for the trial but you have to have it in order to get the device paid for because there has to be a proposal sent, submitted to Medicare in which the speech therapist has to say, 'this device will work for Margaret.' And there's no way you can do that unless you have a trial." So even with "universal" coverage – in Massachusetts – Nancy still had to raise $2,000 to administer the trial so a speech therapist could "prove" that it would benefit Maggie.

And then there was the question of what might constitute a proper trial to secure the evidence that the device would work. Nancy sought to raise $4,000 to extend the trial another four weeks because she felt a shorter period was not long enough for Maggie to demonstrate that she was making progress. She sent letters out to all the folks who had helped her buy her van and raised about $5,000. She was lucky and resourceful. But suppose she were not. To what sort of assistive device would Maggie have had access? Again, access to care – and progress – paradoxically hinged on a mother's tenacity, not the health care system's compassion or regard for Maggie's potentiality.

After the initial four weeks she did well, but in Nancy's estimation, her progress would have been insufficient for Maggie to get coverage for the device. But the extra time helped. By eight weeks, Maggie had qualified and learned how to move her eyes beyond a simple yes or no indication, hold her gaze in place for several seconds, and locate objects with her eye movements.

After the trial in January and February 2010, Robyn wrote the proposal to Medicaid, which was finally accepted in proper form in April. It took until August to get approval and then another month to have the device made. Maggie had been doing very well with a loaner device for two months and then had to go without it for six months, while she waited to get her own device. And here's the most nonsensical detail of this saga: during this entire period *Maggie did not get any speech therapy.* Such barriers to care are beyond explication.

But Nancy would try. Essentially, if the argument was that *My Tobii* was the best vehicle for Maggie to communicate, to continue provision of speech therapy while she was under consideration for the device would undermine the argument that it should be provided. Nancy explains why Maggie "... also didn't get speech therapy because there's like those catch-22s. So in order for Robyn to justify that she needed the *My Tobii*, she had to say this is the best way for Margaret to communicate, which meant that she couldn't continue doing speech therapy during that waiting period because then it would be like saying she doesn't really need the *My Tobii*." Bottom line: "she couldn't get funding for the speech therapy during that waiting period because she was applying for something, for a device."

Nancy paused, "I don't know if Margaret was depressed, but ... what I tried to do during that six months is to keep her really busy. ... So I think she managed to get through that period without being terribly discouraged. And so then she got the machine and it's still slow. She's had ... two months ... everyone, people saw what she could do. I mean, she can make choices with yes and no, she can choose out of fields and select bits on the screen, more for games." Her longer-term goal "is to have her be more facile with this new movement of her eye with dwell time, and for her to expand the range of where she can move her eye around the screen. And ultimately, I mean, I'm trying to get Facebook up on the computer so that ... basically have her be able to choose, 'I want to listen to music, I want to watch a movie, I want to do Facebook, I want to play games.' "

Fundamentally, the plan is to expand her choices from yes and no, to what she wants to do. To regain, as Greg Pearson had done, some elements of his autonomy and self-determination with the help of an assistive device. Nancy understands that this is the next step in the reconstitution or expression of Maggie's personhood, to have "choices so when she clicks on one of those choices then there's something that she can do ... spelling and sending e-mails down the road is a goal. But right now I think choosing letters is beyond her at this point. ..." But she does not think that will be forever.

SACRIFICE, FRUSTRATION, AND LEGACIES

Yet despite this forward gaze, for the first time in our many hours talking about Maggie's story, Nancy was angry and frustrated, even worn out, recounting this story. She had tried so hard and there had been so many barriers to her daughter's care. At best they were illogical; at worst they were insensitive, even cruel. Who could possibly have come up with this schema unless whole classes of individuals were being dismissed as irrelevant and beyond hope?

Nancy summed up her feelings, "I think the hard thing is the waiting part. Like, so here's a person, first she had to wait eighteen months for a diagnosis that was correct. Up until then she wasn't getting speech therapy. ... In other words, when she was in PVS obviously she's not going to getting speech therapy because she can't think. She doesn't have any ability to think. So then you find out that she does, and then she's successful with speech therapy, but then we want her to be *more* successful. And then there's a delay of six months for her to improve."

It was patently unfair and demanded so much of Maggie and Nancy, who had sacrificed so much. She had lost her full time job at AmeriCorps because she was tending to her daughter. She began working there part-time, accepting a much lower level position to accommodate her schedule and eventually losing that employment as well in November 2008 at the height of the recession. She had a bout of pneumonia. She began to collect unemployment insurance until June 2009. When she got a director-level job at AmeriCorps, it was only part-time so she did not qualify for health insurance. To make ends meet, she had to sell her beloved beach house, where she had built a ramp so Maggie could sit and enjoy the sea breeze and the wind in her hair. It had been an exhausting haul.

It was a tough decision to sell the beach house that had been passed down from her great grandparents. It had gained symbolic status in her family, as much a metaphor for adulthood and responsibility as a beloved place

by the sea. The message from her grandparents was, "we want to give this gift
to the next generation. We've enjoyed it, we want to give this gift, so keep it
intact, this is a gift that you pass to the next generation."

It was a legacy that would have to end with Maggie. This was a gift that
Nancy could no longer share. Maggie could neither take on the responsibility
of the house nor make use of it more than a few days a year. It would have
to be sold.

It was a disappointment for Nancy because it also meant that her child
would not have the adulthood *that came with the house*, which generations
of her ancestors had enjoyed. "You know, it's just really a loss. It's just really
sad. And especially knowing that she and I, I mean I, was already preparing
her, I was preparing her to take care of the house. I mean I was showing her
the things that were needed."

She pauses and returns to the present, and how the loss of the house also
represents the forfeiting of Maggie's transition to adulthood, "... so it's interesting, it isn't about money, but in a way part of the lesson is how do you become
a responsible adult? So here's a legacy and here's something for you to take care
of, and here's how you take care of it. So this is how you become a responsible
adult. Like in our family that was part of the legacy. Instead of saying, 'here's
a bunch of money, take care of that.' It's like, 'here's a beautiful home, and it's
special and we want you to give it to your children, so take care of it.'"

Nancy's would be the last generation. And with that realization,
another painful one: Maggie would not have children to continue her family
or this ritual that symbolized continuity with the past, and now rupture with
the future. Long after the fear of death and the shock of disability have subsided, Nancy like other parents of children with severe brain injury has come
to understand that her child's injury has multigenerational consequences. As
she thought about the fate of that beach house, she came to understand that
she had been in denial when it came to thoughts about grandchildren. Now,
"... it was not possible to pretend anymore after a certain time that maybe
she would be well enough to have children. In other words, you can hold on
to that for a while, but then you have to face sort of the reality. That no matter how much Margaret can improve, having children is not going to be part
of her future."

AN EMERGING COLLABORATION

Motherhood will not be part of Maggie's life. That part of her future has been
foreclosed,[12] but her ability to communicate and take an active role in her
recovery has reopened. So even as one aspect of adulthood is lost, another is
nearly regained. Nancy explains how this has evolved. At the start of Maggie's

injury she pushed to get Maggie her due, but now that she is starting to voice an opinion and take some tentative steps toward some semblance of independence, Nancy is pulling back, if ever so slightly.

Nancy explains that at the outset Maggie was totally defenseless and needed a mother's advocacy: "I felt the beginning period, like I had to be right on top, push, I had to be pushing." When others thought she was vegetative, but Nancy thought she was minimally conscious, "... I had to be finding a way to have other people believe that." And later once the diagnosis was clarified and it's determined that "she's in MCS" the questions became "... what can she get? You know, pushing for the speech therapy, getting the eye gaze, the *Eagle Eye* system, getting *My Tobii*. And she's gotten more alert; I guess that's what I was referring to as I pushed her."

But then she corrects herself and acknowledges Maggie's growing role in her own recovery. Her daughter is also partly responsible for some of the recent changes. It is an observation shared by Dr. Schiff who has reminded Nancy that it has not only been maternal exertions that have led to improvements, it has been Maggie too. Nancy notes that "Dr. Schiff says it's not just [my] pushing it's her also, she's getting better. . . ."

It is a time of profound transition from Nancy trying to create opportunities to Maggie starting to take advantage of what her mother had made possible. Together they have begun a passage together where mother and daughter will, in tandem, determine a shared destiny. Although Nancy pushed to get the process this far along, her efforts were but the start of a long journey. That was how it began, "but now in a lot of ways it's that she has to work, she's got to do the work now to be able to communicate."

The good news is that Maggie "wants to do this work." The bad news is the lingering doubt about how long Maggie will be willing or able to sustain the momentum or contend with profound disappointment. Nancy is both elated and fearful of leaving so much in her child's hands, "I don't know, I think part of what my fear is ... this sense of urgency now that she's more alert."

But Nancy appreciates that she must share the space with Maggie. She recognizes that before she was making all the decisions, intuitively guided by a mother's love and their years together. In a poem, she wrote as much. What she "discovered was that the facts were not what guided me but an unswerving clarity that I could understand my daughter's vision unspoken through my love for her and some other mystical understanding." Some of that could now change as Maggie could begin to express herself. The mystical would soon share space with the real: instead of conjuring up what Maggie might think, she could look at her left eye and peer into her soul as her daughter communicated her wishes.

A SECOND ADOLESCENCE

To borrow a helpful developmental analogy, Maggie is now in a second adolescence in the maturation of her recovery. She will have greater opportunities to assume more responsibility for her progress even as Nancy does all she can to sustain her.

That parental responsibility is no less staggering than Nancy's earlier obligations when it was a life and death struggle in the hospital. After taking Maggie so far, the stakes are high and the possibility for disappointment huge. She must continue her dogged advocacy to meet Maggie's needs and Nancy appreciates the responsibility noting: "... we better deliver and give her something so she can communicate."

Whatever the device or tactic, these communication tools "better work." They have to bring her a sense of satisfaction and accomplishment that encourages her to carry on and that also mitigates her isolation. But it is a delicate balance. The tasks should neither be so frustrating so as to exasperate her, nor too simple to be an ineffective vehicle for communication. It is a pragmatic question that prompts Nancy to ask whether the *My Tobii*, is "adequate for her? Is it going to make *her* feel successful? Like, now ... how does she feel? Is she depressed? Is she, is she feeling, like, challenged? ... is she bored?"

The questions are critical because pushing too little will result in continued isolation. Pushing too hard could result in frustration because the task is just too hard for her to accomplish. That is certainly not the objective for one who has suffered so much already. As Nancy cautions: "you don't want her to have a harder life." It is a matter of balance because "you don't want to have her to suffer ... but you've got a goal in mind."

That goal, of course, is progress and small steps toward reliable functional communication, leading to incremental degrees of independence and individuation, much as any child making the passage to adolescence. But Maggie's next phase will not be a typical adolescence because her goals remain unclear and the depth of her recovery uncertain. Her path will follow a *different developmental model* where the milestones are unknown and unmarked. Fundamental questions remain about the pace of her recovery and the aspirations of her parents for its magnitude. How should their hopes be tempered by the biology of her injury and the state of her psyche?

Charting this transition is a considerable challenge because unlike the usual passage from childhood into adulthood, this is a *reemergence into* a maturity that was lost and is now being regained. There is a past in her history that will inform her future in a way not experienced in conventional adolescence. There will be elements of the old and the new mixed into a novel mosaic of the self that neither the past nor present can wholly claim.

Given all this uncertainty, Nancy is looking for "whatever small grain of clarity" she can find, if it exists. Until then, her hopes take her to the heights and her doubts bring her back to ground, "Like someone asked me what do I want now from Margaret ... and it's like ... sure I want her to walk, I want her to sing, I want her to climb a mountainous hill. I'd like her to be able to have a conversation with someone and I'd like to know how she feels, or what she's thinking."

But then reality sets in and speaks of a minimum level of recovery. "I'd like her to have a way to share what she's thinking with whoever she wants to. And I think it's possible ... I mean it's good if she can choose like what shirt to wear, and if she can tell the nurse I'm in pain. ..." And with a more expansive optimism, it would be terrific "for her to go beyond that and be able to choose something herself or say I'd like to learn something about animals, and choose a program."

But the question remains where do her parents set the bar? What is realistic? What aspirations will inevitably lead to disappointment? For now, there is no reassuring Dr. Spock book for these families as they try to navigate a loved one's reemergence into the world, it seems, *for the second time.* That book is yet to be written and that story will not be a simple one. It will be founded upon neuroscience yet done and ethical deliberations about what we owe people like Maggie who remain conscious, but whose depth of understanding, pain, and sequestration from the rest of us we do not yet know.

20 When Consciousness Becomes Prosthetic

It is one of the oldest philosophical questions, knowing the conscious existence of another. As noted earlier, each of us can attest to our own existence but cannot say with certainty that another exists. And this seems to suffice in most cases because those of us who are conscious and can speak and affirm our conscious self can defend our interests and choices. Though it is theoretically suspect, in a practical sense, the communication of one's own consciousness becomes a safeguard of one's prerogatives and rights.

We have, however, seen the horrible consequences for patients who may have been conscious but have been unable to communicate and therefore assert themselves after brain injury. Without the ability to communicate they have been vulnerable from their entry into the emergency room, all the way through the ICU and chronic care. Ignored, neglected, and mistaken as unconscious, they were relegated to custodial care and worse. The entreaties of their loved ones generally went for naught until a few of them were properly diagnosed and shown to be minimally conscious through careful examination and sometimes ancillary neuroimaging tests.

To ensure that the fate of the next generation of minimally conscious patients is better than the current one, neuroscience will need to enable Maggie and others like her to communicate and show that they are here, and deserve a hearing. Science needs to enable them to more fully demonstrate, through their interactions, that they remain part of a human community, a community that is bound together through communication, reminders of our reciprocal obligations to this population of patients.

Advancing an ethical agenda of obligation will require some requisite degree of scientific "proof" of their conscious presence. These "manifestations of self" will need to occur on a more predictive and consistent basis. Only then will there be clarity about society's responsibilities, so that at a minimum a conscious being is never again mistaken for one who is not and that the maximal potential of each patient is achieved.

The importance of such demonstrations cannot be overstated given the legacy of neglect, which has been described, and ongoing concerns about the inflated chronic care costs.[1] In this environment, it is essential that any conflation of vegetative and minimally conscious patients be eliminated so that patients who are in fact conscious are provided with the care that conscious individuals deserve.

DEMONSTRATING (AND FOSTERING) CONSCIOUSNESS: THE MESOCIRCUIT MODEL

To demonstrate their conscious states, some patients will need the help of emerging prosthetic devices, drugs, and neuroimaging tools to facilitate communication. Some will need interventions to more consistently demonstrate their latent capabilities. Others will need them to augment their own intrinsic (if dormant) capabilities. These assistive interventions will serve as a bridge between the patient and the outside world, a barrier that can have its basis in impaired cognition, faulty motor output, or more likely a mix of these two impairments.

For example, in Maggie's case, is she producing thoughts and emotions but having difficulty expressing them because of the damage to her brainstem, that crucial information "super highway" just above the spine? Or, has the damage from the infarctions to her thalamus been so severe as to limit sentience?

The former is a transport question; the latter is one of production. But with damage in *both* her brainstem and her thalamus, she could have some combination of each deficit, making her picture a mixed one between a patient who is somewhere between the minimally conscious and locked-in states.

In this last scenario, her cognitive impairment might be a consequence of a specific circuit mechanism deficit proposed by Niko Schiff and Jerome Posner that alters brain activity after injury. This *mesocircuit*, essential for consciousness, links the thalamus, basal ganglia, and the frontal cortex. In the setting of thalamic injury, it down-regulates, and may shut down, thereby interrupting a complex electrical relationship that is the basis for consciousness.[2,3] This intricate – and enmeshed – relationship once injured can itself be modulated by discrete interventions along its many pathways, thus facilitating consciousness by either inhibiting an inhibition or stimulating an excitatory pathway, or some combination thereof.

In various guises, this sort of circuit manipulation appears to explain the theory behind the effects of deep brain stimulation,[4] mechanisms of recovery after loss of consciousness, and the circuit mechanisms of general anesthesia and deep sleep.[5] It also appears to explain the ability of the sleeping pill Zolpidem (Ambien) to sometimes produce a paradoxical awakening in patients with brain injury.[2,6–9]

There is no more vivid example of the mesocircuit's power than the virtual transformation of George Melendez, the former baseball player who sustained both traumatic and anoxic brain injury after his car spun out of control into a ditch. His story, which was the subject of a *60 Minutes* segment featuring our work at Cornell, is truly remarkable.[10] His mother, Pat Flores, tells of her serendipitous observation when she gave George sleeping pills to help him get to sleep.

They were traveling to San Antonio seeking an alternative therapy for his brain injury. Everyone shared one motel room and George "moaned and yelled all night long." The next day Pat went to the clinic and said, "look, we're not going to last, either you knock him out or you knock us out, but if we don't sleep we can't stay here and do this." And they gave him Ambien.

That night she gave George medicine using his stomach tube. "In about ten minutes my husband had already fallen asleep, I was still watching TV, but kind of noticed there was no sound coming out of George and as I'm turning my head I'm thinking 'wow that medicine is good, it really knocked him out.' "

She laughed as she recalled the potency of the sleeping pill. But then something beyond belief happened: "when I turn around and expecting to see a sleeping George, instead I see a George whose eyes are as wide as I had seen them in the longest time. Since before his accident. And he was just looking intently at everything, and kind of, he was soaking it in. He was looking, and the look on his face was expressive like where am I, what am I doing here? And as I saw that I said 'George!' And he just came out and said 'what?' And I about fell out of that bed. And I woke up my husband and said, 'he just talked! He talked!' And we talked with him until, for a couple of hours until it started fading."

I asked her what they talked about and Pat told me, "Um, mostly asking him 'do you know where you are?' and he said 'no.' And we were telling him and what we were doing there. ... He wasn't doing much talking yet. But he just kept picking at it [his diaper] and looking at me and going, and I go 'what's a matter? You're wondering why that's on?' And I said, 'honey you can't walk, you were in an accident and you can't walk, so I have to put those on so that you don't wet yourself. Ok?' Not happy about it, but he understood why it was on."

The mesocircuit hypothesis helps explain the awakening of patients like George Melendez on Ambien,[2,3] as well as why DBS was effective in Greg Pearson. But most importantly, the theory suggests that we will come to understand, describe, and categorize various brain states by the *circuit disorders* they possess, implicating pathological or dysfunctional components of the brain neuropathways that might be amenable to intervention. For example, Esteban Fridman, a postdoctoral fellow working with Schiff found that the changes in the central thalamus and basal ganglia fit the mesocircuit hypothesis as well.[11]

This circuit-based work is a glimpse of the future and how therapeutics will be designed for patients with disorders of consciousness. So informed scientists and clinicians will be able to manipulate circuit disorder as was done in our DBS in MCS trial. Through that intervention, Greg Pearson achieved functional communication and the ability to express preferences, forever demonstrating his conscious state. Those dramatic changes in brain state are a promissory note for the future and a justification for current resources to sustain research that will help patients like him.

SCANNING FOR AN ANSWER

The demonstration of consciousness will also be made through the use of neuroimaging, scans that show varying degrees of metabolic activity within the brain that are proxies for functional status. One paradigm-changing example was the work of Martin Monti and colleagues using noninvasive approaches, reported in *The New England Journal of Medicine*.[12] Monti and colleagues described a patient who was consistently found to be vegetative on clinical examination before being scanned. Through imaging, however, he was able to answer simple yes/no questions using functional-MRI neuroimaging as a prosthetic communication device. Building upon the passive language neuroimaging methods described in Chapter 10, Monti showed that a vegetative patient – by behavioral criteria – was able to toggle between motor (imagine playing tennis) or spatial imagery (imagine walking around your house) to provide yes/no responses.[12]

The Monti paper raised dramatic ethical questions, not the least of which is the need to reconcile the latent capabilities of a patient deemed vegetative on clinical exam with this volitional ability to communicate by peering within the injured brain. Based on our collective experience and the data presented in the Monti paper this is an exceedingly rare occurrence.

Monti and his colleagues studied fifty-four patients with disorders of consciousness. Clinically, the group included both MCS and VS patients. Although the identification of that one vegetative patient by neuroimaging was a game-changer, it must be taken with several critical caveats. Of the thirty-one patients studied who were in MCS, thirty were effectively identified using the Coma Recovery Scale-Revised (CRS-R) instrument developed by Giacino and Kalmar.[13] This would indicate that the CRS-R is a very sensitive and specific instrument.

In contrast, functional imaging identified only five of fifty-four patients as able to perform command following. This finding is paradoxical because the majority of the higher functioning MCS patients identified clinically at the bedside as being able to follow commands could not do so by neuroimaging criteria. So from a statistical point of view, neuroimaging is neither sensitive nor specific. There would be a bevy of false negative studies as most MCS patients would *not* be identified by these imaging methods.

And most importantly, and lost within the media flurry attending this paper, Monti and colleagues note at the end of their paper that the patient previously found to be consistently in the vegetative state actually fulfilled the criteria for MCS when more intensively examined at the bedside. The authors describe how they made the initial diagnosis and how it was revised both by the scanning process and again by intensive assessment by behavioral criteria thereafter:

> We conducted additional tests in one of the five patients with evidence of awareness on functional MRI, and we found that he had the ability to apply the imagery technique in order to answer simple yes-or-no questions accurately. Before the scanning was performed, the patient had undergone repeated evaluations indicating that he was in a vegetative state, including a month-long specialized assessment by a highly trained clinical team. At the time of scanning, however, thorough retesting at the bedside showed reproducible but highly fluctuating and inconsistent signs of awareness ... findings that are consistent with the diagnosis of a minimally conscious state.[14]

This additional analysis is only partly reassuring because in most all situations this patient would never have been diagnosed as minimally conscious. Few patients will ever be evaluated under current conditions with such intensity. Nonetheless, conceptually, the ultimate diagnosis of MCS is reassuring because it reminds us that the vegetative state is incompatible with engagement with the outside and that when there is consciousness and no motor behavior, it is best to describe such patients as minimally conscious, albeit as *nonbehavioral MCS*. Ultimately, the patient who responded yes and no, was found to be behaviorally in MCS as indicated by his response at the bedside.

So from an ethical analysis, the bedside exam has utilitarian value identifying most of the patients who would turn out to be MCS. But in this case series, neuroimaging had unspeakable deontological value for that one person for whom it made all the difference, by identifying and communicating consciousness where it had not been expected. It was only later identified by behavioral metrics once it *was known to be there.*

Imagine having the ability to communicate, at the level of yes/no responses – and perhaps more – but awaiting some way, some mechanism, to express oneself? Although I am hesitant to engage in hyperbole, I must confess that the analogy that came to mind when I read the Monti paper was of that famous image of the freed Nelson Mandela returning to Robbins Island looking out through the prison's bars that once had confined him.[15] Each had been liberated from an internal exile, one political, the other biological, but each an imprisonment long without the prospect of release. Mandela had to wait for sweeping political changes in his homeland and Monti's subject had to wait for the coalescence of neuroprosthetic technology to allow their respective escapes.[16]

COMMUNICATING WITH MAGGIE?

If the Monti paper was about yes and no, then Maggie's time in the scanner in New York was about yes, no, and *maybe*, reflecting the inconsistency of her response and the *variance* seen when using these methods. This work, published in *Brain* early in 2011, was a project done by Weill Cornell graduate student Jon Bardin under the guidance of Schiff and physicist and neuroimager, Henning Voss.[17]

We used a modified fMRI paradigm like that utilized in England and studied six patients with disorders of consciousness at least at the level of MCS. Each subject was asked to engage in command following, and in deference to Maggie's love of water sports, to imagine that they were swimming. Three of the six subjects produced the mental imagery as seen in the work by Owen and Monti, but two others – who behaviorally are capable of communication at the bedside – did not produce mental imagery that would have been expected.

One subject who had already emerged from MCS noted she had "done" the mental imagery task but *didn't* produce the signal according to the fMRI results. This is a loaded finding and points to the need to disseminate any such technology carefully, lest it be used in lieu of comprehensive bedside evaluation. In the absence of clinical assessment, this patient, in contrast to the Monti patient, might at some point have been labeled as vegetative based on her scan results when there *was* behavioral output. The Monti patient was just the reverse: behaviorally vegetative but in a nonbehavioral MCS state in the scanner.

Maggie was one of the subjects in our study. She produced the activation, but in an interesting twist, did so also robustly outside what is called a region of interest (ROI) – that part of the brain that actually would normally correlate with certain functional tasks. Here, the activation was spatially outside the ROI generally "illuminated" when either thinking about swimming or actually physically engaged in the task. And to further complicate matters, Maggie had variable runs in the scanner, reflecting the intermittent responsiveness Nancy had seen at the bedside.

A more recent analysis by Bardin, Schiff, and Voss points to the methodological need to look beyond the ROI, observing that there is a pattern of responses when the entire brain is considered as the receptive space that suggests an affirmative response.[18] And in a commentary that will accompany this analysis to be published in the *Archives of Neurology*, I note that once this broader spatial template is considered as a locale for a response, the temporal metrics of the response changes.[19] Then, it is important in the scanner – as at the bedside – to take account of slowed responses or the potential for latency lest a "correct" response get lost in the ensuing question.

All of this is to point to the complexity of the brain's adaptive abilities – for example, having a receptive space outside the ROI, and the fallibility of the fMRI to capture the signal of responsive brains.

There is great promise with these methods, but peril remains until we understand mechanisms of recovery and if we fail to appreciate that any response could represent a floor and not the ceiling. Conversely, as we have seen most recently in our *Brain* paper, a nonresponse on imaging is not a definitive negative result and needs to be understood in context of any behavioral data and methodological concerns.

RIGHT TO DIE REDUX

That the Monti patient was not and could not be vegetative, framed the deeper question: If a patient can respond yes or no in the scanner, what more could they do? Of course, a patient who is able to respond to simple yes/no questions might only be able to respond to simple questions and nothing more. Alternately, there could be the potential for so much more, if only enabled.

When asked to speculate about what this technology can and cannot do, for now, I believe a prudential response is warranted because of the aforementioned technical challenges, the infrequency of these responses and our inability to predict when and if they will be manifested. But this edict does not apply to the media, which has been found by the Canadian neuroethicists, Eric Racine and Judy Illes, to overstate the abilities of these new technologies and use incremental progress to ask provocative, hyperbolic questions.[20]

So when the Monti paper was published in February 2010, I was interviewed by *New York Times* correspondent Benedict Carey. I was asked the inevitable question about whether I thought that this new method of communication might help these patients articulate a desire to die. By asking the right-to-die question he made me think of all the historical reasons why this population has so long been neglected, and the paradox, felt by most of us doing this work, that the goal now was to improve the lives of these patients and the families who love them.

It was not about a right to die, although it could be, but rather about a way to make a bad situation better. At least for the population we had studied, it was a way to help those families who had opted *not* to withhold or withdraw care.

Most had made their decisions incrementally, not ideologically. Some had religious objections but most had hoped their loved ones would have done better with the treatment they had received, but it didn't work out that way. They saw glimmers of hope and the early promise of a blossoming of neuroscience and so they stayed the course and hoped for the best. Now with breakthroughs in DBS in MCS and neuroimaging, the question was about preserving the right to die and *affirming the right to care*,[21] the epic struggle that is the focus of these narratives and this book.

In talking with Carey, I tried to balance the importance of neuroimaging as a noninvasive way to study the brain with the crudity of the method and its potential for error and misconstrual. I suggested that, "We've opened up a communication channel with this technique, but in some ways it's like a very bad cell phone connection."[22] In a remarkable quirk of a slow news cycle, my comments were selected as the *Times' Quote of the Day*.

While Monti and colleagues had gained access to the brain, the bandwidth of the connection was still too narrow to be a reliable vector for important conversations. Most of us would prefer to have important conversations on a landline because that technology can accommodate nuance, overlapping conversation, and pretty much ensure that calls will not be dropped. As yet, the equivalent of "landlines" do not exist to communicate with the injured brain. Neuroimaging, as dramatic as it is, still remains the equivalent of a crackling, somewhat unreliable cell phone. There remains many ways that communication can be ruptured – even misleading – at the neural interface.

COMMUNICATING THE CHALLENGES

Prosthetic communication with the injured brain through a neuroimaging vector is a complicated business. Consider what has to occur to produce an intact communication loop. The patient has to understand the question asked, produce the mental images associated with the instructions, hold those images and the yes/no contingent responses in memory, and then produce output back in a timely fashion.[17] At the level of the scanner, it has to capture the brain's activity. And this may not occur because it is not properly calibrated correctly or because the scanner was not patient enough to receive a slow arriving signal. To put the potential for error another way, there might be a signal too weak to be read by the scanner, in a frequency that the scanner cannot recognize or too late to be registered. The potential for a false negative result (when the results erroneously report a negative result in a conscious subject) is staggering. It is so large, in fact, that a negative result does not mean that the patient might not subsequently be found to be conscious.

And even if the scanner operated perfectly without error, we need to recall that misunderstandings still occur for those of us without the neurological challenges of the patients presented here. Even when we are simply talking with each other miscommunication can occur, as Matisse's *The Conversation* reminds us. In the painting, a couple is engaged in what appears to be an awkward exchange. Against a blue background punctuated by a garden scene out the window a man stands stiffly in pajamas while a woman sits in a chair, body forward and head tilted back in a haughty fashion. From this vantage point their efforts at communication do not appear to be going well.

And of course in severe brain injury, the dynamic is even more complex. A conscious patient's response is dependent upon the questions that are asked and the choices that are given. When Maggie, for example, works outside the scanner with a white board and her speech therapists, her response is contingent upon what she is asked and the responses that are supplied to her. If she does not receive the answer she wants, there is a nonresponse that could be catalogued as a lack of interest, misunderstanding, a low arousal state, an effort to get a better response option, or a complete lack of engagement.

Nancy explains, "Well, basically when the speech therapist and then one or two of the aides are also able to help her, they ask her a question that has either a yes/no answer, or even a question ... where she can choose between good or bad, or between different parts of her body. Now what they do is they write questions on a wipe board, she reads the question, and then it broadens the possibility for her. Now she can answer questions that aren't just yes/no but are choices between two different words. Like 'Are you comfortable or uncomfortable?' Or, 'Do you want your position changed, do you want to stay in bed or stay in the chair?' As opposed to just yes and no."

But Nancy carefully notes too, "But of course that's if I ask the right questions. . . ."

LESSONS FROM WENDLAND

The challenge of communicating with MCS patients[23] and its potential consequences become clear in the case of Robert Wendland, which eventually was decided in the California Supreme Court in 2001.[24] After sustaining a traumatic brain injury from a car accident, Mr. Wendland recovered and was in MCS. He lacked decision-making capacity and his wife, Rose, provided ongoing consent for his medical care, including the placement and (multiple) replacements of his feeding tube, which became dislodged on several occasions.

When the feeding tube needed replacement for the fourth time, Rose decided that his situation had gone on long enough and that reinsertion of the tube was inconsistent with Robert's prior wishes. She consulted their children, the patient's brother as well as Mr. Wendland's doctors. All agreed that ongoing treatment was inconsistent with his wishes so she decided to withhold artificial nutrition and hydration with the support of all twenty members of the hospital ethics committee.

When Mr. Wendland's parents sought a restraining order to prevent this withholding of artificial nutrition and hydration, Rose responded by seeking to be named Robert's conservator. Her request was granted and disputed by Mr. Wendland's parents and the case rose up with the courts and was ultimately heard by the California Supreme Court. By then Mr. Wendland had died, but the Court heard the case because of the relevance of the dispute.

To its credit, the Court noted that Mr. Wendland was conscious and did not conflate his diagnosis with the vegetative state and wrote of the effect that a withdrawal of life-sustaining therapy would have on "a conscious conservatee's fundamental rights." They did, however, find that the evidence that Rose Wendland presented about her husband's wishes about living in his current state was not "clear and convincing," the threshold that would have been required to withdraw life-sustaining therapy.

Mr. Wendland had made two comments in which he had "allegedly expressed a desire not to live like a 'vegetable.'" The first one was as he "was recovering from a night's bout of drinking" and the other was after losing his beloved father-in-law. The California Supreme Court cited the logic of a lower trial court in making its ruling about these conversations, again rightly distinguishing MCS from persistent vegetative state (PVS):

> ... neither of these conversations reflect an exact "on all-fours" description of conservatee's present medical condition. More explicit direction just "I don't want to live like a vegetable" is required to justify a surrogate decision-maker terminating the life ... of someone who is not in a PVS.[25]

But what really tipped the scales of justice – and is most important for us as we consider the question of communication with patients who are in MCS – was a 1997 videotape asking Mr. Wendland about his views and preferences. Although the questions were asked using a yes/no board, and not an fMRI scanner, Mr. Wendland's responses and their impact on the court is revealing. His doctor asked him the following questions, as recorded in the trial transcript:

Do you have pain?	Yes.
Do your legs hurt?	No.
Does your buttocks hurt?	No.
Do you want us to leave you alone?	Yes.
Do you want more therapy?	No.
Do you want to get into the chair?	Yes.
Do you want to get back in bed?	No.

Do you want to die?	No answer.
Are you angry?	Yes.
At somebody?	No.[26]

In its deliberations, the California Supreme Court paid special attention to this exchange and the fact that Mr. Wendland did not clearly answer the question about a desire to die. Although the Court noted that "experts dispute the consistency and accuracy of Robert's responses to questions," they felt that his nonresponse to the now operative question was difficult to ignore, especially as he gave "facially plausible 'yes' or 'no' answers to a variety of other questions about his wishes."[27]

Given the doubt cast by his silence to the desire to die question, they found that the required "clear and convincing" evidentiary standard of his wishes had not been met and ruled that they would have denied the motion not to reinsert the tube desired by his conservator, his wife Rose. While the Court limited its ruling to patients who were conscious and did not have an advance directive, the impact of the video interview on Mr. Wendland's prior wishes is troubling. It is quite likely that his prior statements would have allowed a decision to withhold or withdraw life-sustaining therapy when also desired by his conservator, who was also his wife.

But the exchange in the video undercut Robert Wendland's prior wishes, a development that is troubling in light of the impact that prosthetic neuroimaging communication devices might have in the future. Besides the technical fallibility of these devices, we must be concerned about the human element and the distortions that are imposed on normal communication when it becomes one-sided, as was the case in the Monti paper and in our interviews with Maggie.

Patients like Maggie are not yet able to initiate questions. They are wholly dependent upon the questions that are asked. In a less stressful context simply engaged in speech therapy, Nancy recognizes that "conversation" with Maggie is really a one-way street. It is prone to reflect our biases. She told us, "But I would rather she could spell out words herself ... all we're doing is asking her questions. They might not be the *right* questions. And we're letting her choose the answers that *we* think up. They may be the wrong answers."

Nancy recalled when Maggie had her leg cramp while meditating and how they tried to question her about her state of mind and were misled by their *own suppositions* about the response. Nancy was surprised when her daughter finally responded she was "happy" and humbled by the fact that Maggie was really at the mercy of the choices she was given.

At the outset, she asked Maggie: "... are you angry? Are you frustrated? Even calm wasn't the right word ... so we had words she wasn't interested in. She just didn't look at either one, so she was not choosing until I asked her if she was, I think the choice was happy or upset, and she chose happy. And I just was … I guess I was surprised that she would choose the word happy."

Moreover, the answers cannot be all that subtle or nuanced and are reduced to a simple binary, yes or no response. When Maggie replied she was happy though in pain from a leg cramp, there were mixed emotions that no single response could accommodate. Nancy explained, "Well what I guess we didn't ask her 'what are you happy about?' So there was a sequence where she was meditating she was feeling good about that, she said she liked it, she wanted to continue, she felt it helped her, and then she had this movement, posturing that I thought was about emotion, and it turned out she was in pain, but was also happy."

Returning to the Wendland video, there are other ways to explain Wendland's nonresponse.[23] His attention could have been waning; he might have become fatigued or weighing choices. Did he understand the question? His response time – like Maggie's – could have been slow, reflecting a degree of latency often seen in patients with severe brain injury. Or he might have wanted to respond to the question with one of his own, "Who wants to know?" Or perhaps answering "maybe," a choice he was not given.

None of these explanations actually constitute a negative response to the question and thus a nonresponse should neither be taken as dispositive nor undermine prior wishes. And suppose there were an affirmative answer in the scanner? Would there be enough skepticism against that bright flare of a response to reach a level of certainty needed to make such a momentous decision?

Nancy has pondered whether she would ever ask Maggie if she wanted to die and how she would process her response, "… if I asked her, do you think the quality of your life isn't enough. I don't know, what would I do if she said 'no mom, it's not enough.'" She continues, "Would I say—should I ask her would you like to die?" That question, to Nancy seems too much, too extreme and unfair because of her dependency and inability to fully communicate her thoughts, much less her wishes. No, Nancy is reluctant to go there given the breadth and depth of their "discourse." She would not ask that question about a desire to die, "No, it just doesn't feel right to me. It doesn't feel like she's in a position to decide that because she's so vulnerable. I feel like I'd be taking advantage of her."

Pressed on why she viewed it as "taking advantage," she pointed to how one-sided the conversation would be, the power imbalance that occurs when only one conversant can draft the script. She notes, "… the only questions that she can answer are the ones I choose and so they're the only questions. I don't feel like I know what questions she wants me to ask. I just have no idea." There had been many occasions when she misinterpreted Maggie's moods or meanings, "Like so sometimes I think – there was a time where she's like she's moving and I'm thinking she's angry whatever or she's in pain or ... I was trying to interpret what I saw in Margaret and ... it turned out that she just wanted to go back to bed. Like it wasn't a big [deal] ... it wasn't a what you call it ... [an] ethical crisis or some sort of metaphysical like dilemma like I want to die, like I'm so depressed." It was just a desire to go to bed, to stretch a leg, to work out a cramp.

Nancy is cautious, "Whereas I might have interpreted it as something larger. It was just I'm tired, I want to go to bed." The tendency is to ascribe deeper meanings to what might be a trivial choice and this could take on dangerous implications when seeking to answer a big question like a desire to die. She has learned not to ask big questions because the answers will only breed ambiguity, given the current state of their communicative channel.

And that seems wise. With the technology's narrow bandwidth and the patient's inability to more fully participate by initiating or nuancing responses, the best that can be expected are responses indicative of assent or dissent, not informed consent or refusal. At least for now, while neuroprosthetic communication is an advance over the status quo, it does not yet have the sufficient degree of robustness to serve as a communication channel to articulate a preference to live or die.

Until that level of sophistication is reached, it is important that this technology is not inappropriately used to "become a routine arbiter of whether or not life-sustaining therapy be withdrawn."[23] A patient's previously articulated preferences or advance care planning should guide care and should not be undercut by this emerging technology, which will inevitably be brought forward in family disputes like Schiavo or Wendland. In these contentious situations the technology is likely to offer information that is unclear, uncertain, or unobtainable, often undercutting previous attempts by the patient to exercise their civil rights by articulating their views in advance.

It would be ironic, and indeed counterproductive, if early neuroprosthetic devices designed to foster the civil rights of patients and restore their autonomy and voice, were used to undermine authentic patient choice and silence prior preferences because technical deficiencies fostered doubt and confusion. But this is only a temporary caution because it is more than likely than not, that this technology matures to the point to restore decision-making capacity to many who now lack it.

And with this restoration will come the return of autonomous choice to the patient and the regained expression of their self-determination. Until then, we will have to craft mosaic choices utilizing what was known about the patient's prior wishes and the available expressions from the patient weighed against the choices voiced by the surrogate decision maker. Ironically, surrogate decision making will be made more complicated in the early phases of prosthetically assisted communication, seeking to integrate the reemerging voice of the patient without violating their prior wishes or placing them in avoidable harm because of misconstruals.

21 The Rights of Mind

Was Nancy comforted that Maggie had begun to communicate? Less than I thought she would be. I had expected that she would be thrilled that Maggie had reached this longed-for elusive milestone. But in fact, Nancy was incredibly frustrated, even alarmed that Maggie had access to communication as infrequently as she did.

It seemed that Maggie's ability to communicate, as intermittent as it, was most dependent upon the reciprocal skill of a speech therapist who visits Middleboro three times a week. According to Nancy, she "is the only one who communicates with her."

So was it comforting that at least it happened on those occasions?

Nancy tells us, "I mean it's comforting to know that it can happen, but kind of frightening to know that it only happens a few times a week when the speech therapist is with her. ..." And then, "... not regularly, partly because Margaret hasn't been consistent ..." in her pattern of communication. Sometimes the therapist shows up and Maggie won't communicate. Other times when she might, the therapist is not there.

Imagine the scenario, first you learn that your daughter is conscious and not vegetative, that she can understand and sometimes communicate. Then you discover that those precious opportunities are limited to but a few hours a week. And in those other moments, you suspect that she might be able to communicate, if given the opportunity. But until that happens, she is silenced.

Nancy is frustrated and she believes that Maggie is as well. She also thinks that her daughter is angry and depressed too. Nancy told us, "So I mean I'm frustrated ... how can I really be happy about what's happening with Margaret when it's so limited. ..." Like many patients with disorders of consciousness, Maggie finds herself wholly dependent upon others and/or machinery to regain her voice, to have the ability to communicate with others. To express a thought, tell us she is in pain or hungry, or tell someone that she loves them – all of that self-expression is dependent upon the resources necessary to pay a speech therapist (or support a run in the scanner). It is time consuming, laborious, and intermittent, requiring expertise and patience working in tandem. Without that partnership – the affirmative actions on others upon whom they depend – these folks are completely or mostly silenced. Even Nancy's communication with Maggie is dependent and enhanced when the therapist is in the room. Without all this support it is ominous and dark: the image of conscious, sentient individuals who remain unable to give voice to their active minds.

BRAIN INJURY ON THE MARGINS

At the outset of this study I tended to think about the care of the minimally conscious as if it were simply an entitlement issue. As such, I thought that the quality of patients' assessment and ongoing care could be ameliorated by directing more resources to the problem through reimbursement reform. Medical necessity and its ill-suited relationship with brain injury seemed like a logical first step down that road. And even now, I have no doubt that harmonizing time frames of recovery and reimbursement streams would advance care, decrease capricious denials, and lead to rehabilitation trials of appropriate duration. But, as I have asserted earlier, I am not convinced that reimbursement reform will happen without fundamentally changing how we view the minimally conscious, their needs, and their place in society.

Here's an example of their marginalization: Over a decade since MCS became a diagnostic category there still is no reliable epidemiological data on the incidence and prevalence of the minimally conscious state. The most cited estimate of prevalence is that there are between 112,000 and 280,000 adult and pediatric patients in MCS in the United States.[1] Unfortunately, this study was an *estimate* from a heterogeneous group of patients and does not represent actual demography.

With a then Cornell medical student Maria Master, Joseph Giacino, and Cornell colleague Linda Gerber, I tried to build upon this earlier study by examining a number of regional and state-based brain injury registries to esti-mate this epidemiology. Our paper was called, "The Minimally Conscious State: A Diagnosis in Search of an Epidemiology," echoing Jennett and Plum's description of PVS as a syndrome without a name.[2]

It was an incredibly challenging study to do because many of the instru-ments that measured functional status conflated disability with impaired consciousness. For example, a patient who could not speak because he or she was on a ventilator might be conscious or not and receive a lower score because of a lack of motor output, for example, vocalization. And depending upon the assumptions we used, for example, life expectancy, which can be determined by a patient's clinical state or decisions to withdraw care by sur-rogates, we got inconsistent and ambiguous results.[2]

Our bottom line conclusion was that prospective, longitudinal epide-miological studies needed to be done in order to identify these patients, know where they were in the health care system, and meet their needs.[2] An Institute of Medicine (IOM) Exploratory Meeting on Disorders of Consciousness chaired by Dr. Kathy Foley, a neurologist at Memorial Sloan-Kettering Cancer Center and leading palliative care expert, made the same recommendation for epidemiological data, but the IOM was unable to secure congressional funding for a formal blue-ribbon report.[3]

That these funds could not be secured is understandable if we consider how little is spent on brain injury at the federal level. Although the incidence of traumatic brain injury is 1.5 to 2.0 million persons per year in the United States with a prevalence of 2.5 to 6.5 million individuals left with some degree of impairment, the allocation for the Reauthorization of the Traumatic Brain Injury Act for 2008 was $106 million dollars with total costs of $1.5 billion over the 2008–12 period.[4] And the ongoing debate on the federal deficit and entitlement spending is only going to make matters worse.

But large epidemiological studies are necessary to give validity to the claim that these patients deserve a hearing and that their care is not categorically futile. Only large-scale studies will demonstrate that this is a population in need of scientific engagement and clinical services and provide the road map for the construction of serious public policy, which can only be suggested by this narrative study.

The argument for epidemiological, population-based studies for the minimally conscious state (MSC), first made in the IOM Exploratory Meeting report published in *Neurology* in 2007,[3] is now made all the more compelling because of the epidemiological work of neuropsychologist Risa Nakase-Richardson.

In 2012, Dr. Nakase-Richardson, and her colleagues from the National Institute on Disability and Rehabilitation Research (NIDRR) Traumatic Brain Injury Model Systems Programs (TBIMS), found that 68 percent of traumatic brain injury (TBI) patients on in-patient rehabilitation services regained consciousness, and of those, 23 percent emerged from posttraumatic amnesia.[5] In addition, 19.6 percent of participants regained functional independence. Over time, they were able to live "without in-house supervision." A slightly smaller number (18.7 percent) had the potential to be employed in either a market-based or sheltered setting.[5]

These are notable findings because the data was collected from twenty NIDDR Model System Programs from a data base of 9,028 patients. Only 396 subjects were eligible for enrollment because they were categorically unconscious upon entry into rehabilitation. If the subjects' data set was incomplete, or if there was even minimal evidence of command following, they were excluded from prospective study. In addition, their degree of impairment had to be very significant upon enrollment. Enrollees had to have a Glasgow Coma Scale (GCS) less than six upon arrival in the emergency department and the actual cohort had an average GCS equal to three, the lowest value consistent with life.

Nakase-Richardson and her coauthors also found that patients made "significant" progress two years after TBI and more modest improvement for up to five years thereafter. Although a small cohort, this finding argues strongly for the longitudinal assessment of patients beyond the acute care setting to ensure that there is an accurate tracking of the patient's functional status over time. This will help mitigate the aforementioned problem of misdiagnosis.

In the aggregate, these NIDDR TBIMS data belie the prevailing nihilism directed at this population and discount the stories presented here as somehow unique or an exception to the rule. In point of fact, two-thirds of very severely injured patients regain consciousness and nearly 20 percent regain functional independence.

OVERCOMING NEURONAL SEGREGATION

The Nakase-Richardson and colleagues data is an advance in the argument, but it is only a start toward having a comprehensive demographic picture of this population and their needs. The fact that this basic epidemiological information is wanting, at this advanced date, speaks to the continued marginalization of this population.

The lack of such basic epidemiological knowledge about patients with disorders of consciousness suggests that they remain outside the health care system and out of our collective gaze. They remain invisible to policy makers and not of sufficient interest to warrant the cost of an accurate and formal epidemiology, essential to even initiating a plan to meet their needs.

It could be said that this cohort of patients remain segregated from mainstream medical care. *Segregation is a hard word, and I invoke it advisedly.* But if we reflect back on the trajectory of care we have just traversed with patients and their families it becomes clear that these patients suffer from a different standard of care than the rest of us. Because of prevailing social attitudes about severe brain injury and skepticism about any prospect of recovery, the care of these patients is often deemed futile even before one could honestly know.

Mrs. Waters, the mother of Jimmy who was hit by a car before being deployed as a Marine to Iraq summed up the problem. She put it frankly, "You're not seeing people who are brain injured ... on the street. They're not going to baseball games, they're unseen and unheard. And that's the problem. People in wheelchairs, they're out and about. They have jobs ... you kind of can't mess with ... people who are aware of their surroundings ... when do you see people like Jimmy except in an institutional environment? ...

They're the unseen and unheard ... and even the people who were supposed to help him really didn't want to help him."

As this volume attests, the resources that attend to the care of these patients fall off after their acute survival is assured, and at that point their marginalization begins. Families of patients who do not recover quickly enough are often encouraged to withhold or withdraw care, and sometimes become organ donors even before they have had the chance to declare themselves prognostically. Those who do not recover quickly or robustly enough are placed in chronic care facilities. Sometimes these referrals are, as John Whyte and colleagues have alleged, the product of systematic exclusion from rehabilitation programs based on insurance criteria that do not fit the biology of the MCS.

When patients end up in chronic care, families find that they are often ill-equipped and unable to provide needed medical care. There, patients are left to suffer from a degree of neglect that can only be believed when it's recounted in such a stereotypic manner by so many respondents. And so segregated, these patients often regain consciousness while in chronic care facilities, only to remain misdiagnosed for years. There they remain, in their beds, discounted and distanced from any prospect of a proper diagnosis much less any benefit stemming from nascent scientific innovation occurring far away in academic centers.

Now that progress in neuroscience has made us aware of the potential for these diagnostic errors, it is no longer acceptable to plead ignorance and say that one did not know of the errors of omission, of the neglect. At this point, there is a collective responsibility to not misdiagnose a conscious individual and to put in safeguards designed to prevent diagnostic error or its perpetuation over time. At the very least, those organizations that have oversight over the care of these patients (the Joint Commission and the National Committee for Quality Assurance, among others) should advance standards that call for the screening of patients diagnosed as vegetative for the reemergence of consciousness at appropriate clinical milestones after injury. Evaluation one year after injury might make the most sense for an initial screen of injuries following trauma, cardiac arrest, and vascular injuries.

But more is required than merely enhancing diagnostic accuracy. This should be a minimal first step, indeed it should be the norm and expectation. More aspirationally, we need to break down the forces of neuronal segregation that have too long marginalized these patients and deprived them of compassionate care, much less a proper diagnosis and access to emerging treatments and diagnostic paradigms.

This requires an ethical argument because neuronal segregation has become such an entrenched feature of how we care for the minimally conscious. To overcome it we must do more than argue about entitlements and health care benefits, we must affirm the recognition and engagement of consciousness as a civil right, rights that are fundamental and neither discretionary nor mere entitlements.

Instead, we must appreciate that it is an ethical imperative to view consciousness as a civil right when it is present. We must acknowledge that patients who are minimally conscious must be properly diagnosed because it is simply wrong to segregate a brain injured, but conscious, person from those who know them and love them by keeping them in chronic care facilities far from their homes and diagnostic accuracy. And it is equally wrong to deprive them access to proper rehabilitation, emerging drugs, or neuroprosthetic interventions that might foster their recoveries or ability to engage with others.

To perpetuate patterns of neurosegregation, given what we now know about the potential of the minimally conscious patient, is simply unethical. It is unethical because it is cruel to deprive a conscious individual the opportunity to experience human companionship and community. That possibility is extinguished when consciousness, that spark of personhood, upon which our collective relationships hinge, is overlooked or ignored. When that happens it might as well be extinguished.

Whether it is snuffed out through an error of omission or willful neglect, the failure to properly diagnose consciousness or sustain its emergence is not an option but a moral obligation. It is a responsibility that makes engagement possible. For with a failure to identify a person as conscious, there is no reason to try and communicate. And with that omission comes a failure to engage and continued exile from a human community, marked by shared communication. Simply stated, without being properly identified as conscious these patients will not be as fully integrated into society as might be possible. Instead, they will continue to be segregated and set apart from others with whom they might have been able to relate.

The importance of such integration is a point stressed by the 2006 UN Convention on the Rights of Persons with Disabilities. That venerable document clearly states that persons with disabilities should "have access to ... support services ... necessary to support living and inclusion in the community, and *to prevent isolation or segregation from the community*" (italics added).[6]

Just consider the thought experiment and imagine yourself in the bed, mistaken as unconscious when you were not, perhaps barely recognizing the maternal gaze directed toward you as you are unable to convey evidence of your presence. Like Maggie, we might imagine you yearning to be acknowledged as there, as present. And like her, once recognized, you might remember to be exuberant in moving your one moving eye, up and down, the morning after you were rediscovered, never wanting to be mistaken as being absent again.

No, to meet the needs of patients like Maggie, and all those her story represents, something more fundamental than entitlement reform needs to occur. These patients need to be recognized, their place in society secured and the status of their civil rights affirmed. For these reasons, we can no longer view their medical needs as discretionary but ethically compelling, especially any technological advances that might restore their ability to be reintegrated into society through the provision of voice, the ability to make contact and communicate with others.

RIGHTS, COMMUNICATION, AND COMMUNITY

Writing in support of the UN Universal Declaration of Human Rights, the philosopher Richard McKeon addressed the role technology and science might have in promoting communication and free speech.[7] In a prescient essay, written in 1948, entitled, "The Philosophical Bases and Material Circumstances of the Rights of Man," McKeon traces the history of the right to free speech from the contractarians of the eighteenth century and envisions a future when science and technology might need to be invoked to preserve this natural right. In that future, he argues, the preservation of free and unencumbered speech will only remain, or become, possible through the achievement of social and economic rights made possible by science and technological progress.[8] McKeon links the freedom of communication and thought to advances in science and technology that might hinder expression:

> The advancement of science and technology, which gave rise, as a result of changes consequent to it, to the problem of economic and social rights, has had a direct effect in the new significance that has been given to a fourth set of rights – the freedom of communication and thought.[9]

But McKeon's essay can also be read as using science in the service of securing the right to freedom of communication and thought, of voice.

In this articulation of a right dependent upon the proper use of emergent technologies, McKeon anticipates the dependence of severely brain-injured patients whose freedom of communication and expression of thought will hinge completely on technologies like deep brain stimulation, neuroimaging, brain computer interfaces, or pharmacologic agents. If there is a "fourth set of rights" essential for free thought and communication then these technologies must become available to allow for the voices of these patients to be resecured.

McKeon is blunt about the indispensability of science to these fundamental rights. He notes that "unless economic and social rights are first secured, civil and political rights are an empty sham and pretense."[9] In this vein, modern-day society is obliged to help the injured reclaim their voice through medical technology because it is an economic and social right that is instrumental to a fundamental right: the ability to communicate with each other.

This right to communication – and community – remains central to the aforementioned UN Convention on the Rights of Persons with Disabilities. It notes a "general obligation" "to undertake or promote research and development of, and to promote the availability and use of new technologies, including information and communications technologies. Mobility aids, devices and assistive technologies, suitable for persons with disabilities, giving priority to technologies at an affordable cost. ..."[6] This obligation also includes the promotion of research toward the development of these devices and the training of professionals "to better provide the assistance and services guaranteed by those rights."[6]

TECHNOLOGIES AND CAPABILITIES

Inviolable access to neuroprosthetic technology, and enabling medical care and rehabilitation, can also be asserted through a "capabilities" argument, discourse which in some respects has superseded more traditional appeals to human rights. The capabilities approach was initially advanced by the economist and Nobel Laureate, Amartya Sen, who spoke of the limitations of negative rights if their achievement did not sufficiently result in justice.[10] For example, if the granting of negative rights resulted from the lifting of a societal prohibition but the removal of this infringement left the newly enfranchised still disempowered, the new right would be hollow and theoretical.[10] Sen argued that something more instrumental was needed to link rights to constructive action and the *capability* to do something, to function, to achieve a good or fulfill a need,[11] or in the philosopher's Sridhar Venkatapuram's more recent formulation, to fulfill a goal.[12,13]

Sen importantly notes that rights and opportunities must be understood within a practical context with an eye to action, especially in the context of disability. At a keynote address at the World Bank conference on disability in 2004,[14] Sen noted that, "An understanding of the moral and political demands of disability is important not only because it is such a widespread and impairing feature of humanity, but also because the tragic consequences of disability can be substantially overcome with determined societal help and imaginative intervention. ..."[15]

Invoking Sen's work on disability, Venkatapuram also notes that individuals with disabilities may need additional help and resources "converting resources into pursuing their plans of life."[16] And so it is if we argue for the rights of patients with disorders of consciousness. Without the capability to actualize these rights, the delegation of rights will be worthless and an exercise in theory. For these patients to communicate, to reestablish connections severed by injury, they will need to be recognized as first having this right and then acknowledged as in need of having the capability necessary to realize that right.

Whether one invokes McKeon's early rights language, or the more recent capabilities arguments of authors like Sen and Venkatapuram, the point is clear. Access to neuroprosthetic technologies, drugs, and devices that might restore functional communication cannot be viewed as a mere entitlement to be funded or cut, a benefit to be shaved in a tight budget year, or a service at the margins. It cannot be about economics as Patrisha Wright, a disability advocate asserted when the question was one of access: "Would we ask what the cost/benefits are of putting black people on a bus?"[17]

Instead, these needs have an essential moral quality in establishing an inherent human right, or better yet, fostering capability: to use communication to form and be part of human community; to embrace the dispossessed so that once again they might enjoy the warmth and solidarity of human companionship, experiences grounded, in large part, in the restoration of voice and functional communication.

In short, it becomes an argument in favor of integration over segregation. If individuals who might be able to communicate are denied the resources to do so, they are then denied access to being maximally integrated into society.

HABLE CON ELLA

Community and communication: Although this linkage is yet to be apprehended by policy makers and the public at large, it has entered into our artistic consciousness in the brilliant work of Pedro Almodovar in the Academy Award–winning film *Hable con Ella [Talk or Speak with Her]*, erroneously translated from the Spanish as *Talk to Her*.[18,19] The story is of two women, a bullfighter and ballerina, who have sustained severe brain injury and appear vegetative. One dies and the other survives and regains the ability to communicate, buttressed by the "affections" of an orderly whose boundary violation leads him to jail. But Almodovar does not sanction the orderly who he names *Benigno*, the good. I believe this is because Almodovar recognizes that Benigno alone appreciated that communication is a reciprocal linkage that builds human community, hence the key preposition in the original title. We talk *with* each other and not *to* each other.

Almodovar appreciated the centrality of relationality and the importance of communication in realizing these bonds so central to human community[20,21] and overcoming what he describes as "a world full of obstacles."

As Almodovar told *The Guardian* in a 2002 interview, the opening scene of *Hable con Ella* depicts these two women as "walking around blind and sleeping walking." His intent: "From that moment on, I am telling the audience that there are going to be two women with closed eyes who will be facing this world full of obstacles . ..."[22] How right he was! To paraphrase Freud's reflections on the Oedipus Complex, sometimes the scientist discovers what the artist already knew.[23]

FUTURE IN THEIR BONES

Despite the evidence shared in previous chapters about the scientific advances that have occurred over the past two decades, advancing an argument for a right to the recognition of, or fostering of, consciousness might sound far-fetched and illusory given the state of present technology. After all, the restoration of voice, as in our DBS study, remains something that has only been achieved in research settings, and on rare occasions. I acknowledge that. But it has been done, proof of principle has been demonstrated, and there is no reason to think that progress will not continue.

I would like you, the reader to imagine, if you will, what will be possible if this research proceeds apace and the technology progresses, as will inevitably occur. And if we do not prepare our moral selves for this technological capability, we will be ill-prepared to share this advance with those who need it.

C. P. Snow, the British scientist and novelist who wrote of the two cultures that divide the sciences from the humanities, also famously observed that "scientists have the future in their bones."[24] And in this context, it is hard for many of us in the field not to imagine a time when communicative abilities will be restored for many patients with disorders of consciousness. Already the progress is significant: the development of DBS and neuroimaging has shown – and drug trials with the flu drug Amantadine and the sleeping pill Zolpidem will likely soon show[25–31] – that some hope is on the way.

Indeed, if past is prologue, work done over the past decade heralds great advance and progress. But it also portends peril because society still does not view the needs of this population with the urgency, or respect, that it deserves. It is long past time to reflect upon our biases so that as progress is made, society will appreciate its obligation to make it available and accessible to patients in need. Like C. P. Snow, we have to take a forward view and embrace the expectation that technology will provide a means for the minimally conscious to harness their residual cognitive capacities and express their love, hopes, and fears.

To the skeptics and those who claim that the argument put forward here is premature, let me respond – once again – with the sage comments of Professor Sen. Speaking on disability at the World Bank in 2004, Sen reminded us of our collective potential for clever and humane intervention and warned of our predilection for societal lassitude: "Given what can be achieved through intelligent and humane intervention, it is amazing how inactive and smug most societies are about the prevalence of the unshared burden of disability."[15]

FROM THE AMERICANS WITH DISABILITIES ACT TO OLMSTEAD

Inactivity and smugness. Yes, that remains the challenge. Before we can articulate the rights of patients in the minimally conscious state, much less equip them with the capabilities to improve their lot, society needs to first be awakened so as to affirm the rights of this population.

This will be a political process, a *rights movement*, that will gradually transform attitudes and views so that ultimately citizens will ask themselves, how did we treat those people as we did? Why didn't we appreciate their needs? And then, collectively we will be able to admit what we failed to do and acknowledge they deserve no less than any other conscious person.

Admitting how we have fallen short and affirming what remains to be done is neither a trivial act of confession nor statement of intent. It is nothing less than an acknowledgment that these people, so long sequestered and placed to the side, are in fact part of our civil society and that they are deserving of the rights and protections afforded other citizens, the inclusive rights of citizenship.

These rights should be enjoyed by those with severe brain injury, not only because of what the UN Convention maintains, but what the Americans with Disabilities Act (ADA) asserts.[32] The ADA was landmark legislation passed by Congress and signed into law by President George Herbert Walker Bush in 1990. It was intended to prohibit discrimination against persons with disabilities and ensure equal opportunity in employment (Title I) as well as access to public entities such as state and local government services including transportation (Title II), public accommodations, commercial facilities (Title III), and telecommunications (Title IV).[33] Title V contains miscellaneous provisions including an antiretaliation codicil.

In 1999, the ADA was upheld – some analysts have said that it was even strengthened – when the U.S. Supreme Court heard *Olmstead v. L.C.*, which was a challenge to Title II.[34] The case involved two women, Lois Curtis and Elaine Wilson who each had developmental and psychiatric disabilities. Both women were mentally retarded, with Ms. Curtis also diagnosed with schizophrenia and Ms. Wilson, a personality disorder. They were both voluntarily hospitalized in a state psychiatric hospital in Georgia for treatment. But once their conditions stabilized each asked that they be transferred to a community facility, a request that their treatment professionals thought appropriate to their condition. Despite this judgment, they remained institutionalized. The state of Georgia cited the cost of community care as a defense. Ms. Curtis filed suit alleging that their confinement violated Title II of the ADA. Ms. Wilson quickly followed suit.

Their question has been *our question*, the central issue of this book, the marginalization and segregation of patients with severe brain injury from the mainstream. Although the stories I told are unique and the science of MCS cutting edge, in the end, the story I was trying to tell was not novel. It had been told many times before, when people who were deaf, were excluded as deaf and dumb or when the blind were thought infirmed. No, this saga about MCS is just another chapter in the evolution of disability rights. Their treatment, their pattern of isolation and marginalization is straight out of the proverbial play book, acknowledged by one scholar who noted, "perhaps the word that best describes the historical treatment of persons with disabilities is *separation*" (italics in original).[35]

It was not until I had completed writing this story about MCS did I realize it was the newest chapter in a longer text, and not a novel volume in itself. This theme of segregation has long been part of the saga of the disability rights movement. Indeed, with the help of Commissioner Chai Feldblum of the Equal Opportunity Employment Commission, a disability rights legal scholar who was a key drafter of the ADA, I came to see that the tension between segregation and integration had also long been the fundamental challenge of the disability rights community, as most notably played out in *Olmstead*.[36]

And in *Olmstead*, that history was also repeating itself. Specifically, could Ms. Curtis and Ms. Wilson be compelled to be separated from society, that is segregated in a psychiatric hospital, when a less restrictive community venue was deemed by their doctors as a reasonable and safe alternate? Although people with disabilities like Curtis and Wilson had long been discriminated against, this time there was hope – because of the ADA. The law would seem to be on their side because Congress had been explicit in its legislative intent. In uncharacteristically frank language, the drafters of the ADA acknowledged the history of marginalization and segregation, of people with disabilities.

That history is complex and itself woven into the fabric of the civil rights movement. Jim Crow laws led to the segregation of people with disabilities as they had maintained the separation of the races. Disability theorist, Jacqueline Vaughn Switzer, observes that "The similarity between the Jim Crow laws of the South and the prejudice against disabled people has been noted by several authors, most of whom cite policymakers' belief that such segregation at the time was considered benign and beneficial."[37] Legal scholar Timothy Cook points out that these parallel practices of segregation were based on perceptions of inferiority and superiority, a categorization operationalized through segregative practices:

> Our government's systematic segregation and exclusion of those thought to be inferior and unfit, of course, was not limited to persons with disabilities. Indeed, the far better known and understood official apartheid in the country has been based on race, especially after the Supreme Court in 1896 gave the states *carte blanche* authority to establish "separate-but-equal" government services in *Plessy v. Fergusson*. The Jim Crow system established after *Plessy* and the government-supported, systematic segregation of persons with disabilities during precisely the same period were no mere coincidences of historical events. The historical record abounds with evidence that disability discrimination emanated from the same attitudes and prejudices fomenting at the turn of the century regarding race. Public officials felt that a solution regarding disability, equal to the severity and the magnitude of the "problem" of racial mixing, was imperative.[38]

In drafting the ADA, Congress's intent was to rewrite that history and it said so explicitly in the legislation. And the authors of the ADA specifically made note of the question of segregation in explaining their legislative intent. Simply stated, Congress saw a "mandate for the elimination of discrimination against individuals with disabilities" precisely because "historically, society has tended to isolate and segregate individuals with disabilities, and, despite some improvements, such forms of discrimination against individuals with disabilities continue to be a serious and pervasive social problem."[39]

Professor Feldblum in an analysis of the antidiscrimination provision of the ADA squarely places the law within the context of civil rights. She notes that:

> The second antidiscrimination concept of the ADA is presumed on the assumption that with disabilities have a *civil right* to be considered part of the societal norm. This approach itself is revolutionary because it contrasts sharply with the traditional approach "of doing special things" for people with disabilities based on a charity model. ... Indeed, one of the striking aspects of the second concept of antidiscrimination is that it requires affirmative activities on the part of employers and business *not* as part of a "help the handicapped" program, but rather as a response to the legitimate demands of a group whose civil rights have traditionally been denied.[40]

So contextualized, the courts found in favor of the plaintiffs. The Federal District Court first hearing *Olmstead* agreed with the plaintiffs and found that "unnecessary institutional segregation constitutes discrimination *per se*, which cannot be justified by a lack of funding." Justice Ruth Bader Ginsburg writing for the majority of the Supreme Court agreed.[41] She noted by way of context that, "Congress explicitly identified unjustified 'segregation' of persons with disabilities as a form of discrimination." And most critically the Court upheld the key "integration regulation" of the ADA nestled within Title II that requires a "public entity [to] administer ... programs ... in the most integrated setting appropriate to the needs of qualified individuals with disability."[42] It also upheld the appeals court ruling that states could not invoke budgetary concerns when it came to ADA compliance unless the expenditure would be "so unreasonable given the hundreds of demands of the state's mental health budget that it would fundamentally alter the services it provides." That wasn't the case for the state of Georgia and the two women were granted their request to live in the community.

AN "OLMSTEAD-LIKE ARGUMENT"

Appreciating how the lived experiences of MCS patients and their families fit into this larger sociocultural and legal context would have been more readily apparent to one who came to these questions from fields like disability studies or the law. But for me it was something of a revelation. Indeed, when I made civil rights argument for MCS patients it often went ignored or was met with annoyance and arrogant self-assurance that I was wrong. The prevailing view was that people who were the focus of my advocacy did not have the need, much less the right to these rights. Finding an affirming set of arguments in the disability literature, notably Chai Feldblum's notion that I had been making an "Olmstead-like argument," has been a welcome and affirming development. It has led the way to additional scholarship justifying the further integration of people with MCS into society and has provided interdisciplinary validation of arguments originating in the medical model and patient narratives presented here.

But even as there is agreement amongst scholarly approaches, people with disorders of consciousness push the limits of an Olmstead-like formulation and suggest that inclusion and integration can transcend place. For those with disorders of consciousness, it is not so much about living in the community but being *part* of that community. Here, community is not just a physical place but also about relationships with others, made possible by communication. Here, community is achieved not by just placement but enablement, by providing MCS patients with the means, skills, or tools to make connections with others. And when provided with this capability to communicate, community is rebuilt.

This benefit is not solely for patients in MCS. Their reentry into a community marked by communication benefits others too. If we recall the joy felt by Angilee Wallis when Terry rejoined the conversation or when Corinth Pecco took Greg shopping, it becomes apparent that the benefits of integration were, as in the case of school desegregation, widely cast.

And so invoking the next iteration of an "Olmstead-like" decision, we could and should ask, if familial and social integration is possible, as it was with Greg Pearson and Terry Wallis and may be for so many others if they obtain even *currently* existing cognitive rehabilitation. If so, then would not efforts to block access to these means to the achievement of a person's highest degree of integration – "the most integrated setting appropriate" – to their station, would that not constitute a violation of Title II of the ADA?

And would it not be a violation of their civil rights because, absent the restoration of functional communication, they would need to be maintained in a more restrictive environment? What is the difference between the litigants in Olmstead's release to a less segregated venue, than perhaps giving a patient like Greg Pearson the ability to be cared for at home with proper assistance?

And would not policies like medical necessity that limits the length of time patients receive rehabilitation based on *somatic* evidence of improvement become even more legally problematic when the metric used to assess progress in these patients is ill-suited to the measurement of their improvement? Might it not be the object of a class-action suit against a discriminatory federal policy that denies needed services to patients who are inappropriately assessed for their medical condition? That is, might it be better to assess the neurological improvements (which likely predate behavioral manifestations of the progress necessary under medical necessity) to receive continued funding for care?

Long before a patient *shows* signs of improving behaviorally, his brain may demonstrate changes that herald recovery. But medical necessity is a construct that presupposes *motor function*, a kind of ability that would discriminate against those who cannot move, who cannot respond to a command because they cannot control their limbs. For some minimally conscious patients, the failure to properly assess their minds could lead to the assumption that they were not conscious, when their nonresponse was due to a lack motor function.

Either way, withholding or prematurely terminating rehabilitative services would result in the perpetuation of the segregative and restrictive policies suffered by the plaintiffs in Olmstead. Not providing (as some criteria seem to do), or prematurely curtailing the rehabilitative services (as medical necessity does) that would allow patients to be better integrated with their families, and in some circumstances live with them, would seem to violate the stated objective of the ADA, as forcefully affirmed in Olmstead, to overcome the legacy of *segregation* – now Congress's word, not mine – that has been foisted upon people with disabilities.

WHAT IS OWED?

In an era of fiscal scarcity, one needs to acknowledge limits. The expectation is not for special treatment, but parity. First in the realm of the quality of diagnosis. Nowhere else in medicine would diagnostic error rates of the scope seen with disorders of consciousness be tolerated. At a minimum, patients who are minimally conscious deserve not to be mistaken as vegetative, especially at key junctures like when the appellation of permanence is applied. Second, those who are minimally conscious who are able to perceive pain should be entitled to adequate pain and symptom management. Discomfort and distress should be evaluated with the recognition that these patients are especially vulnerable because they can experience pain but they may not be able to communicate their distress.

Reasonable efforts at the restoration of functional communication, as understood within the financial parameters set out by Olmstead, should be made. By this, I do not suggest that everyone gets a neuroprosthetic device, like a deep brain stimulator, or hours in the fMRI scanner in order to communicate. Instead, I would suggest low-cost remedies like adequate physical therapy, drug trials with active agents like Amantadine and Zolpidem, and the provision of low-tech devices like communication boards. The use of expensive and still investigational functional neuroimaging can and should be done, in specialized centers, to clarify the diagnosis and help to better ascertain the presence of consciousness when reliable behavioral assessments like the use of the Coma Recovery Scale-R are inconclusive.

Resources should also be directed to family support. These families courageously struggle under a tremendous burden, experiencing something akin to a prolonged and complicated bereavement. They need respite care, in-house nursing services and psychological support, services that might be seen as an expanded role for community hospice programs.[43]

Adequate resources should be directed to basic, translational and epidemiological research.[3] At the basic level, support should be directed to research that will elucidate mechanisms of recovery from severe brain injury. Funding should also be made available to foster the development of neuroprosthetic devices and drugs, a challenge because patients with disorders of consciousness have been viewed as an orphan population not worthy of sustained corporate investment and been complicated by regulatory challenges.[44,45]

These efforts should be coupled with cost-benefit analyses that look at how these interventions might decrease fixed custodial costs already in the system by increasing a patient's functional status. For example, should

DBS for MCS move beyond proof of principle, and the success seen in Greg Pearson's case be replicated, one could study whether the fixed costs associated with the complications of his pre-DBS state (bed sores, blood clots, pneumonia, and malnutrition) might be offset by the *medical* benefits of DBS. Neuromodulation allowed him to eat by mouth, become more mobile and tell doctors when he felt unwell, thus decreasing risks of medical complications and expediting medical attention.[46] All of these benefits offset medical costs.

Finally, this research agenda should be complemented by a comprehensive epidemiological assessment of the scope of need of this population.[3] Remarkably, we still do not have credible data on how many people are in MCS in the United States. This metric will be necessary for any serious public policy planning.[2]

BEYOND OLMSTEAD

The prior section would seem to constitute a modest policy agenda that should be in our collective reach. But I am under no illusions that it will be readily achieved because even now, people with disorders of consciousness have not been viewed as the beneficiaries of the ADA or Olmstead.

Commenting on the passage of the ADA, disability scholar Jacqueline Vaughn Switzer noted that the work had only begun. She observed that, "Just as the landmark case *Brown v. Board* in 1954 failed to produce immediate desegregation of the nation's schools, passage of nondiscriminatory legislation has failed to put an end to stereotypes that still characterize people with disabilities."[47] The rights articulated in the ADA, and affirmed in Olmstead, not only need to be societally reenforced for those who have been recognized as objects of discrimination, they *also* need to be seen as applicable to those in MCS, patients for whom the ADA first seemed irrelevant.

As I have argued, MCS patients have been so marginalized, so segregated from the medical – and legal mainstream – that they seem to have fallen beyond the coverage of the disability rights movement and the ADA. It is not that the ADA could not offer some protection. I would think it could. Instead it was a question of applicability. Until now, to my knowledge, no one has made an ADA claim for this population. Indeed, if these patients had come under the protection of the ADA much of what has been reported here would be deemed inconsistent with prevailing law. Their care, their neglect, their segregation, would be seen in violation of its provisions.

Moreover, these omissions would have been covered by a self-righteous media, ever eager to recount a tale of victimization. But that has not happened. Their story has somehow gone untold and unnoticed because, somewhere in our collective consciousness, it was felt unimportant and unworthy of attention because those with disorders of consciousness remained simply, "the disabled," not "people with disabilities."[48]

That is they remained anonymous, without recognition of their person-hood. And without that key acknowledgment, they were deemed as illegiti-mate objects of laws designed to protect *people*. Like groups before them, this is not the only time in the struggle for civil rights that individuals were not recognized as being eligible to enjoy the rights held by the dominant class. Throughout history, exclusion has been a sad, but recurrent pattern in the widening circle of those given basic civil rights.

From women suffragettes at Seneca Falls, to civil rights workers at the bridge at Selma, to early gay rights activists at Stonewall, our nation's history speaks to marginalized groups having to appeal for rights enjoyed in full by other citizens: the right to vote; integration; marriage. These were rights that were taken for granted by the majority but had to be secured for minority groups first thought disqualified or ineligible.

Writing a review of Linda Hirshman's *Victory*,[49] a chronicle of the gay rights movement, Rich Benjamin places these cycles of advocacy and struggle into a helpful historical context. Enfranchisement of those with severe brain injury falls into this line of civil rights struggles. He observes how marginal-ized groups have worked:

> Ever since the Enlightenment, when intellectuals articulated the crucial promises of the modern liberal state – security, liberty and self-governance – society's dispossessed have struggled to claim these rights as their own. The gay and lesbian movement, like the black civil rights and women's movements, has from its earliest days sought security (protection from violence and discrimination), freedom (inalienable human and group rights) and self-governance (the ability to participate effectively in political and economic life).[50]

Benjamin's comment is instructive. Civil rights movements are familiar in retrospect but shockingly absurd or even outrageous before they successfully achieve their goals and convert the mainstream to their cause.

Disability advocates place their efforts within this larger American Civil Rights lineage, often drawing parallels, sometimes even with good humor. One activist was to have said, "Black people fought for the right to ride in the front of the bus. We're fighting for the right to get on the bus."[51] And as early as 1980, ADA proponent, Justin Dart, asserted that what was needed was a "strong, highly visible, comprehensive civil rights law."[52] And that is what occurred, with one scholar noting that "two ground breaking statues – the Rehabilitation Act of 1973 and the ADA of 1990 – exemplify the civil rights model ...", most notably, "the ADA, which has often been referred to as the most significant civil rights legislation in U.S. history."[53]

But the achievement of this success took a different path for disabil-ity activists. In a sense they had the greater challenge because the fight was invisible and unseen. In his definitive history, *No Pity, People with Disabilities Forging a New Civil Rights Movement*, Joseph P. Shapiro observes that:

> ... disability rights constituted a steath civil rights movement. Although its activists pointed to the black, women's, and gay rights movements as models, unlike those causes, the disability rights movement had never filled the streets with tens of thousand protesters. It had no Martin Luther King, Jr., to bring it together, no Betty Friedan to write its manifesto. It had no unifying touchstone moment of courage or anger like the Montgomery Bus Boycott, the Freedom Rides of the Stonewall riots. There was virtually no attention from the public or press. The fight for disability civil rights was a largely invisible, almost underground, movement.[54]

Shapiro worries that the stealthiness of the movement, while effective, had an important liability: it may have failed to rally society to its cause in a persuasive and enduring manner. Presciently in the years before the *Olmstead* challenge, he asked, "What happens when Congress grants a new group minority rights, but society has little understanding that those rights have been awarded or why they are needed?"[55] When these rights were won "without dramatic Freedom Rides, church bombings or 'I have a Dream' speech to stir the conscience of a guilty nation?"[56] It was a serious concern, all the more so because he envisioned that the ADA, "which promised integration, will have more impact than any civil rights law since the 1964 act that banned discrimination against blacks, women, and ethnic and religious minorities."[56]

One consequence of the successful but stealthy disability rights movement is that some people with disabilities were excluded and left behind. The impact of the ADA and even *Olmstead* has not yet dug deeply enough into the nation's conscience and reached the plight of people with disorders of consciousness. They were simply overlooked. Absent a broader and deeper consensus, patients who did not fit society's perceptions of disability were simply not viewed as disabled. Very sick, gravely wounded? Yes. Labeled as terminally ill and seen as better off dead, as the *Not Yet Dead* disability activist group's name implies?[57] Perhaps.

But are people with MCS disabled in the way that the ADA would be relevant to them? To date, the answer to that question is a pointed ... no. They just did not fit that category and hence have not yet received the hard fought protections enjoyed by other people with disabilities. They were victims of a category error.

Segregation is predicated on a category error and thus it is important to be sure that we address all the ways in which people with disabilities might be mistakenly classified, or overlooked. One fundamental way in which this occurs is to fail to see disabled people as fully human, as the late Justin Dart, a leading disability activist and architect of the ADA observed. Speaking to the incompleteness of a stealth disability movement and lingering biases Dart noted that, "Our society is still infected by an insidious, now almost unconscious, assumption that people with disabilities are less than fully human and therefore are not entitled to the respect, the opportunities, and the services and support systems that are available to other people as *a matter of right*" (italics added).[58]

REREADING BROWN

So empowered by the ADA and *Olmstead*, let us then reread *Brown v. Board* as a *matter of right*. When it was written it was all about race. But now, in the context of the ADA and *Olmstead*, its mandate can be seen as more expansive: the abolition of the separate but equal doctrine and education as it relates to those people who are minimally conscious.

In the post-*Olmstead* era, what are the lessons embedded in *Brown v. Board* beyond racial integration? Read in this new light, one of emergent disability rights, *Brown* can be particularly helpful because it addresses *education* and child development.

Decades before Sen articulated the relationship between rights and capabilities, the Warren Court drew the link between civil rights and education's ability to give young people the opportunity to live productive lives:

> Today, education is perhaps the most important function of state and local governments. Compulsory school attendance laws and the great expenditures for education both demonstrate our recognition of the importance of education to our democratic society. It is required in the performance of our most basic public responsibilities, even service in the armed forces. It is the very foundation of good citizenship. Today it is a principal instrument in awakening the child to cultural values, in preparing him for later professional training, and in helping him to adjust normally to his environment. In these days, it is doubtful that any child may reasonably be expected to succeed in life if he is denied the opportunity of an education. Such an opportunity, where the state has undertaken to provide it, is a right that must be made available to all on equal terms.[59]

Presciently, the Warren Court affirmed the relationship between the achievement of civil rights and the provision of an enabling educational experience, which would provide children with the preparation that they would need. Over time, this relationship between rights and capabilities, as provided by education, has become emblematic of the civil rights movement. It has been seen as a means toward upward mobility, a means to break down generations of segregation and has been encapsulated in the well-known advertising campaign of the United Negro College Fund: "*a mind is a terrible thing to waste."* That slogan, which speaks to how civil rights have been enabled by access to education, is reminiscent of Sen's capabilities, which when reframed toward those in the minimally conscious state also points to the developmental capacity of injured brains to recover and regain ground, if properly assisted. Education for the young and rehabilitation for the brain injured are more closely linked if recovery from brain injury is viewed in a developmental frame. That is, an unfolding process that occurs as a process of an evolving biology from a new set point determined by the patient's injury.

If we reconsider the possible axonal sprouting, and clear structural changes in the brain, seen in Terry Wallis's nearly two decades after his injury, we see echoes of an earlier developmental process.[60] From infancy on through childhood and adolescence, the sprouting and pruning of connections between neurons occurs as a way to organize and connect the growing brain to itself.[61] Has something similar occurred in the setting of severe brain injury? Has a developmental process been reharnessed to become a reparative one? At this juncture we do not know. But there is emerging information from animal models that there may be a link. For example, there is evidence that wound healing following damage to the rat neocortex is accompanied by axonal sprouting and that this is motivated by stem cells, perhaps linking brain repair to early developmental biology.[62]

The first time around, this process is developmental. After an injury, the process is regenerative, or at least recuperative in which the patient begins their recovery *later* in life and with a different set of goals in mind. As I suggested earlier, the process is a recapitulation of an earlier developmental one, which education is meant to assist and complement.

So why not alter our framework and recast rehabilitation done after injury as a sort of re-education? Might this have implications for how experts think about rehabilitation after injury? Would it not make good sense for early age educators who work with the developing brain to compare notes with those who seek its recovery? I suspect that much common ground could be found on techniques and methods geared toward the promotion of verbal fluency, motor skills, and socialization through such dialogue across traditional silos of knowledge.

The invocation of education as analogy or metaphor may seem far-fetched but the brain injury literature is rife with commentary by survivors who speak of knowing something once and then having to relearn the task after their injury. Bob Woodruff of ABC News told me he had to relearn some words he had forgotten and refile others that he had misplaced.[63] He spoke of it as an educational task of learning (old) now new vocabulary and organizing it in a way that he could retrieve and access it.

His comments are reminiscent of those of Trish Meili, the Central Park Jogger, who wrote in her remarkable memoir how she had to relearn math after having been a financial analyst for Smith Barney.[64] So too, did Claudia Osborn, a physician who sustained a brain injury in her frontal lobe affecting her decision-making abilities. She recalled she once knew medicine and had to relearn much of what she once knew, ultimately becoming an abstract painter.[65]

Reconceptualizing rehabilitation as a kind of late-life education might also raise the question of how much time is necessary to achieve pedagogical goals and how many resources are needed. Might not the school day be extended for those who are recovering, progressively over time, accommodating for fatigue and other mitigating factors? Let us think about what the young child must accomplish in the early years of school and how long it takes to reach early milestones. It becomes obvious that anyone who has to regain lost abilities in conventional rehabilitation is spending but a fraction of the time necessary to achieve these same goals, altering expectations that the process will take months and years and not weeks.

Given this mix of biology and brain injury narratives, it makes some sense to view early childhood education and brain injury rehabilitation as somehow linked, where insights in one area might illuminate challenges in the other. And if education works for the progressively maturing brain, might not a similar model work for recovering minds as it retraces familiar but long forgotten milestones like command following, expressive speech, and ambulation? This recapitulation of an earlier developmental process is made necessary by the setback of injury. Like the education of a child, brain injury rehabilitation's purpose is to help an individual meet progressive functional goals and to maximize one's potential, a point also made by the UN Convention on Disability, which speaks to the "full development of human potential" through an "inclusive education system at all levels."[6]

The education of children with disabilities is also guaranteed under the 1990 Individuals with Disabilities Education Act (IDEA), which furthers the link between the civil rights movement and disability rights.[66] In the view of disability scholars Doris Zames Fleischer and Freida Zames, it "extends to children with disabilities the principle of equality of educational opportunities underlying the landmark 1954 Supreme Court decision in *Brown v. Board of Education*."[67] This federal "special education" statute extends educational benefits to youth with disabilities up to age twenty-one. If we come to understand rehabilitation in a more educational frame, might not the IDEA become a template for expanding these educational rights to older individuals in MCS whose recovery process is in essence a reprise of an earlier developmental process? Might not the distinction between developmental and acquired disability become irrelevant when it comes to the provision of educational benefits?

But there is more embedded in the *Brown* decision than questions about educational policy – it also speaks to the emotional burden of segregation on the psyche of those who are separated. It was an argument, of course predicated on race, but one that has relevance to emotional needs of whatever group is excluded on an arbitrary or discriminatory basis. Writing of the enduring psychological impact of this practice, the Supreme Court observed that:

> To separate them from others of similar age and qualifications solely because of their race generates a feeling of inferiority as to their status in the community that may affect their hearts and minds in a way unlikely ever to be undone.[59]

Whether the placement of young survivors of brain injury into nursing homes typically serving the elderly will leave similar psychological scars and "feelings of inferiority," we cannot know. But we do know that many of the mothers interviewed for this volume intuited a difference between these facilities and ones serving younger patients. Nancy Worthen, Mary Waters, Shirley Green, and others sought to find placement for their children with their own generational cohort, where they weren't expected to experience the decline of a patient with dementia in the next bed.

Nancy memorably characterized Middleboro as, "a *dorm of young people. They just happen to all be brain injured.*" She told me that, Maggie is "in a room with a woman who has a very similar stroke to Margaret's, who is young. She has a baby daughter whose name is Margaret, which is kind of fun, because the little girl comes in and people say 'Margaret' and Margaret turns her head. And they've gotten to know her, so there's a social connection just within her room, with her roommate and her roommate's friends and family. ..." Unlike all the other places she had been, Maggie now "actually has two or three people in the nursing home who are her peers who come and visit her because now they know her and they know her story and so they talk with her. I'm not ... saying that couldn't happen in a nursing home with elderly people, but they have more in common because they're recovering."

Nancy's reflections, and those of fellow mothers, reflect the same moral intuition held by the Warren Court: it could be argued that housing young brain-injured patients in nursing homes serving the elderly is ethically and legally comparable to the segregation of black children in inferior schools or the mentally retarded in a psychiatric hospital, as argued in *Brown* and *Olmstead*, respectively.

When the Senate passed the ADA, Senator Ted Kennedy said it was "a historic step in the long journey to complete the unfinished business of America to bring full civil rights and fair opportunity to" all citizens.[68] Rereading canonical texts like *Brown* is a step in completing that journey to equality for those who are only now seen as entitled to make it.

22 A Call for Advocacy

When Lyndon Johnson nominated Thurgood Marshall to the Supreme Court as its first black justice, Marshall thanked the president for being in command of history. He told LBJ, "You didn't wait for the times. You made them."[1] Robert Caro, Johnson's biographer, feels that Marshall's gratitude to the president was not for his elevation to the court but rather for Johnson's forward-looking stance on American civil rights.[1]

To date, we have been waiting for the times to change before we change our attitudes and practices toward those who are minimally conscious. Ours is a moment of history that calls to collectively take control. We need to make the times our own and respond to what interdisciplinary study in the neurosciences and the medical humanities is teaching us about the experiences of those in a minimally conscious state. It is time that *rights come to mind.*

To do this we must build upon the disability rights movement with its deep debt to its predecessor movements and affirm consciousness as a right that must be recognized, respected, and enabled. It will foster productive science and rectify societal deficiencies that remain untenable, if not inhumane. The goal is a nascent social movement that will place the needs of these patients and families on the legislative agenda, so that in a bipartisan fashion they can be fully protected under the law and receive the care and support that they need.

To begin we need our generation of Freedom Riders, those who won't wait for the times but make them their own. These advocates will join in the long march of a new civil and disability rights struggle. Like their predecessors they will be motivated by a sense of what is right and the need to rectify injustice. But their journey will be different.

Although they will sit in solidarity with those who were turned away, they will not march over bridges, arms linked together. Instead they will cross into spaces that are as fraught but seldomly seen. Their vigil will be at a bedside in chronic care and not a lunch counter in a five and dime, but their cause is the same: overcoming segregation and the promotion of the civil rights of those who have too long been out of society's gaze.

Like their predecessors, today's Freedom Riders will need fortitude to sustain the effort, because the kind of reform that will be required can neither be achieved quickly, nor solely by those who are directly affected.

Broadening the scope of advocacy is essential. Families cannot do it alone. They don't have time for protest. They are worn down and do not have the energy, much less the resources, to run – or even walk – for a cure. Mary Waters, the mother of Jimmy who was struck by a car just before he was to deploy to Iraq as a Marine, told us that caring for her son is "like having an extra job just doing this."

Their long vigil leads to fatigue, defeatism, and depression, and often feelings of going alone, unaided by external support.[2] These struggles can lead to bankruptcy in up to 5 percent of families,[3] with those on Medicaid being especially vulnerable.[4] All of this compounds the trauma of the original injury and makes families less available for outside advocacy.[5]

Family members are frankly too burdened by caregiving to engage in the social action necessary to initiate and sustain a social movement. Theirs is a solitary sort of advocacy,[6] fought at a microeconomic level trying to get their sons or daughters, husbands or wives an extra hour of rehab each week, a diagnostic study, or a rudimentary prosthetic device.

Their advocacy is personal, not political, making sure their loved ones are turned in bed so they don't get bedsores. Sitting vigil in chronic care, so that pain is recognized and treated. They have a hard time leaving the bedside for the larger political fight and have difficulty delegating caregiving to others. Nancy speaking of Maggie said, "... if I were to leave her advocacy to a social worker alone, to answer the questions alone, I would feel neglectful. Because I know my daughter better ... I think a social worker ... can never be the same as the family's passion and love. . . ."

So therein lies the challenge: we neither see the patients who are sequestered in chronic care, nor hear from their families because they are consumed by the provision of and support at the bedside. What we do see are the patients that have seemingly done well.

We are grateful for the heroic recoveries of ABC's Bob Woodruff [7] and more recently Congresswoman Gabby Giffords,[8] but their stories, once picked up by the media, only tend to dichotomize outcomes and ongoing difficulties. Media accounts are bifurcated: one is either beyond hope or has a miraculous recovery. Such reports minimize the longitudinal struggles of most patients with brain injury who remain somewhere between the extremes and need ongoing care and concern. But they are never the focus. Instead we are left with hopeful rhetoric and coverage that belies the difficult reality between the superficial coverage, allowing us to deny unmet needs and burdens.

It was a moment for celebration when Gabby Giffords first returned to Congress and a bitterly divided House brought a unity of applause and words of thanks for her recovery.[8] A far better tribute would be for our political leadership, and the public at large, to recognize the true challenge brain injury represents for Ms. Giffords and others who have been injured in both civilian and military life.

We must recall that every success story carries a legacy of challenge, and that for every success story there are many whose potential has not been achieved, whose conscious selves are ignored for want of attentive and sustained care. We need only remember the fate of Bob Woodruff whose high-profile injury did not protect him from the specter of neglect.

Days away from nursing home placement, six weeks into his stay at Bethesda Naval Hospital because he was not making overt medical progress and remained unconscious, Woodruff was himself almost a casualty of medical necessity and about to be dispatched to a nursing home.[9] Even someone of his stature and fame was not immune to the forces of discharge planning and cost containment.

But then, days before he was about to be sent out of the hospital, Bob awakened to greet his wife, Lee. He asked her, "Hey, Sweetie where've you been?"[9] That same question should be asked of each of us as we contemplate the rights, liberties, and care that are owed to those amongst us with severe brain injury.[10] They and their families deserve a civil rights movement that they are too burdened to lead.

That is a responsibility that the rest of us must help them bear.

Epilogue

As I write these final words in January 2013, we are between visits. Maggie and Nancy Worthen have just left New York, and Dustin Manwiller is to come soon. Dustin was last in New York in 2008 and our team is eager to see him in person again. We are now seeing up to a couple of patients a month, and it has become almost like having house guests as patients and families come and go.

And for us the most amazing thing is how things seem to change with time, a passage that we still cannot readily predict, though we try. This chronicle is but a chapter in lives that will continue to evolve even as this narrative ends. That is how it should be because one of the messages I have sought to convey is that the injured brain is not static but a dynamic entity, whose biology if properly understood and harnessed has recuperative powers we might only imagine. So as I conclude, let me provide an update on the lives of some of the courageous patients and families you have come to know.

THE FUTURIST

Let me start where so much of this story began, in Arkansas, and with Terry Wallis. I last spoke to Angilee in October 2012 when a news reporter wanted to interview the family. She turned them down, but shared with me how Terry was doing. With a mother's joy, she told me, "He's learned so much," though she admitted, "he still has bad memory problems."

Although he is "more aware of time now," "he still thinks he's a teenager" even though he is forty-nine. But now, when his parents ask him what year it is, he won't answer. Not just because he does not know it but because "he refuses to accept it," thinking he can "not be that old."

But things are changing. For the first time he is aware of the passage of time and how his needs might evolve over the hours. Remarkably, although he is generally stuck in the present, he is anticipating the future. Angilee noticed this at nighttime when she and her husband Jerry would go to sleep. Terry would "holler" at them and ask, "And what if I need you? What am I supposed to do?"

It does not sound like much, but this is something he could not do when he was mired in his eternal present, when he could not conceptualize time. That simple request, that concern of his at bedtime represents the reemergence of a planning function that is wholly dependent on a sense of time.

Now, nearly thirty years after his car accident, though, his world is still 1984, the past is slowly receding. And most importantly, Terry is looking forward, albeit tenuously, into the future.

THE ARTIST

Maggie was far more responsive than when we last saw her in November 2010, and Nancy was more optimistic. Her responses with her one functioning eye were quicker, and she noticed when people came into her room. It was an obvious improvement over the past several years.

Following a hard patch, things were getting better. Nancy explained that it was because she and Maggie are able to do art therapy together. With the aid of an art therapist, Jeannie Bestoso, who she met at a conference on brain injury, Nancy makes art with Maggie, making her daughter positively happy. At first Maggie and the therapist "made these little clay pots that were very crude." But no matter, they were Margaret's, "her hands were on the clay."

The pride of ownership comes through in Nancy's recounting of how her daughter, never much for art, has found solace and companionship with her mother in this true collaboration. Working together, Nancy directs the brush or sculpts the clay with her hand over Maggie's, which while immobile, feels the swoop of the painted canvass or texture of the wet earth between her fingers.

It can make Maggie joyous and emotional. She seems to love this activity more than the time she struggles to use the computer screen to spell out words with her eye movements. She detests the computer, according to Nancy, but loves the painting, the brushes, the pencils, and the chance to go to do art by the seaside and the beach, "where she could see the water."

Maggie expresses her pleasure with a heightened degree of emotionality. How can Nancy be so sure of Maggie's reaction? It is "just the fact that she's responsive. In other words the fact that she's excited enough and involved enough that she laughs or cries ... to *me* it is a strong indication that she's involved. And then when I open her eyes she's looking at the painting. I mean, she's looking at what's happening as she sees her hand doing it. She doesn't always attend to what is happening. But there are times when I see her and she's really looking at her hand touching the paper." Then, she continues in a more sober tone, "it is hard because sometimes you want to see things but I guess ... it's ... she doesn't give the indication that she doesn't want to do it. She gives the indication that she does."

Paul, Maggie's father, is convinced that art has been a game changer for his daughter. Nancy tells me that Paul "would say that the art has changed her life totally." It has made her more expressive and communicative. And although Nancy is more conservative in her assessment she admits that Maggie's quality of life over the last six months is the best it has been since she had her stroke. No small confession for a woman who has been so tempered and balanced in her assessment of the road she and her daughter are traveling. But she is quick to remind me that "... it's not a happy thing. It's not happy. There isn't anything beautiful or happy about it."

Notwithstanding the reflective comments that bring her back to the ultimate trauma she has experienced as a mother, Nancy seems more at peace with her world. She has reconciled herself to Maggie's second childhood. "It's not what I expected." She wanted "to have grandchildren but I'm not going to so I have Margaret and ... maybe that's why there's a certain degree right now of feeling satisfied because she seems to be moving ahead. I can feel really good that I've done everything I could possibly do."

And in the moment, she and Maggie are having fun. And even more importantly, she and her daughter are creating beautiful things. With a mother's pride she tells me, "I think they are lovely." And most meaningfully, after all these years, they are being productive together. With some pride she notes, "We have fun together. It's created I think a way for Margaret and I to be together that for me is productive. Like it is actually productive because we actually make paintings that I think are pretty. And so just the fact that it's productive for me and her together."

Their shared artworks have been printed up as cards and Nancy has even started a small business selling the reproductions online and at craft fairs. She has yet to sell the original artwork because "they are too valuable."

THE DIARIST

It will be five years since we last saw Dustin. Like Maggie, his accident was in 2006 and like her, Dustin communicates by making use of his one functioning eye. In his case, he relies on his retained sight to read and direct his gaze toward a letter board hooked up to a computer that allows him to spell out his thoughts. The computer keeps track of the direction of his head and creates written text for others to read.

Dustin has come a long way since his near-death experiences in a nursing home described in Chapter 9 when he had autonomic instability and central hyperthermia, or intractably high fevers. With fevers to 106 degree Fahrenheit and a barely palpable blood pressure, his uncle, a doctor at the hospital told his brother that his son was not going to make it. But he did.

And that is not all he persevered. He survived his accident in significant pain because a hip fracture was never repaired. Kathie, Dustin's mom recalls that the doctors at the receiving hospital told her that "broken bones don't kill you." In a sweeping indictment of what she and her son experienced, she sums up their experience in an e-mail sent to us in 2009:

> Ultimately, the doctors at [the hospital] just didn't believe Dustin would survive, and after he amazed us all by making it through, they always thought he would be in a vegetative state the rest of his life (even telling us we would need to evaluate his quality of life). So why set broken bones, if someone is going to spend the remainder of their life staring into space? Now, because his hip was never set and healed turning in, Dustin has pain and orthopedic issues that may have been avoided. I just don't understand why doctors would go to the extremes they did to save Dustin's life (and don't get me wrong—we are grateful for everything) and then just write him off as another brain injury.

He went on, without treatment until he had a tendon release to rectify the "orthopedic issues" because his hip fracture was not initially repaired. Then, in 2010, he finally had it fixed. The surgery has brought relief and allowed him to sit comfortably in a chair.

But the most heart-wrenching act: when he developed a bad keratopathy and conjunctivitis in that one working eye, that eye upon which he would read the letter board and let the letter board read him, a nursing home ophthalmologist performed a tarsorrhaphy – a surgical procedure in which the eyelids are closed shut – with the hope of quelling the infection and protecting the cornea. In applying that treatment, the ophthalmologist had inadvertently sealed off Dustin's contact with the world.

Like the hip fracture that caused so much pain, his ability to see was written off. His one way to connect with the world was taken from him. His reality was a long way from the legal theory behind anything resembling an Olmstead-like argument urging maximal integration into society. He was essentially written off and shut in. It just didn't matter.

But it did. Because shortly thereafter, Dustin was found to have the ability to communicate, in much the same way as Maggie is starting to demonstrate. But unlike Maggie, Dustin could move his head and was, as his mother once wrote us in an e-mail, "a computer geek."

All he needed was a brain computer interface (BCI) that would allow him to use a track board and his recovering mind would do the rest. But like Maggie's access to *My Tobii*, the delays and bureaucracy were untenable. His mother wrote us in 2009 that "his occupational and speech therapists have submitted to Medicaid for his equipment, but of course it seems he'll be a senior citizen before they come through."

So enter Shawniqua Williams, then a Cornell medical student (and MIT engineering graduate), to the rescue. With a little bit of ingenuity and some expenditures at Radio Shack, Shawniqua set the family up with a "head mouse" and a system, freely available on the web, that Dustin could use. His mother described the method in an e-mail, "The system that Dustin uses to write now scans top to bottom, he hits the switch when it's at the line he wants and then it scans left to right until it hits the letter he wants. It also has a word prediction capacity. If he sees the word he wants he can just hit the word. When he is done typing, he hits the switch to return to the message window and it speaks what he just typed."

And since then, well he's become a diarist, sending us e-mails. The first one was on January 18, 2010: "I just added your email address an im dustin manwiller I m doing well. ...." A couple of days later, he had progressed to use a joystick to choose the letters writing us, "Now I use my hand instead of my head to use computer."

Shortly thereafter Kathie wrote to tell us how this little bit of technology had changed their lives, "It's very cool and he loves telling us what his plans for the day are, what he wants DVR'd, what he wants to watch and when on TV, when he wants to be in his bed and what time he wants his TV to shut off. He can also control the TV through his computer. There is still so much we haven't even touched on yet."

Dustin has been a frequent writer communicating through e-mail capturing his experiences and desires: "I send emails to say what i want." His one-line aphorisms, simple yet profound, when one recalls their origin. The simplicity of "I use this computer to say a lot" belies the alternative of where he would be and what he would do if he did not have access to this technology. In a word: silence.

That is not to say that all his musings are profound. Like any young man, much of it is about TV ("Monday at 8 p.m. Is family guy") and the foods he hopes to again be able to eat ("When i am out of my wheel chair lets eat real food").

But much of it is also about recalling the past and acknowledging his limitations: "Before i got in my car accident I was a good artist" or "I just found out that I am not working at blockbuster." Sometimes he writes about friendship and love, "I miss having you as a friend," even "I really like seeing you because everything look great and i want to date you."

On November 23, 2011 he wrote to his listserv, "Happy thanksgiving everyone. IM thankful for films food and talkshows and everyone that loves me good bye and thanksgiving is tomorrow and everyone should be thankful."

Our most recent e-mail was December 15, 2012, he wrote to us of his excitement about coming to New York:

"Hello going sounds really good because i can show you what i can
do now"
We can't wait. ...

A SMALL LIFE

By the time Maggie and Nancy came to New York in late November 2012, we had begun to see patients at the Rockefeller University Hospital under the aegis of the Consortium for the Advanced Study of Brain Injury (CASBI) between Weill Cornell Medical College and the Rockefeller University. Maggie was one of the first subjects we admitted to Rockefeller.

I last saw her the morning of November 29 and was immediately taken by her awareness of my entry into her room. Unlike her prior visit, she quickly noted my presence and was paying attention to what I had to say.

Having learned the day before of her love of art and her dislike of the computer, I sought to see if she could express her preferences to me, if I asked the proper set of questions. When I asked her about the computer, which her mother described as her modern-day nemesis, there was a blank stare. No enthusiasm, no passion.

In contrast, I got her attention when I said, "Maggie, I hear you are a pretty good artist." And when I asked her if she liked to paint with her mother, she looked down with her left eye with a vigorous swoop I had not seen before. She even tried to vocalize, something she had not done at our last visit. Although it was but a downward glance, the intensity of its assertion verged on the poetic, an expression of intent and interest, totally absent when we were discussing the computer interface.

When I think back on the encounter, I will long see that one eye tucked deeply down when she expressed herself. It was an exclamation point that convinced me that there was so much more she wanted, and needed to say, and so much more that we needed to do to help her communicate. Although I am gratified that we helped to identify her conscious self and her capabilities, it still saddened me that we could not bypass the lack of motor output that hinders her from more fully expressing herself.

It is possible that Maggie's next chapter will be a BCI that links her brain directly to a computer to give voice to her mind within. But that will be the subject for another time, and a decision that will have to take account of the potential burdens and benefits of such an intervention.

But for now, I'll close with Nancy's reflections, not on where Maggie is going, but where she is, her journey to the present, and the consolation of what has already been accomplished. As she reflected on the past six years she recalls the progression of her thinking. At the outset, she thought she would have to assess Maggie's quality of life and withdraw care, if she was still vegetative in a year. "But then it still wasn't a year and they said she was in vegetative state." But she "couldn't do it because *I didn't believe it.*" Eighteen months later, "we come here then we find out okay, so she can communicate." And then the realization "it's not enough to just move your eye."

And then the accommodation and altered expectations. Yes, moving one's eye is not enough, "But it's enough to have a life, even a small life. And I guess I feel that she and I were creating this smaller life that was enough. It is enough. She has people that love her. She has relationships. Now she has something productive that she can do ... and a family that loves her. A lot of people don't have even that."

"So ... I don't know, I think a small life is okay."

Notes

1   DECISIONS

1. Giacino J, Childs N, Cranford R, Jennett B, Katz D, Kelly JP, Rosenberg JH, Whyte J, Zafonte RD, Zasler ND. The minimally conscious state: Definition and diagnostic criteria. *Neurology* 2002 58(3):349–53.

2   THE INJURY

1. Fins JJ, Hersh J. Solitary advocates: The severely brain injured and their surrogates. In *Patients as policy actors (critical issues in health and medicine)*, ed. Hoffman B, Tomes N, Grob R, Schlessinger M. New Brunswick, NJ: Rutgers University Press, 2011. Pp. 21–42.
2. Fins JJ. A review of Woodruff L and B: In an instant: A family's journey of love and healing. *JAMA* 2007 297(23):2642–3.
3. Woodruff L, Woodruff B. *In an instant: A family's journey of love and healing.* New York: Random House, 2007.
4. Consensus conference. Rehabilitation of persons with traumatic brain injury. NIH Consensus Development Panel on Rehabilitation of Persons with Traumatic Brain Injury. *JAMA* 1999 282(10):974–83.

3   COMING TO TERMS WITH BRAIN INJURY

1. Fins JJ, Plum F. Neurological diagnosis is more than a state of mind: Diagnostic clarity and impaired consciousness. *Arch Neurol* 2004 61(9):1354–5.
2. Penfield W. *The mystery of the mind.* Princeton, NJ: Princeton University Press, 1978.
3. Barondess J. Personal communication with: Joseph J Fins. April 2003.
4. Evans, HH. High tech vs. "high touch": The impact of medical technology on patient care. In *Sociomedical perspectives on patient care*, ed. Clair JM, Allman RM. Lexington: The Press of University of Kentucky, 1993. Pp. 82–95.
5. Osler W. *The principles and practice of medicine.* New York: Appleton,1892.
6. Reiser SJ. The technologies of time measurement: Implications at the bedside and the bench. *Ann Intern Med* 2000 132(1):31–6.
7. Racine E, Bar-Ilan O, Illes J. fMRI in the public eye. *Nat Rev Neurosci* 2005 6(2):159–64.

8. Fins JJ. Neuroethics, neuroimaging and disorders of consciousness: Promise or peril? *Trans Am Clin Climatol Assoc* 2011 122:336–46.
9. Posner JB, Saper CB, Schiff ND, Plum F, eds. *Plum and Posner's diagnosis of stupor and coma*. 4th edition. New York: Oxford University Press, 2007.
10. Giacino JT, Kalmar K, Whyte J. The JFK Coma Recovery Scale-Revised: Measurement characteristics and diagnostic utility. *Arch Phys Med Rehabil* 2004 85(12):2020–9.
11. A definition of irreversible coma. Report of the Ad Hoc Committee of the Harvard Medical School to Examine the Definition of Brain Death. *JAMA* 1968 205(6):337–40.
12. Fins JJ. Constructing an ethical stereotaxy for severe brain injury: Balancing risks, benefits, and access. *Nat Rev Neurosci* 2003 4:323–7.
13. Beecher HK. Ethical problems created by the hopelessly unconscious patient. *N Engl J Med* 1968 278:1425–30.
14. Fins JJ. Ethics of clinical decision making and communication with surrogates. In *Plum and Posner's diagnosis of stupor and coma*, ed. Posner JB, Saper CB, Schiff ND, Plum F. 4th edition. New York: Oxford University Press, 2007. Pp. 376–85.
15. Fins JJ, Miller FG, Acres CA, Bacchetta MD, Huzzard LL, Rapkin BD. End-of-life decision-making in the hospital: Current practices and future prospects. *J Pain Symptom Manage* 1999 17(1):6–15.
16. Fins JJ. *A palliative ethic of care: Clinical wisdom at life's end*. Sudbury, MA: Jones and Bartlett Publishers, 2006.
17. Fins JJ. The ethics of modulating consciousness: The imperative of minding time. *Prog Brain Res* 2009 177:371–82.
18. Penfield W. The significance of the Montreal Neurological Institute. In *Neurological biographies and addresses*, ed. Milford H (Foundation Volume, Published for the Staff, to commemorate the Opening of the Montreal Neurological Institute, of McGill University). London: Oxford University Press, 1936.
19. Ibid., pp. 42–3.
20. Fins JJ. A leg to stand on: Sir William Osler and Wilder Penfield's "neuroethics." *Am J Bioeth* 2008 8(1):37–46.
21. Fins JJ. "Humanities are the hormones": Osler, Penfield and "neuroethics" revisited. *Am J Bioeth* 2008 8(1):5–8.

4 THE ORIGINS OF THE VEGETATIVE STATE

1. Jennett B, Teasdale G, Braakman R, Minderhoud J, Knill-Jones R. Predicting outcome in individual patients after severe head injury. *Lancet* 1976 1(7968):1031–4.
2. Plum F, Posner JB. *The diagnosis of stupor and coma*. 2nd edition. Philadelphia, 1972.

3. At the time of Dr. Plum's death in 2010, Dr. Posner said that the identification of the locked-in state was "all Fred" according to Dr Schiff. Whether this is false modesty on the part of Dr. Posner or was generosity on behalf of Dr. Plum is hard to discern. What is known is that in the 1972 *Lancet* article on PVS, Dr. Plum gives Dr. Posner co-credit for the identification of the locked-in state.

4. Reis DJ, Posner JB, eds. *Frontiers of neuroscience, a symposium in honor of Fred Plum*. New York: New York Academy of Sciences, 1994.

5. Jennett B, Plum F. Persistent vegetative state after brain damage: A syndrome in search of a name. *Lancet* 1972 1 (7753):734–37.

6. Schiff, ND. Personal communication with: Joseph J Fins. December 13, 2010.

7. In the matter of Karen Quinlan, Supreme Court of New Jersey. 70 N.J. 10, 355 A.2d 677 (1976).

8. Quinlan J, Quinlan JD. *Karen Ann: The Quinlans tell their story*. Garden City, NY: Doubleday & Co., 1977.

9. Cantor N. Twenty-five years after Quinlan: A review of the jurisprudence of death and dying. *J Law Med Ethics* 2001 29(2):182–96.

10. Richmond C. Fred Plum. *Lancet* 2010 376(9739):412.

11. Fins JJ, Schiff ND. The after-life of Terri Schiavo. *Hastings Cent Rep* 2005 35(4):8.

12. Brown D, Murray S. Schiavo autopsy released [Internet]. *The Washington Post*. June 16, 2005. [Accessed August 4, 2011.] Available from: http://www.washingtonpost.com/wpdyn/content/article/2005/06/15/AR2005061500512.html.

13. Drane JF. *More humane: A liberal catholic bioethics*. Edinboro, PA: Edinboro University Press, 2003.

14. Wefing JB. *The life and times of Richard J. Hughes: The politics of civility*. New Brunswick, NJ: Rivergate Books, 2009.

15. Ibid., p. 256.

16. Fins JJ. Rethinking disorders of consciousness: New research and its implications. *Hastings Cent Rep* 2005 35(2):22–4.

17. Laureys S, Faymonville ME, Peigneux P, Damas P, Lambermont B, Del Fiore G, Degueldre C, Aerts J, Luxen A, Franck G, Lamy M, Moonen G, Maquet P. Cortical processing of noxious somatosensory stimuli in the persistent vegetative state. *Neuroimage* 2002 17(2):732–41.

18. Fins JJ. Neuroethics and neuroimaging: Moving towards transparency. *Am J Bioeth* 2008 8(9):46–52.

19. Fins JJ. *A palliative ethic of care: Clinical wisdom at life's end*. Sudbury, MA: Jones and Bartlett Publishers, 2006.

20. Fins JJ. Lessons from the injured brain: A bioethicist in the vineyards of neuroscience. *Camb Q Healthc Ethics* 2009 18(1):7–13.

21. Fins JJ. Neuroethics, neuroimaging and disorders of consciousness: Promise or peril? *Trans Am Clin Climatol Assoc* 2011 122:336–46.

22. *Roe v. Wade*. 410 U.S. 113, 93 S.Ct. 705, 35 L.Ed 2nd 147 (1973).

23. Fins JJ. Constructing an ethical stereotaxy for severe brain injury: Balancing risks, benefits, and access. *Nat Rev Neurosci* 2003 4(4):323–7.

5 A SHIFT SINCE QUINLAN

1. Fins JJ. Rethinking disorders of consciousness: New research and its implications. *Hastings Cent Rep* 2005 35(2):22–4.
2. Fins JJ. Being conscious of their burden: Severe brain injury and the *Two Cultures* challenge. Proceedings from Disorders of Consciousness, 87th Annual Conference of the Association for Research in Nervous and Mental Disease. *Ann NY Acad Sci* 2009 1157:131–47.
3. Brody H. *The healer's power*. New Haven, CT: Yale University Press, 1992.
4. Wijdicks EFM, Rabinstein AA. The family conference: End-of-life guidelines at work for comatose patients. *Neurology* 2007 68(14):1092–4.
5. Fins JJ. *A palliative ethic of care: Clinical wisdom at life's end*. Sudbury, MA: Jones and Bartlett Publishers, 2006.
6. Callahan D. When self-determination runs amok. *Hastings Cent Rep* 1992 22(2):52–5.
7. Posner JB, Saper CB, Schiff ND, Plum F, editors. *Plum and Posner's diagnosis of stupor and coma*. 4th edition. New York: Oxford University Press, 2007.
8. Black K. *In the shadow of polio*. Cambridge, MA: Da Capo Press, 1996.
9. Plum F, Lukas DS. Studies on respirators: (1) the effect of the Monaghan portable respirator on ventilatory insufficiency in acute poliomyelitis. *Trans Am Neurol Assoc* 1950 51:272–3.
10. Black K. *In the shadow of polio*. Cambridge, MA: Da Capo Press, 1996. P. 124.
11. NYPH WCMS: Fred Plum archives, Box 2, undated ms, circa late 1970s.
12. Fins JJ. Affirming the right to care, preserving the right to die: Disorders of consciousness and neuroethics after Schiavo. *Palliat Support Care* 2006 4(2):169–78.
13. Fins JJ, Pohl BA. Neuro-palliative care and disorders of consciousness. In *Oxford Textbook of palliative medicine*, ed. Hanks G, Cherny NI, Christakis NA, Fallon M, Kassa S, Portenoy RK. Oxford: Oxford University Press, 5th edition. In press.

6 MAGGIE'S WISHES

1. Meili T. *I am the Central Park jogger: A story of hope and possibility*. New York: Scribner, 2003.
2. Condition of participation for hospitals, 42 CFR, Volume 3 Part 482, Subpart C (1986).
3. Fins JJ. Severe brain injury and organ donation: A call for temperance. *Virtual Mentor* 2012 14(3):221–6.
4. Gibbs BJ. Medicare conditions of participation for organ donation: An early assessment of the new donation rule. Office of Inspector General, Department of Health and Human Services. Washington, DC: 2000. OEI-01-99-00020. [Accessed July 24, 2012.] Available from: http://www.sharenj.org/healthcare_professionals/pdf/Medicare%20Conditions.pdf.
5. Christakis N. *Death foretold: Prophecy and prognosis in medical care*. Chicago: University of Chicago Press, 2001.

6. Fins JJ, Master MG, Gerber LM, Giacino JT. The minimally conscious state: A diagnosis in search of an epidemiology. *Arch Neurol* 2007 64(10):1400–5.

7   SOMETHING HAPPENED IN ARKANSAS

1. Parker-Pope T. The happy marriage is the "me" marriage [Internet]. *The New York Times*. December 31, 2010. [Accessed July 16, 2013.] Available from: http://www.nytimes.com/2011/01/02/weekinreview/02parkerpope.html?scp=1&sq=couples%20relationships&st=cse.
2. Fins JJ. Futility in clinical practice: Report on a congress of clinical societies. *J Am Geriatr Soc* 1994 42(8):861–5.
3. Fins JJ, Solomon MZ. Communication in intensive care settings: The challenge of futility disputes. *Crit Care Med* 2001 29 (2 Suppl.):N10–N15.
4. Booth CM, Boone RH, Tomlinson G, Detsky AS. Is this patient dead, vegetative, or severely neurologically impaired? Assessing outcomes for comatose survivors of cardiac arrest. *JAMA* 2004 291(17):870–9.
5. Suppes A, Fins JJ. How relationships shape medical decision making. Presented at the International Association of Relationship Research, Chicago, IL. July 2012.
6. Suppes A, Fins JJ. Surrogates expectations in severe brain injury. *Brain Inj.* 2013 27(10):1141–7.
7. Goldenberg S. Terry talks. *The Guardian* (London). July 11, 2002: Sect. Guardian Features: 2.
8. Schiff ND, Fins JJ. Hope for "comatose" patients. *Cerebrum* 2003 5(4):7–24.
9. Vallis M. Man wakes up from coma, thinks Reagan is president. *National Post.* July 10, 2003: Sect. A:1.
10. Man speaks after 10-year silence. [Internet] CNN. July 8, 2003. [Accessed July 16, 2013.] Available from: http://edition.cnn.com/2003/US/South/07/07/mute.no.more/.

8   FROM PVS TO MCS

1. Medical aspects of the persistent vegetative state (1). The Multi-Society Task Force on PVS. *N Engl J Med* 1994 330(21):1499–1508.
2. Medical aspects of the persistent vegetative state (2). The Multi-Society Task Force on PVS. *N Engl J Med* 1994 330(22):1572–9.
3. Medical aspects of the persistent vegetative state (1). The Multi-Society Task Force on PVS. *N Engl J Med* 1994 330(21):1499–1508. P. 1501.
4. Jennett B. *The vegetative state: Medical aspects, ethical and legal dilemmas.* Cambridge: Cambridge University Press, 2002. Pp. 63–4.
5. Giacino JT, Ashwal S, Childs N, Cranford R, Jennett B, Katz DI, Kelly JP, Rosenberg JH, Whyte J, Zafonte DO, Zasler ND. The minimally conscious state: Definition and diagnostic criteria. *Neurology* 2002 58(3):349–53. Pp. 350–1.

6. Jennett B, Plum F. Persistent vegetative state after brain damage: A syndrome in search of a name. *Lancet* 1972 1 (7753):734–7.
7. Jennett B, Bond M. Assessment of outcome after severe brain damage. *Lancet* 1975 1(7905):480–4.
8. Ibid., p. 483.
9. Giacino JT, Kezmarsky MA, DeLuca J, Cicerone KD. Monitoring rate of recovery to predict outcome in minimally responsive patients. *Arch Phys Med Rehabil* 1991 72(11):897–901.
10. Giacino JT, chair. Head Injury- ISIG Committee Minutes. June 2, 1992.
11. Winslade WJ. *Confronting traumatic brain injury*. New Haven, CT: Yale University Press, 1998. Pp. 125–40.
12. Culhane C. Rehabilitation facilities hit in congressional hearing. American Medical News [Internet]. March 12, 1992. [Accessed August 5, 2011.] Available from: http://business.highbeam.com/137033/article-1G1-12055429/rehabilitation-facilities-hit-congressional-hearing.
13. Winslade WJ. *Confronting traumatic brain injury*. New Haven, CT: Yale University Press, 1998. P. 131.
14. Giacino JT, Kalmar K. The vegetative and minimally conscious states: A comparison of clinical features and functional outcome. *J Head Trauma Rehabil* 1997 12(4):36–61.
15. Giacino JT, Kalmar K. Diagnostic and prognostic guidelines for the vegetative and minimally conscious states. *Neuropsychol Rehabil* 2005 15(3/4):166–74.
16. Bernat JL. Questions remaining about the minimally conscious state. *Neurology* 2002 58(3):337–8.
17. Coleman D. The minimally conscious state: Definition and diagnostic criteria. *Neurology* 2002 58(3):506–7.
18. Fins JJ, Schiff ND. The minimally conscious state: Definition and diagnostic criteria. *Neurology* 2002 59(9):1473.
19. I am indebted to this metaphor first used by Ben Carey. See, Carey B. Inside the injured brain, many kinds of awareness [Internet]. *The New York Times*. April 5, 2005. [Accessed August 5, 2011.] Available from: http://www.nytimes.com/2005/04/05/health/05coma.html?pagewanted=1&sq=joseph%20fins&st=cse&scp=17.
20. Fins JJ. Clinical pragmatism and the care of brain damaged patients: Toward a palliative neuroethics for disorders of consciousness. *Prog Brain Res* 2005 150:565–82.
21. Goldenberg S. Terry talks. *The Guardian* (London). July 11, 2002: Sect. Guardian Features: 2.
22. Fins JJ, Master MG, Gerber LM, Giacino JT. The minimally conscious state: A diagnosis in search of an epidemiology. *Arch Neurol* 2007 64(10):1400–5.
23. Schnakers C, Vanhaudenhuyse A, Giacino J, Ventura M, Boly M, Majerus S, Moonen G, Laureys S. Diagnostic accuracy of the vegetative and minimally conscious state: Clinical consensus versus standardized neurobehavioral assessment. *BMC Neurol* 2009 9:35.

24. Andrews K, Murphy L, Munday R, Littlewood C. Misdiagnosis of the vegetative state: Retrospective study in a rehabilitation unit. *BMJ* 1996 313(7048):13–16.
25. Childs NL, Mercer WN, Childs HW. Accuracy of diagnosis of persistent vegetative state. *Neurology* 1993 43:1465–7.
26. Wilson FC, Harpur J, Watson T, Morrow JI. Vegetative state and minimally responsive patients – regional survey, long-term case outcomes and service recommendations. *NeuroRehabilitation* 2002 17(3):231–6.
27. I am grateful to Dr. Jerome B. Posner for originally making this analogy.
28. Löwenberg B, Downing JR, Burnett A. Acute myeloid leukemia. *N Engl J Med* 1999 341(14):1051–62.
29. Licht JD. Acute promyelocytic leukemia–weapons of mass differentiation. *N Engl J Med* 2009 360(9):928–30.

9   LEAVING THE HOSPITAL

1. Thompson HJ, Pinto-Martin J, Bullock MR. Neurogenic fever after traumatic brain injury: An epidemiological study. *J Neurol Neurosurg Psychiatry* 2003 74(5):614–19.
2. Zussman R. *Intensive care: Medical ethics and the medical profession.* Chicago: The University of Chicago Press, 1992.
3. Bosk CL. *Forgive and remember: Managing medical failure.* 2nd edition. Chicago: The University of Chicago Press, 2003.
4. Wanzer SH, Adelstein SJ, Cranford RE, Federman DD, Hook ED, Moertel CG, Safar P, Stone A, Taussig HB, van Eys J. The physician's responsibility toward hopelessly ill patients. *N Engl J Med* 1984 310(15):955–9.
5. Livingston DH, Tripp T, Biggs C, Lavery RF. A fate worse than death? Long-term outcome of trauma patients admitted to the surgical intensive care unit. *J Trauma* 2009 67(2):341–8.
6. Klonoff PA. A therapist experiential model of treatment for brain injury. *Bull Menninger Clin* 2011 75(1):21–45.
7. Yetman L. Neuroscience nurses caring for family members of patients with acquired brain injury in acute ward settings: Nursing defensively in a double bind. *Can J Neurosci Nursing* 2008 30(4):26–33.
8. Gosseries O, Demertzi A, Ledoux D, Bruno MA, Vanhaudenhuyse A, Thibaut A, Laureys S, Schnakers C. Burnout in healthcare workers managing chronic patients with disorders of consciousness. *Brain Inj* 2012 26(12):1493–9.
9. Van den Broek MD, Lye R. Staff stress in head injury rehabilitation. *Brain Inj* 1996 10(2):133–8.
10. Heffernan DS, Vera RM, Monaghan SF, Thakkar RK, Kozloff MS, Connolly MD, Gregg SC, Machan JT, Harrington DT, Adams CA Jr, Cioffi WG. Impact of socioethnic factors on outcomes following traumatic brain injury. *J Trauma* 2011 70(3):527–34.
11. Hoffman JM, Donoso Brown E, Chan L, Dikmen S, Temkin N, Bell KR. Change in inpatient rehabilitation admissions for individuals with traumatic brain injury

after implementation of the medicare inpatient rehabilitation facility prospective payment system. *Arch Phys Med Rehabil* 2012 93(8):1305–12.

12. Keenan A, Joseph L. The needs of family members of severe traumatic brain injured patients during critical and acute care: A qualitative study. *Can J Neurosci Nursing* 2010 32(3):25–35.

13. Turner BJ, Fleming J, Ownsworth T, Cornwell P. Perceived service and support needs during transition from hospital to home following acquired brain injury. *Disabil Rehabil* 2011 33(10):818–29.

14. Turner BJ, Fleming JM, Ownsworth TL, Cornewll PL. The transition from hospital to home for individuals with acquired brain injury: A literature review and research recommendations. *Disabil Rehabil* 2008 30(16):1153–76.

15. Whyte J. Personal communication with: Joseph Fins. May 28, 2013. Accompanying e-mail to the author detailing the history of the Disorders of Consciousness Special Interest Group of the NIDDR Traumatic Brain Injury Model Systems communications with McKesson concerning their admission criteria for acute rehabilitation.

16. McKesson [Internet]. [Accessed May 31, 2013.] Available from: http://www .mckesson.com.

17. Hammergren JH [Internet]. [Accessed May 31, 2013.] Available from: http://www.mckesson.com/about-mckesson/our-company/executive-officers/ john-h-hammergren/.

18. McKesson InterQual evidence-based clinical content [Internet]. [Accessed May 31, 2013.] Available from: http://www.mckesson.com /payers/decision-management/interqual-evidence-based-clinical-content/ interqual-evidence-based-clinical-content/.

19. Hagen C, Malkmus D, Durham P. *Levels of cognitive function.* Downey, CA: Rancho Los Amigos Hospital, 1972.

20. Canedo A, Grix M, Nicoletti J. An analysis of assessment instruments for the minimally responsive patient (MRP): Clinical observations. *Brain Inj* 2002 16(5):453–61.

21. National Institute on Disability and Rehabilitation (NIDDR) [Internet]. [Last updated May 16, 2013; accessed June 2, 2013.] Available from: http://www2 .ed.gov/about/offices/list/osers/nidrr/index.html.

22. Schnakers C, Vanhaudenhuyse A, Giacino J, Ventura M, Boly M, Majerus S, Moonen G, Laureys S. Diagnostic accuracy of the vegetative and minimally conscious state: clinical consensus versus standardized neurobehavioral assessment. *BMC Neurol* 2009 9:35.

10 HEATHER'S STORY

1. "The afterlife of Terri Schiavo: Rethinking disorders of consciousness." Annual Ethics Conference, Carilion Health Care System, October 26, 2007, Roanoke, VA.

2. Prachar TL, Mahanes D, Arceneaux A, Moss BL, Jones S, Conaway M, Burns SM. Recognizing the needs of family members of neuroscience patients in an intensive care setting. *J Neurosci Nurs* 2010 42(5):274–9.

3. Fins JJ. A 38-year-old man with a secondary leukemia who needs setting of goals of care. In *Palliative and end-of-life pearls*, ed. Heffner JE, Byock I. Philadelphia: Hanley and Belfus, 2002. Pp. 174–6.

4. Wynia MK, Cummins DS, VanGeest JB, Wilson IB. Physician manipulation of reimbursement rules for patients: between a rock and a hard place. *JAMA* 2000 283(14):1858–65. *Arch Phys Med Rehabili* 2008 89:182–7.

5. Fins JJ. Minds apart: Severe brain injury. In *Law and neuroscience: Current legal issues*, ed. Freeman M. New York: Oxford University Press, 2010. Pp. 367–84.

6. Nolan JP, Soar J. Postresuscitation care: Entering a new era. *Current Opin Crit Care* 2010 16(3):216–22.

7. Choi HA, Badjatia N, Mayer SA. Hypothermia for acute brain injury–mechanisms and practical aspects. *Nat Rev Neurol* 2012 8(4):214–22.

8. Levy DE, Bates D, Carronna JJ, Cartlidge NE, Knill-Jones RP, Lapinski RH, Singer BH, Shaw DA, Plum F. Prognosis in nontraumatic coma. *Ann Intern Med* 1981 94(3):293–301.

9. Wijdicks EF, Hijdra A, Young GB, Bassetti CL, Wiebe S. Quality Standards Subcommittee of the American Academy of Neurology. Practice parameter: prediction of outcome in comatose survivors after cardiopulmonary resuscitation (an evidence-based review): Report of the quality standards subcommittee of the American Academy of Neurology. *Neurology* 2006 71:1535–7.

10. Blondin NA, Greer DM. Neurologic prognosis in cardiac arrest patients treated with therapeutic hypothermia. *Neurologist* 2011 17(5):241–8.

11. American Heart Association. CPR Statistics [Internet]. [Updated June 2011; accessed on August 22, 2012.] Available from: http://www .heart.org/HEARTORG/CPRAndECC/WhatisCPR/CPRFactsandStats/ CPR-Statistics_UCM_307542_Article.jsp.

12. Merchant RM, Yang L, Becker LB, Berg RA, Nadkarni V, Nichol G, Carr BG, Mitra N, Bradley SM, Abella BS, Groeneveld PW. American Heart association get with the guidelines-resuscitation investigators: Incidence of treated cardiac arrest in hospitalized patients in the United States. *Crit Care Med* 2011 39(11):2401–6.

13. Kern KB. Optimal treatment of patients surviving out-of-hospital cardiac arrest. *JACC Cardiovasc Interv* 2012 5(6):597–605.

14. Halpern NA, Pastores SM. Critical care medicine in the United States 2000–2005: An analysis of bed numbers, occupancy rates, payer mix, and costs. *Crit Care Med* 2010 38(1):65–71.

15. Arguments in this section derive from: Fins JJ. Disorders of consciousness and disordered care: Families, caregivers and narratives of necessity. *Arch Phys Med Rehabil* 2013; doi: 10.1016/j.apmr.2012.12.028.

16. Berube J, Fins J, Giacino J, Katz D, Langlois J, Whyte J, Zitnay GA. *The Mohonk Report: A report to Congress improving outcomes for individuals with disorders of consciousness*. Charlottesville, VA: National Brain Injury Research, Treatment & Training Foundation, 2006.

17. McNamee S, Howe L, Nakase-Richardson R, Peterson M. Treatment of disorders of consciousness in the Veterans Health Administration polytrauma centers. *J Head Trauma Rehabil* 2012 27(4):244–52.

11 NEUROIMAGING AND NEUROSCIENCE IN THE PUBLIC MIND

1. Katz J. *The silent world of doctor and patient*. New York: Free Press, 1986.
2. Pearce JM. Walter Edward Dandy (1886–1946). *J Med Biogr* 2006 14(3):127–8.
3. Fins JJ. Lessons from the injured brain: A bioethicist in the vineyards of neuroscience. *Camb Q Healthc Ethics* 2009 18(1):7–13.
4. Fins JJ. Rethinking disorders of consciousness: New research and its implications. *Hastings Cent Rep* 2005 35(2):22–4.
5. Kinner HC, Korein J, Panigrahy A, Dikkes P, Goode P. Neuropathological findings in the brain of Karen Ann Quinlan – the role of the thalamus in the persistent vegetative state. *N Engl J Med* 1994 330:1469–75.
6. Cantor N. Twenty-five years after Quinlan: A review of the jurisprudence of death and dying. *J Law Med Ethics* 2001 29(2):182–96.
7. Cranford RE. Medical futility: Transforming a clinical concept into legal and social policies. *J Am Ger Soc* 1994 42(8):894–8.
8. Annas GJ. The "right to die" in America: Sloganeering from Quinlan and Cruzan to Quill and Kevorkian. *Duquesne Law Rev* 1996 34(4):875–97.
9. Annas GJ. Foreword: Imagining a new era of neuroimaging, neuroethics and neurolaw. *Am J Law Med* 2007 33(2–3):163–70.
10. The following section is an expanded discussion of neuroimaging in disorders of consciousness which originally appeared as: Fins JJ. Neuroethics and neuroimaging: Moving towards transparency. *Am J Bioeth* 2008 8(9):46–52.
11. Plum F, Schiff ND, Ribary U, Llinas R. Coordinated expression in chronically unconscious persons. *Philos Trans R Soc L B Biol Sci* 1998 353(1377):1929–33.
12. Schiff ND, Ribary U, Plum F, Llinas R. Words without mind. *J Cogn Neurosci* 1999 11(6):650–6.
13. Schiff, ND, Ribary, U, Plum, F, Llinas, R. Human oscillatory brain activity near 40 Hz: Correlation with cognitive temporal binding and alteration during long term unconsciousness. Abstract presented at Society for Neuroscience 26th Annual Meeting (172.12).
14. Schiff ND. E-mail to: Joseph Fins. April 6, 2011.
15. Bates D. The vegetative state and the Royal College of Physicians guidance. *Neuropsychol Rehabil* 2005 15(3–4):175–83.
16. Royal College of Physicians. The vegetative state: Guidance on diagnosis and management. Report of a working party. London: Royal College of Physicians, 2003.

17. Menon DK, Owen AM, Williams EJ, Minhas PS, Allen CMC, Boniface SJ, Pickard JD. Cortical processing in persistent vegetative state. Wolfson Brain Imaging Centre Team. *Lancet* 1998 352(9123):200.
18. Schiff ND, Plum F. Cortical function in the persistent vegetative state. *Trends Cogn Sci* 1999 3(2):43–4.
19. Menon DK, Owen Am, Pickard JD. Response from Menon, Owen and Pickard. *Trends Cogn Sci* 1999 3(2):44–6.
20. Schiff ND, Ribary U, Moreno DR, Beattie B, Kronberg E, Blasberg R, Giacino J, McCagg C, Fins JJ, Llinas R, Plum F. Residual cerebral activity and behavioural fragments can remain in the persistently vegetative brain. *Brain* 2002 125(Pt. 6):1210–34.
21. Laureys S, Faymonville ME, Peigneux P, Damas P, Lambermont B, Del Fiore G, Degueldre C, Aerts J, Luxen A, Franck G, Lamy M, Moonen G, Maquet P. Cortical processing of noxious somatosensory stimuli in the persistent vegetative state. *Neuroimage* 2002 17(2):732–41.
22. Cassell E. *The nature of suffering.* New York: Oxford University Press, 2004.
23. Schiff ND, Rodriguez-Moreno D, Kamal A, Kim K, Giacino J, Plum F, Hirsch J. fMRI reveals large scale network activation in minimally conscious patients. *Neurology* 2005 64(3):514–23.
24. Hirsch J, Ruge MI, Kim KH, Correa DD, Victor JD, Relkin NR, Labar DR, Krol G, Bilsky MH, Souweidane MM, DeAngelis LM, Gutin PH. An integrated functional magnetic resonance imaging procedure for preoperative mapping of cortical areas associated with tactile, motor, language, and visual functions. *Neurosurgery* 2000 47(3):711–21.
25. Fins JJ. Neuroethics, neuroimaging and disorders of consciousness: Promise or peril? *Trans Am Clin Climatol Assoc* 2011 122:336–46.
26. Parts of this section are based on: Fins JJ. Affirming the right to care, preserving the right to die: Disorders of consciousness and neuroethics after Schiavo. *Palliat Support Care* 2006 4(2):169–78.
27. Wallis C. The twilight zone of consciousness. *Time Magazine.* October 27, 2003:43–4.
28. MacKeen D, Rabin R. States of awareness. *Newsday.* October 26, 2003.
29. Authority for the governor to issue a one-time stay to prevent the withholding of nutrition and hydration from a patient, HB 35E (2003).
30. Supreme Court of Florida. No. SC04-925 Jeb Bush, Governor of Florida, et al., Appellants, vs. MICHAEL SCHIAVO, Guardian of Theresa Schiavo, Appellee. September 23, 2004.
31. In the Circuit Court for Pinellas County, Florida. Circuit Civil Case No. 03-008212-CI-20. Michael Schiavo, Petitioner as Guardian of the person of Theresa Marie Schiavo vs. Jeb Bush, Governor of the State of Florida and Charlie Crist, Attorney General of the State of Florida, Respondents.
32. Goodnough A. Comatose woman's case heard by Florida court, law passed to prolong life is at issue. *The New York Times.* September 7, 2004: Sect. A:14.
33. Long P. Supreme Court refuses to take governor's appeal in Schiavo case. *The Miami Herald.* January 24, 2005.

34. Wolfson J. Defined by her dying, not her death: The guardian ad litem's view of Schiavo. *Death Stud* 2006 30(2):113–20.

35. Goldsmith S. Cover photo. *U.S. News & World Report* 2005 138(12): cover.

36. Annas GJ. "Culture of life" politics at the bedside–the case of Terri Schiavo. *N Engl J Med* 352(16):1710–15.

37. Fins JJ. In: Hamilton J. Schiavo autopsy: damage, no abuse [transcript]. All Things Considered. National Public Radio. June 15, 2005. [Accessed August 6, 2011.] Available from: http://www.npr.org/player/v2/mediaPlayer.html?action= 1&t=1&islist=false&id=4705007&m=4705008.

38. Bill Frist's balancing act [Internet]. *US News and World Report*. March 27, 2005. [Accessed July 11, 2013.] Available from: http://www.usnews.com/usnews/news/ articles/050404/4culture.b.htm.

39. Weldon D. Statement on House floor [transcript]. This Week with George Stephannopolous. ABC. March 27, 2005.

40. Carey B. For parents, the unthinkability of letting go [Internet]. *The New York Times*. March 20, 2005. [Accessed August 6, 2011.] Available from: http://www .nytimes.com/2005/03/20/weekinreview/20carey.html?scp=5&sq=joseph%20 fins%20schiavo&st=cse.

41. Bush v. Schiavo, 885 So. 2d 321, 325 (Fla. 2004).

42. Bumiller E. Supporters praise Bush's swift return to Washington. *The New York Times*. March 21, 2005: Sect. A:15.

43. Hulse C, Kirkpatrick DD. Congress passes and Bush signs Schiavo measure. *The New York Times*. March 21, 2005: Sect. A:1.

44. Kirkpatrick DD, Stolberg SG. How family's cause reached the halls of Congress. *The New York Times*. March 22, 2005: Sect. A:1.

45. Shepherd L. *If that ever happens to me: Making life and death decisions after Terri Schiavo*. Chapell Hill: University of North Carolina Press, 2009.

46. President's statement on Terri Schiavo [Internet]. National Right to Life. March 17, 2005. [Accessed July 16, 2013.] Available from: http://www.nrlc.org/ euthanasia/Terri/WHstatement031705.html.

47. Carey B. New signs of awareness in some brain-injured patients. *The New York Times*. February 8, 2005: Sect. A:1.

48. Winslade W. *Confronting traumatic brain injury*. New Haven, CT: Yale University Press, 1998.

49. Jackson T. E-mail to: Joseph J Fins. March 5, 2005. 5:05 p.m.

50. Weller BJ. E-mail to: Joy Hirsch. February 9, 2005. 4:59 p.m. Courtesy Dr. Joy Hirsch.

51. Fins JJ. Mind and matter: Ethical challenges of deep brain stimulation [transcript]. Dana Foundation. Dana Center. November 22, 2008.

52. Fins JJ, Plum F. Neurological diagnosis is more than a state of mind: Diagnostic clarity and impaired consciousness. *Arch Neurol* 2004 61:1354–5.

53. Zimmer C. What if there is something going on in there [Internet]. *New York Times Magazine*. September 28, 2003. Correction appended, October 19, 2003.

[Accessed April 12, 2011.] Available from: http://query.nytimes.com/gst/fullpage
.html?res=9503E0D71E3AF93BA1575AC0A9659C8B63&&scp=12&sq=
joseph%20fins&st=cse.

54. Fins JJ. *A palliative ethic of care: Clinical wisdom at life's end.* Sudbury,
MA: Jones and Bartlett Publishers, 2006.

55. Fins JJ. Affirming the right to care, preserving the right to die: Disorders
of consciousness and neuroethics after Schiavo. *Palliat Support Care* 2006
4(2):169–78.

56. Owen AM, Coleman MR, Boly M, Davis MH, Laureys S, Pickard JD. Willful
modulation of brain activity in disorders of consciousness. Detecting awareness
in the vegetative state. *Science* 2006 313(5792):1402.

57. Carey B. Vegetative patient shows signs of awareness, study says [Internet].
The New York Times. September 7, 2006. [Accessed April 20, 2011.] Available
from: http://www.nytimes.com/2006/09/07/health/07cnd-brain
.html?sq=schiavo%20adrian%20owen&st=cse&adxnnl=1&scp=1&adxn
nlx=1303304802-mMjjqWTWRjSWMY/VEMfoug.

58. Fins JJ. Border zones of consciousness: Another immigration debate? *Am J Bioeth*
2007 7(1):51–4.

59. Osler W. The leaven of science. In *Aequanimitas: With other addresses to
medical students, nurses and practitioners of medicine.* Philadelphia: P.
Blakiston's Son & Co, 1904.

60. Fins JJ, Illes J, Bernat JL, Hirsch J, Laureys S, Murphy E. Neuroimaging and
disorders of consciousness: Envisioning an ethical research agenda. *Am J Bioeth*
2008 8(9):3–12.

61. Carey B. Trace of thought is found in "vegetative" patient [Internet]. *The
New York Times.* February 3, 2010. [Accessed August 6, 2011.] Available
from: http://www.nytimes.com/2010/02/04/health/04brain
.html?scp=4&sq=adrian%20owen&st=cse.

62. Medical aspects of the persistent vegetative state (1). The Multi-Society Task
Force on PVS. *N Engl J Med* 1994 330 (21):1499–508.

63. Medical aspects of the persistent vegetative state (2). The Multi-Society Task
Force on PVS. *N Engl J Med* 1994 330 (22):1572–9.

64. Supplemental material to: Owen AM, Coleman MR, Boly M, Davis MH, Laureys
S, Pickard JD. Willful modulation of brain activity in disorders of consciousness.
Detecting awareness in the vegetative state. *Science* 2006 313(5792):1402.

65. Fins JJ, Schiff ND. The after-life of Terri Schiavo. *Hastings Cent Rep* 2005
35(4):8.

66. Fins JJ, Schiff ND. Shades of gray: New insights from the vegetative state.
Hastings Cent Rep 2006 36(6):8.

67. Pickard. Personal communication with: Joseph Fins. Cambridge. 2007.

68. Firestein S. *Ignorance: How it drives science.* New York: Oxford University
Press, 2012.

69. Holmes OW. *Borderlines of knowledge in some provinces of medical knowledge.*
Boston: Ticknor and Fields, 1862.

12 CONTRACTURES AND CONTRADICTIONS: MEDICAL NECESSITY
AND THE INJURED BRAIN

1. Banja J. Patient advocacy at risk: Ethical, legal and political dimensions of adverse reimbursement practices in brain injury rehabilitation in the U.S. *Brain Inj.* 1999 13(10):754–8.
2. Woodruff L, Woodruff B. *In an instant: A family's journey of love and healing.* New York: Random House, 2007.
3. Exclusions from coverage and Medicare as secondary payer, 42 U.S.C. 1395y(a)(1) (A) (2010).
4. Miller NW. What is medical necessity? *Physician's News Digest.* August 14, 2002. [Accessed March 10, 2011.] Available from: http://www.physiciansnews .com/2002/08/14/what-is-medical-necessity/.
5. World Health Organization. International classification of diseases (ICD) [Internet]. [Accessed December 20, 2012.] Available from: http://www.who.int/ classifications/icd/en/.
6. Gosseries O, Bruno MA, Chatelle C, Vanhaudenhuyse A, Schnakers C, Soddu A, Laureys S. Disorders of consciousness: What's in a name? *NeuroRehabilitation* 2011 28(1):3–14. doi: 10.3233/NRE-2011-0625.
7. MCG, formerly Milliman Care Guidelines [Internet]. [Accessed July 12, 2013.] Available from: http://www.milliman.com/expertise/healthcare/products-tools/ milliman-care-guidelines/.
8. Granger CV, Carlin M, Diaz P, Dorval J, Forer S, Kessler C, Melvin JL, Miller LS, Riggs RV, Roberts P. Medical necessity: Is current documentation practice and payment denial limiting access to inpatient rehabilitation? *Am J Phys Med Rehabil* 2009 88(9):755–65.
9. Arango-Lasprilla JC, Ketchum JM, Cifu D, Hammond F, Castillo C, Nicholls E, Watanabe T, Lequerica A, Deng X. Predictors of extended rehabilitation length of stay after traumatic brain injury. *Arch Phys Med Rehabil* 2010 91(10):1495–1504.
10. Buntin MB. Access to postacute rehabilitation. *Arch Phys Med Rehabil* 2007 88(11):1488–93.
11. Reiser SJ. The technologies of time measurement: Implications at the bedside and the bench. *Ann Intern Med* 2000 132(1):31–6.
12. Fins JJ. Clinical pragmatism and the care of brain damaged patients: Toward a palliative neuroethics for disorders of consciousness. *Prog Brain Res* 2005 150: 565–82.
13. Stinneford KM, Kirschner KL. Concepts of medical necessity in rehabilitation. *Top Stroke Rehabil* 2004 11(2):69–76.
14. Fins JJ. Vowing to care. *J Pain Symptom Manage* 2002 23(1):54–7.
15. Cohen R. Get a divorce [Internet]. *The New York Times.* July 28, 2002. [Accessed June 4, 2011.] Available from: http://www.nytimes.com/2002/07/28/ magazine/28ETHICIST.html.
16. Sheldon JR, Straube DM. *Disability, divorce, SSI, and Medicaid: Using creative alimony, child support and property settlements to maximize SSI, ensure*

Medicaid eligibility, and create funding for assistive technology. Buffalo, NY: Neighborhood Legal Services, Inc., 2008.

17. Bauby JD. *The diving bell and the butterfly.* New York: Alfred A Knopf, 1997.
18. Tavalaro J, Tayson R. *Look up for yes.* New York: Kodansha International, 1997.
19. Consensus conference. Rehabilitation of persons with traumatic brain injury. NIH Consensus Development Panel on Rehabilitation of Persons with Traumatic Brain Injury. *JAMA* 1999 282(10):974–83.
20. Pear R. Settlement eases rules for some Medicare patients [Internet]. *The New York Times.* October 22, 2012. [Accessed October 26, 2012.] Available from: http://www.nytimes.com/2012/10/23/us/politics/settlement-eases-rules-for-some-medicare-patients.html?_r=1.
21. GLENDA JIMMO, K.R. by her guardian Kenneth Roberts, Miriam Katz, Edith Masterman, Mary Patricia Boitano, National Committee to Preserve Social Security and Medicare, National Multiple Sclerosis Society, Parkinson's Action Network, Paralyzed Veterans of America, American Academy of Physical Medicine and Rehabilitation, Alzheimer's Association, United Cerebral Palsy, and Rosalie McGill, on behalf of themselves and all others similarly situated, Plaintiffs, v. Kathleen Sebelius, in her official capacity as Secretary of Health and Human Services, Defendant. Case No. 5:11-cv-17. United States District Court, D. Vermont. October 25, 2011.
22. Editorial. A humane Medicare rule change [Internet]. *The New York Times.* October 23, 2012. [Accessed October 25, 2012.] Available from: http://www.nytimes.com/2012/10/24/opinion/a-humane-medicare-rule-change.html.
23. Zasler N, Katz D, Zafonte R, editors. *Brain injury medicine.* 2nd edition. New York: Demos Medical, 2013.
24. Schiff ND, Fins JJ. Hope for "comatose" patients. *Cerebrum.* 2003 5(4):7–24.
25. Patient Protection and Affordable Care Act, Public Law 111–148, 124 Stat. 119 (March 23, 2010).
26. Department of Health and Human Services, et al., *Petitioners v. Florida, et al.* USC 11–398 (August 12, 2011).
27. This section draws on a presentation entitled "Neuroethics, brain injury rehabilitation and health care reform: An historical and future perspective" which was presented at The Craig Hospital 2012 Brain Injury Summit. Beaver Creek, Colorado. January 11, 2012 as well as a manuscript: Fins JJ. "Disorders of consciousness and disordered care: Families, caregivers and narratives of necessity." *Arch Phys Med Rehabil* 2013; doi: 10.1016/j.apmr.2012.12.028.
28. Connors S, D'Orsie S. Brain Injury Association of America [Internet]. [Accessed February 14, 2012.] Available from: http://www.biaw.org/_literature_78393/Health_Care_Reform_article.
29. Pascrell B. (D-NJ) Ensure brain injury patients can access comprehensive rehabilitation through health care reform. [Letter to fellow House Members.] April 7, 2011.
30. Carusone P. Letter to the Honorable Kathleen Sebelius, Secretary Health and Human Services. April 7, 2011.

31. Pascrell W. Keynote Address. The 2nd federal interagency conference on traumatic brain injury. March 10, 2006. Bethesda, MD.
32. Bilmes L, Stiglitz J. The economic costs of the war in Iraq. An appraisal three years after the beginning of the conflict. Cambridge, MA: National Bureau of Economic Research. February 2006. Working Paper #12054.
33. Cooper H, Stolberg SG. Obama declares end to combat operations in Iraq [Internet]. *The New York Times.* August 31, 2010. [Accessed October 14, 2012.] Available from: http://www.nytimes.com/2010/09/01/world/01military .html?pagewanted=all&_r=0.
34. Goldberg M. Testimony before the house committee on veteran affairs. October 17, 2007.
35. Dr. James Kelly (Intrepid Center). Personal communication with: Joseph J Fins. Craig Hospital Brain Injury Summit, Beaver Creek, Colorado. January 19, 2012.
36. Shear MD, Wheaton S, Zeleny J. Giffords's return marks moment of unity in divided house [Internet]. *The New York Times.* August 1, 2011. [Accessed January 6, 2013.] Available from: http://thecaucus.blogs.nytimes .com/2011/08/01/giffords-return-marks-moment-of-unity-in-divided-house/.
37. CNN Wire Staff. Giffords leads crowd in pledge at vigil marking one year since shooting [Internet]. [Accessed January 6, 2013.] Available from: http://www.cnn .com/2012/01/08/us/arizona-shooting-anniversary/index.html.
38. Wheaton S. When injuries to the brain tear at hearts. *The New York Times.* January 10, 2012: Sect. D:1.
39. Luft HS. Becoming accountable – opportunities and obstacles for ACOs. *N Engl J Med* 2010 363(15):1389–91.
40. Berkowitz SA, Miller ED. Accountable care at academic medical centers – Lessons from Johns Hopkins. *N Engl J Med* 2011 364(7):e12. doi: 10.1056/ NEJMp1100076.
41. Kastor JA. Accountable care organization at academic medical centers. *N Engl J Med* 2011 364(7):e11. doi: 10.1056/NEJMp1013221.
42. Fins JJ. Disorders of consciousness and disordered care: families, caregivers and narratives of necessity. *Arch Phys Med Rehabil* 2013; doi: 10.1016/j. apmr.2012.12.028.
43. Fins JJ. "Wait, wait – don't tell me"... tuning in the injured brain. *Arch Neurol* 2012 69(2):158–60.
44. McNamee S, Howe L, Nakase-Richardson R, Peterson M. Treatment of disorders of consciousness in the Veterans Health Administration polytrauma centers. *J Head Trauma Rehabil* July–August 2012 27(4):244–52. doi: 10.1097/ HTR.0b013e31825e12c8. Review.
45. Berube J, Fins J, Giacino J, Katz D, Langlois J, Whyte J, Zitnay GA. *The Mohonk Report: A report to Congress improving outcomes for individuals with disorders of consciousness.* Charlottesville, VA: National Brain Injury Research, Treatment & Training Foundation, 2006.
46. Polytrauma blast-related injuries. Family care map for the polytrauma system of support [Internet]. [Accessed December 21, 2012.] Available from: http://www .polytrauma.va.gov/support/training-and-education.asp.

47. US Department of Veteran Affairs. Family care map [Internet]. [Accessed December 21, 2012.] Available from: http://www.hsrd.minneapolis.med.va.gov/FCM/default.asp.
48. US Department of Veteran Affairs. Affordable Care Act and the Veterans Health Administration [Internet]. [Accessed December 21, 2012.] Available from: http://www.va.gov/health/aca.asp.
49. Lammi M, Smith VH, Tate RL, Taylor CM. The minimally conscious state and recovery potential: A follow-up study 2–5 years after traumatic brain injury. Arch Phys Med Rehabil 2005 86(4):746–54.
50. Nakase-Richardson R, Whyte J, Giacino JT, Pavawalla S, Barnett SD, Yablon SA, Sherer M, Kalmar K, Hammond FM, Greenwald B, Horn LJ, Seel R, McCarthy M, Tran J, Walker WC. Longitudinal outcome of patients with disordered consciousness in the NIDRR TBI Model Systems Programs. J Neurotrauma January 1, 2012 29(1):59–65. doi: 10.1089/neu.2011.1829. Epub 2011 Aug 4.
51. Taylor CM, Aird VH, Tate RL, Lammi MH. Sequence of recovery during the course of emergence from the minimally conscious state. Arch Phys Med Rehabil 2007 88(4):521–5.
52. Fins JJ. The ethics of modulating consciousness: The imperative of minding time. Prog Brain Res. 2009 177:371–82.
53. Oxford English Dictionary. Chronic, adj. [Internet]. [Accessed July 12, 2013.] Available from: http://www.oed.com/view/Entry/32570?redirectedFrom=chronic#eid.

13 MINDS, MONUMENTS, AND MOMENTS

1. Fins JJ. Severe brain injury? Is it just a matter of time? Temporal markers of discovery and recovery. III International Conference on Coma & Consciousness. Salerno, Italy. July 7, 2010. See also, Garcia-Ballester L. Introduction: Practical medicine from Salerno to the Black Death. In Practical medicine from Salerno to the Black Death, ed. Garcia-Ballester L, French R, Arrizabalaga J, Cunningham A. Cambridge: Cambridge University Press, 1994.
2. DiGregorio S, Granese MT. Forever overhead. Opening lecture, III International Conference on Coma & Consciousness. Salerno, Italy. July 4, 2010.
3. Saint Augustine. Confessions. Radice B, ed. New York: Penguin Books, 1978.
4. This section on Terry Wallis and the eternal present is based on "Minding Time," a Phi Beta Kappa address delivered by Dr. Fins at Wesleyan University May 23, 2009. It is excerpted and modified here with permission of the university. http://newsletter.blogs.wesleyan.edu/2009/05/23/fins-82-delivers-phi-beta-kappa-address/
5. Voss HU, Uluc AM, Dyke JP, Watts R, Kobylarz EJ, McCandliss BD, Heier LA, Beattie BJ, Hamacher KA, Vallabhajosula S, Goldsmith SJ, Ballon D, Giacino JT, Schiff ND. Possible axonal regrowth in late recovery from minimally conscious state. J Clin Invest 2006 116(7):2005–11.
6. Mukherjee P, McKinstry RC. Diffusion tensor imaging and tarctography of human brain development. Neuroimaging Clin N Am 2006 16(1):19–43.

7. Winslade W. *Confronting traumatic brain injury.* New Haven, CT: Yale University Press, 1998.

8. Ibid., pp. 78–9.

9. Heidegger M. *Being and time.* Macquarrie J, Robinson E, translators. New York: HarperPerennial, 2008.

10. Gracia Guillén D. Personal communication with: Joseph J Fins. Madrid, Spain. Fundacion Zubiri. November 11, 2012.

11. Fins JJ. Rethinking disorders of consciousness: New research and its implications. *Hastings Cent Rep* 2005 35(2):22–4.

12. Flier FJ, de Vries Robbé PF. Nosology and causal necessity; the relation between defining a disease and discovering its necessary cause. *Theor Med Bioethics* 1999 20(6):577–588.

13. Berlinski D. *Tour of the calculus.* New York: Vintage Books, 1997.

14. Christakis NA. Prognostication and bioethics. *Daedalus* 18(4):197–214.

15. Medical aspects of the persistent vegetative state (1). The Multi-Society Task Force on PVS. *N Engl J Med* 1994 330 (21):1499–1508.

16. Medical aspects of the persistent vegetative state (2). The Multi-Society Task Force on PVS. *N Engl J Med* 1994 330 (22):1572–9.

17. Soanes C, Stevenson A, eds. *Persistent. Concise Oxford English Dictory.* 11th edition. New York: Oxford University Press, 2008.

18. J Bernat. E-mail to: Joseph Fins. May 20, 2011.

19. Fins JJ. Ethics of clinical decision making and communication with surrogates. In *Plum and Posner's diagnosis of stupor and coma,* ed. Posner JB, Saper CB, Schiff ND, Plum F. 4th edition. New York: Oxford University Press, 2007. Pp. 376–85.

20. Whyte J, Katz D, Long D, et al. Predictors of outcome in posttraumatic disorders of consciousness and assessment of medical effects: A multicenter study. *Arch Phy Med Rehabil* 2005 86(3):453–62.

21. Jennett B. *The vegetative state: Medical aspects, ethical and legal dilemmas.* Cambridge: Cambridge University Press, 2002. Pp. 63–4.

22. Blake R. *The day Donny Herbert woke up.* New York: Harmony Books, 2007.

23. Fins JJ. A review of: Blake R, the day Donny Herbert woke up. *JAMA* 2008 299(8):959–60.

24. Schiff ND, Rodriguez-Moreno D, Kamal A, Kim KH, Giacino JT, Plum F, Hirsch J. fMRI reveals large-scale network activation in the minimally conscious state. *Neurology* 2005 64(3):514–23.

25. Laureys S, Faymonville ME, Degueldre C, Fiore GD, Damas P, Lambermont B, Janssens N, Aerts J, Franck G, Luxen A, Moonen G, Lamy M, Maquet P. Auditory processing in the vegetative state. *Brain* 2000 123(8):1589–601.

26. Schiff ND. Modelling the minimally conscious state: Measurements of brain function and therapeutic possibilities. *Prog Brain Res* 2005 150:473–93.

27. Edelman GM. *Bright air, brilliant fire.* New York: Basic Books, 1992.

28. Rucker RVB. *Geometry, relativity and the fourth dimension.* Mineola: Dover, 1977.

29. Fins JJ. Clinical pragmatism and the care of brain damaged patients: Toward a palliative neuroethics for disorders of consciousness. *Prog Brain Res* 2005 150:565–82.

30. Luauté J, Maucort-Boulch D, Tell L, Quelard F, Sarraf T, Iwaz J, Boisson D, Fischer C. Long-term outcomes of chronic minimally conscious and vegetative states. *Neurology* 2010 75(3):246–52.

31. Estraneo A, Moretta P, Loreto V, Lanzillo B, Santoro L, Trojano L. Late recovery after traumatic, anoxic, or hemorrhagic long-lasting vegetative state. *Neurology* 2010 75(3):239–45.

32. Bernat JL. The natural history of chronic disorders of consciousness. *Neurology* 2010 75(3):206–7.

33. Owen AM, Coleman MR, Boly M, et al. Willful modulation of brain activity in disorders of consciousness: Detecting awareness in the vegetative state. *Science* 2006 313(5792):1402.

34. Supplemental material to: Owen AM, Coleman MR, Boly M, et al. Willful modulation of brain activity in disorders of consciousness: Detecting awareness in the vegetative state. *Science* 2006 313(5792):1402.

35. Fins JJ, Schiff ND. Shades of gray: New insights from the vegetative state. *Hastings Cent Rep* 2006 36(6):8.

36. Di HB, Yu SM, Weng XC, et al. Cerebral response to patient's own name in the vegetative and minimally conscious states. *Neurology* 2007 68(12):895–9.

37. Fins JJ, Illes J, Bernat JL, Hirsch J, Laureys S, Murphy E. Neuroimaging and disorders of consciousness: envisioning an ethical research agenda. *Am J Bioeth* 2008 8(9):3–12.

38. Whyte J and Myers R. Incidence of clinically significant responses to zolpidem among patients with disorders of consciousness: A preliminary placebo controlled trial. *Am J Phys Med Rehabil* 2009 88(5):410–18.

39. Parts of this section are based on: Fins JJ. Affirming the right to care, preserving the right to die: Disorders of consciousness and neuroethics after Schiavo. *Palliat Support Care* 2006 4(2):169–78.

40. Fins JJ. Constructing an ethical stereotaxy for severe brain injury: Balancing risks, benefits, and access. *Nat Rev Neurosci* 2003 4:323–7.

41. Fins JJ. *A palliative ethic of care: Clinical wisdom at life's end*. Sudbury, MA: Jones and Bartlett Publishers, 2006.

42. Schiff ND. Recovery of consciousness after brain injury: A mesocircuit hypothesis. *Trends Neurosci* January 2010 33(1):1–9.

14 HEADS AND HEARTS, TOIL AND TEARS

1. Fins JJ. Ethics of clinical decision making and communication with surrogates. In *Plum and Posner's diagnosis of stupor and coma*, ed. Posner JB, Saper CB, Schiff ND, Plum F. 4th edition. New York: Oxford University Press, 2007. Pp. 376–85.

2. Snyder L; American College of Phsicians, Ethics, Professionalism, and Human Rights Committee. American College of Physician Ethics Manual: 6th edition. *Ann Internal Med* 2012; 156(1_Part_2):73–104.
3. American College of Physicians, Ethics, Professionalism and Human Rights Committee. American College of Physicians Ethics Manual. 5th edition. Philadelphia: The American College of Physicians, 2005.
4. The National Commission for the Protection of Human Subjects of Biomedical and Behavioral Research. The Belmont report: Ethical principles and guidelines for the protection of human subjects of research. U.S. Department of Health, Education, and Welfare. *Fed Regist* April 18, 1979 44(76):23192–7.
5. Evans JH. *The history and future of medical ethics: a sociological view.* New York: Oxford University Press, 2012.
6. Jones JH. *Bad blood, the Tuskegee syphilis experiment.* New York: The Free Press, 1993.
7. The National Research Act, Pub. L. 93–348, 88 Stat (July 12, 1874).
8. Jonsen A. *The birth of bioethics.* New York: Oxford University Press, 1998.
9. Committee on Quality of Health Care in America, Institute of Medicine. To err is human: Building a safer health system. Kohn LT, Corrigan JM, Donaldson MS, editors. Washington, DC: National Academies Press, 2000.

15   WHAT DO FAMILIES WANT?

1. Fins JJ, Illes J, Bernat JL, Hirsch J, Laureys S, Murphy E. Neuroimaging and disorders of consciousness: Envisioning an ethical research agenda. *Am J Bioeth* 2008 8(9):3–12.
2. Fins JJ, Shapiro Z. Neuroimaging and neuroethics: Clinical and policy considerations. *Curr Opin Neurol* 2007 20(6):650–4.
3. Wallace SE. The needle in the haystack: International consortia and the return of individual research results. *J Law Med Ethics* 2011 39(4):631–9.
4. Wolf SM, Lawrenz FP, Nelson CA, Kahn JP, Cho MK, Clayton EW, Fletcher JG, Georgieff MK, Hammerschmidt D, Hudson K, Illes J, Kapur V, Keane MA, Koenig BA, Leroy BS, McFarland EG, Paradise J, Parker LS, Terry SF, Van Ness B, Wilfond BS. Managing incidental findings in human subjects research: Analysis and recommendations. *J Law Med Ethics* 2008 36(2):219–48. P. 211.
5. Illes J, Kirschen MP, Edwards E, Bandettini P, Cho MK, Ford PJ, Glover GH, Kulynych J, Macklin R, Michael DB, Wolf SM, Grabowski T, Seto B. Practical approaches to incidental findings in brain imaging research. *Neurology* 2008 70(5):384–90.
6. Richardson HS. *The ancillary-care obligaions of medical researchers.* New York Oxford University Press, 2013.
7. Fins JJ. A review of Moral Entanglements: The Ancillary-Care Obligations of Medical Researchers by Henry S. Richardson. New York: Oxford Univerity Press, 2012. *Notre Dame Philosophical Reviews.* May 19, 2013 [Internet]. [Accessed

May 19, 2003.] Available from: http://ndpr.nd.edu/news/40053-moral-entanglements/.

8. Reilly P. When should an investigator share raw data with the subjects. *IRB* 1980 2(9):4–5.

16   DEEP BRAIN STIMULATION IN MCS

1. Kuhn TS. *The structure of scientific revolutions.* Chicago: University of Chicago Press, 1970.

2. Carey B. New signs of awareness in some brain-injured patients. *The New York Times.* February 8, 2005: Sect. A:1.

3. Davey, Matthew. ACT (Australian Capital Territory) Memorial [Internet]. [Accessed October 31, 2012.] Available from: http://www.memorial.act.gov.au/person.php?id=138.

4. Hovell D. United in grief [Internet]. Army: The Soldiers's Newspaper. [Accessed October 31, 2012.] Available from: http://www.defence.gov.au/news/armynews/editions/1118/topstories/story01.htm.

5. Penfield W. *The mystery of the mind.* Princeton, NJ: Princeton University Press, 1978.

6. Fins JJ. A leg to stand on: Sir William Osler and Wilder Penfield's "neuroethics." *Am J Bioeth* 2008 8(1):37–46.

7. Snow CP. *The two cultures and the scientific revolution.* New York: Cambridge University Press, 1959.

8. Fins JJ, de Melo Martin I. C.P. Snow's *Two Cultures* fifty years later: An enduring problem with an elusive solution. *Technol Soc* 2010 32(1):1–4.

9. Fins JJ. C.P. Snow at Wesleyan: Liberal learning and the origins of the "third culture." *Technol Soc* 2010 32(1):10–17.

10. Penfield W. Epileptic automatism and the centrencephalic integrating system. *Res Publ Assoc Res Nerv Ment Dis* 1952 30:512–28.

11. Jasper HH. Wilder Penfield: His legacy to neurology. The centrencephalic system. *Can Med Assoc J* 1977 116(12):1371–2.

12. The Nobel Prize in physiology or medicine 1981: Roger W. Sperry, David H. Hubel, Torsten N. Wiesel [Internet]. [Accessed November 1, 2012.] Available from: http://www.nobelprize.org/nobel_prizes/medicine/laureates/1981/.

13. Walshe FMR. The brain-stem conceived as the highest level of function in the nervous system; with particular reference to the automatic apparatus of Carpenter (1850) and to the centrencephalic integrating system of Penfield. *Brain* 1957 80(4):510–39.

14. Schiff ND. *Wilder Graves Penfield: Philosophy, physiology and the mystery of the mind [senior thesis].* Stanford, CA: Stanford University; 1987.

15. Notable figures [Internet]. Montreal Neurlogical Institute and Hospital, McGill University. [Last updated June 26, 2012; accessed June 20, 11.] Available from: http://www.mni.mcgill.ca/about/notable/.

16. Fins JJ. Deep brain stimulation: Ethical issues in clinical practice and neurosurgical research. In *Neuromodulation*, ed. Krames E, Peckham PH, Rezai A. London: Elsevier, 2009. Pp. 81–91.
17. Fins JJ. Deep brain stimulation. In *Encyclopedia of bioethics*, Post SG, Editor-in-Chief. 3rd edition. Volume 2. New York: MacMillan Reference, 2004:629–34.
18. Speelman JD, Bosch DA. Resurgence of functional neurosurgery for Parkinson's disease: A historical perspective. *Mov Disord* 1998 13(3):582–8.
19. Benabid AL, Pollak P, Louveau A, Henry S, de Rougemont J. Combined (thalamotomy and stimulation) stereotactic surgery of the VIM thalamic nucleus for bilateral Parkinson disease. *Appl Neuorphysiol* 1987 50(1–6):344–6.
20. Fins JJ, Schachter M. Investigators, industry and the heuristic device. Ethics, patent law and ethical innovation. *Account Res* 2001 8(3):219–33.
21. Blank RH. *Brain policy*. Washington, DC: Georgetown University Press, 1999.
22. The Deep-Brain Stimulation for Parkinson's Disease Study Group. Deep-brain stimulation of the subthalamic nucleus or the pars interna of the globus pallidus in Parkinson's disease. *N Engl J Med* 2001 345(13):956–63.
23. Kumar R, Lozano AM, Kim YJ, Hutchinson WD, Sime E, Halket E, Lang AE. Double-blind evaluation of subthalamic nucles deep brain stimulation in advanced Parkinson's disease. *Neurology* 1998 51(3):850–5.
24. Cohadon F, Richer E, Rougier A, Deliac PH, Loiseau H. Deep brain stimulation in cases of prolonged post-traumatic unconsciousness. In *Neurostimulation: an overview*, ed. Lazorthes Y, Upton ARM. Mt Kisco, NY: Futura Publishers, 1985. Pp. 247–50.
25. Tsubokawa T, Yamamoto T, Katayama Y, Hirayama T, Maejima S, Moriya T. Deep-brain stimulation in a persistent vegetative state: Follow up results and criteria for selection of candidates. *Brain Inj* 1990 4:315–27.
26. Hosobuchi Y, Yingling C. The treatment of prolonged coma with neurostimulation. In *Electrical and magnetic stimulation of the brain and spinal cord*, ed. Devinsky O, Beric A, Dogali M. New York: Raven Press, Ltd., 1993: 247–52.
27. Giacino JT, Ashwal S, Childs N, Cranford R, Jennett B, Katz DI, Kelly JP, Rosenberg JH, Whyte J, Zafonte DO, Zasler ND. The minimally conscious state: Definition and diagnostic criteria. *Am Acad Neurol* 2002 58(3):349–53.
28. Schiff ND, Giacino JT, Fins JJ. Deep brain stimulation, neuroethics and the minimally conscious state: Moving beyond proof of principle. *Arch Neurol* 2009 66(6):697–702.
29. Lockman J, Fisher RS. Therapeutic brain stimulation for epilepsy. *Neurol Clinic* 2009 27(4):1031–40.
30. Schiff ND, inventor; Cornell Research Foundation (Ithaca, NY), assignee. Deep Brain Stimulation Method. US Patent 5938688. August 17, 1999.

17   MENDING OUR BRAINS, MINDING OUR ETHICS

1. Fins JJ. Ethics rounds: An introduction to the series. *J Pain Symptom Manage* 1998 15(2):134–5.

2. Dantz B. Case presentation: Pain, suffering and the unconscious patient. *J Pain Symptom Manage* 1999 17(4):301.
3. Miller FG, Fins JJ, Snyder L. Assisted suicide and refusal of treatment: Valid distinction? *Ann Intern Med* 2000 132(6):470–5.
4. Schiff ND. Commentary: Neurobiology, suffering and unconscious brain states. *J Pain Symptom Manage* 1999 17(4):303–4.
5. This ethical analysis is drawn in part from: Fins JJ. Justice, clinical research and the minimally conscious state. The President's Bioethics Commission. (By invitation.) New York. May 18, 2011.
6. Tsubokawa T, Yamamoto T, Katayama Y, Hirayama T, Maejima S, Moriya T. Deep-brain stimulation in a persistent vegetative state: Follow up results and criteria for selection of candidates. *Brain Inj* 1990 4:315–27.
7. Hosobuchi Y, Yingling C. The treatment of prolonged coma with neurostimulation. In *Electrical and magnetic stimulation of the brain and spinal cord*, ed. Devinsky O, Beric A, Dogali M. New York: Raven Press, Ltd., 1993: 247–52.
8. Rothman DJ, Rothman SM. *The Willowbrook wars*. New Brunswick, NJ: Aldine Transaction, 2005.
9. Jones J. *Bad blood: The Tuskegee syphilis experiment*. New and expanded edition. New York: Free Press, 1993.
10. Beecher HK. Ethics and clinical research. *N Engl J Med* 1966 274(24):1354–60.
11. The National Research Act, Pub. L. 93–348, 88 Stat (July 12, 1874).
12. Jonsen AR. *The birth of bioethics*. New York: Oxford University Press, 1998.
13. The National Commission for the Protection of Human Subjects of Biomedical and Behavioral Research. The Belmont report: Ethical principles and guidelines for the protection of human subjects of research. DHEW Publication No. (OS) 78-0012. Washington, DC: U.S. Government Printing Office, 1978.
14. Evans JH. *The history and future of medical ethics: A sociological view.* New York: Oxford University Press, 2012.
15. Preminger BA. The case of Chester M. Southam: Research ethics and the limits of professional responsibility. *Pharos Alpha Omega Alpha Honor Med Soc* 2002 65(2):4–9.
16. Fins JJ. A proposed ethical framework for interventional cognitive neuroscience: A consideration of deep brain stimulation in impaired consciousness. *Neurol Res* 2000 22(3):273–8.
17. Fins JJ, Bacchetta MD, Miller FG. Clinical pragmatism: A method of moral problem solving. *Kennedy Inst Ethics J* 1997 7(2):129–45.
18. Carmichael M. Healthy shocks to the head. *Newsweek*. June 24, 2002:56–8.
19. The future of mind control. *The Economist*. May 25, 2002.
20. El-Hai J. The lobotomist. *The Washington Post Magazine*. February 4, 2001:16–31.
21. El-Hajai J. *The lobotomist: A maverick medical genius and his tragic quest to rid the world of mental illness*. Hoboken, NJ: John Wiley & Sons, 2005.
22. Herbert W. Psychosurgery redux. *US News & World Report*. November 3, 1997:63–4.

23. Midgley M. Biotechnology and monstrosity: Why we should pay attention to the "yuk factor." *Hastings Cent Rep* 2000 30(5):7–15.
24. Psychosurgery. *Lancet* 1972 2(7767):69–70.
25. Matthew SJ, Yudofsky SC, McCullough LB, Teasdale TA, Jankovic J. Attitudes toward neurosurgical procedures for Parkinson's disease and obsessive-compulsive disorder. *J Neuropsychiatry Clin Neurosci* 1999 11(2):259–67.
26. Fins JJ. From psychosurgery to neuromodulation and palliation: History's lessons for the ethical conduct and regulation of neuropsychiatric research. *Neurosurg Clin N Am* 2003 14(2):303–19.
27. Raju TNK. The Nobel chronicles. 1949: Walter Rudolf Hess (1881–1973); and Antonio Egas Moniz (1874–1955). *Lancet* 1999 353(9160):1281.
28. Damasio AR. Egas Moniz, pioneer of angiography and leucotomy. *Mt. Sinai J Med* 1975 42(6):502–13.
29. Tierney AJ. Egas Moniz and the origins of psychosurgery: A review commemorating the 50th anniversary of Moniz's Nobel Prize. *J Hist Neurosci* 2000 9(1):22–36.
30. Jasper HH. A historical perspective: The rise and fall of prefrontal lobotomy. *Adv Neurology* 1995 66:97–114.
31. Diefenbach GJ, Diefenbach D, Baumeister A, West M. Portrayal of lobotomy in the popular press: 1935–1960. *J Hist Neurosci* 1999 8(1):60–9.
32. Valenstein ES. *Great and desperate cures: The rise and decline of psychosurgery and other radical treatments for mental illness.* New York: Basic Books, 1986.
33. Koppell BH, Rezai AR. The continuing evolution of psychiatric neurosurgery. *CNS Spectr* 2000 5(10):20–31.
34. Gaylin WM, Meister JS, Neville RC, editors. *Operating on the mind: The psychosurgery conflict.* New York: Basic Books, 1975.
35. Perlstein R. *Nixonland: The rise of a president and the fracturing of America.* New York: Scribner, 2008.
36. Delgado JM, Anshen RN, eds. *Physical control of the mind: Toward a psychocivilized society.* New York: Harper and Row, 1969.
37. Delgado JMR. Social rank and radio-stimulated aggressiveness in monkeys. *J Nerv Ment Dis* 1967 144(5):383–90.
38. Delgado JMR. Aggression and defense under cerebral radio control. *UCLA Forum Med Sci* 1967 7:171–93.
39. Delgado JMR. Implantation of multilead electrode assemblies. Technical Documentary Report, ADL-TDR. United States Aeromedical Research Laboratory, Holloman Airforce Base, N.M. March 1969:1–19.
40. Osmundsen JA. "Matador" with a radio stops wired bull: Modified behavior in animals subject of brain study. *The New York Times.* May 17, 1965: Sect. A:1.
41. Crichton M. *Terminal man.* New York: Knopf. 1977.
42. Mark VH, Ervin FR. *Violence and the brain.* New York: Harper and Row, 1970.
43. Mark VH. Brain Surgery in aggressive epileptics. *Hastings Cent Rep* 1973 3(1):1–5.

44. Medical News. Debate over benefits and ethics of psychosurgery involve public. *JAMA* 1973 225(8):913–14.
45. National Commission for the Protection of Human Subjects of Biomedical and Behavioral Research. Research involving those institutionalized as mentally infirm: report and recommendations. Washington, DC: US Dept of Health, Education, and Welfare; 1978.
46. The National Commission for the Protection of Human Subjects of Biomedical and Behavioral Research. Use of psychosurgery in practice and research: report and recommendations of National Commission for the Protection of Human Subjects of Biomedical and Behavioral Research. *Fed Regist* 1977 May 23 42(99):26318–32.
47. Blatte H. State prisons and the use of behavior control. *Hastings Cent Rep* 1974 4(4):11.
48. Donnelly J. The incidence of psychosurgery in the United States, 1971–1973. *Am J Psychiatry* 1978 135(12):1476–80.
49. Culliton BJ. Psychosurgery: National commission issues surprisingly favorable report. *Science* 1976 194(4262):299–301.
50. Fins JJ. The ethical limits of neuroscience. *Lancet Neurol* 2002 1(4):213.
51. Fins JJ. Constructing an ethical stereotaxy for severe brain injury: Balancing risks, benefits and access. *Nat Rev Neurosci* 2003 4(4):323–7.
52. National Bioethics Advisory Commission. Research involving persons with mental disorders that may affect decision-making capacity: Vol. 1, report and recommendations of the National Bioethics Advisory Commission. Rockville, MD: National Bioethics Advisory Commission; December 1998.
53. Fins JJ. Justice, Clinical research and the minimally conscious state. The President's Bioethics Commission. (By invitation.) New York. May 18, 2011.

18   IT'S STILL FREEDOM

1. Fins JJ, Giacino J, Rezai A, Schiff N. Ethical insights from a neuromodulation trial to restore function in the minimally conscious state. Abstract presented at Society for Neuroscience 36th Annual Meeting. October 2006.
2. Fins JJ. A proposed ethical framework for interventional cognitive neuroscience: A consideration of deep brain stimulation in impaired consciousness. *Neurol Res* 2000; 22(3):273–8.
3. Fins JJ, Miller FG. Enrolling decisionally incapacitated subjects in neuropsychiatric research. *CNS Spectr* 2000 5(10):32–42.
4. Fins JJ. Constructing an ethical stereotaxy for severe brain injury: Balancing risks, benefits and access. *Nat Rev Neurosci* 2003 4(4):323–7.
5. Fins JJ. From psychosurgery to neuromodulation and palliation: History's lessons for the ethical conduct and regulation of neuropsychiatric research. *Neurosurg Clin N Am* 2003 14(2):303–19.
6. Miller FG, Fins JJ. Protecting human subjects in brain research: A pragmatic perspective. In *Neuroethics: Defining the issues in theory, practice and policy*, ed. Illes, J. New York: Oxford University Press, 2005.

7. Fins JJ. Deep brain stimulation. In *Encyclopedia of bioethics*, Post SG, Editor-in-Chief. 3rd edition. Volume 2. New York: MacMillan Reference, 2004:629-34.

8. Schiff ND, Fins JJ. Hope for "comatose" patients. *Cerebrum* 2003 5(4):7-24.

9. Fins JJ, Schiff ND. Conflicts of interest in deep brain stimulation research and the ethics of transparency. *J Clin Ethic*. 2010 21(2):125-32.

10. Fins JJ. Deep brain stimulation, free markets and the scientific commons: Is it time to revisit the Bayh-Dole act of 1980? *Neuromodulation* 2010 13(3):153-9.

11. Fins JJ, Mayberg HS, Nuttin B, Kubu CS, Galert T, Strum V, Stoppenbrink K, Merkel R, Schlaepfer T. Neuropsychiatric deep brain stimulation research and the misuse of the humanitarian device exemption. *Health Aff (Millwood)* 2011 30(2):302-11.

12. Ambrose S. *Undaunted courage: Merriwether Lewis, Thomas Jefferson and the opening of the American west*. New York: Simon & Schuster, 1997.

13. Fins JJ. Lessons from the injured brain: A bioethicist in the vineyards of neuroscience. *Camb Q Healthc Ethics* 2009 18(1):7-13.

14. Lewis and Clark trail [Internet]. [Accessed July 15, 2013.] Available from: http://lewisandclarktrail.com/section4/wacities/chinook/index.htm.

15. Giacino JT, Kalmar K, Whyte J. The JFK Coma Recovery Scale-Revised: measurement characteristics and diagnostic utility. *Arch Phys Med. Rehabil* 2004 85(12):2020-9.

16. Schiff ND, Giacino JT, Kalmar K, Victor JD, Baker K, Gerber M, Fritz B, Eisenberg B, O'Connor J, Kobylarz EJ, Farris S, Machado A, McCagg C, Plum F, Fins JJ, Rezai AR. Behavioral improvements with thalamic stimulation after severe traumatic brain injury. *Nature* 2007 448(7153):600-3

17. A Discussion about brain stimulation [Internet]. Charlie Rose Show. PBS. 2007. Available from: http://www.charlierose.com/view/interview/8627.

18. Parfit D. *Reasons and persons*. New York: Oxford University Press, 1986.

19. Faden R, Beauchamp T. *A History and theory of informed consent*. New York: Oxford University Press, 1986.

20. Kemode F. *The sense of an ending*. New York: Oxford University Press, 2000.

21. I am grateful to Professor Andy Szegady-Mazak for his suggesting Kemode's work in connection with a question about the *Diver of Paestum* (see Chapter 12).

22. Fins JJ. A proposed ethical framework for interventional cognitive neuroscience: A consideration of deep brain stimulation in impaired consciousness. *Neurol Res* 2000 22(3):273-8.

23. Glannon W. Neurostimulation and the minimally conscious state. *Bioethics* 2008 22(6):337-45.

24. Gillett G. Minimally conscious states, deep brain stimulation and what is worse than futility. *J Bioeth Inq* 2011 8(2):145-9.

25. Thomas L. *The lives of a cell: Notes of a biology watcher*. New York: The Viking Press, 1974.

26. Dewey J. The quest for certainty. In *The later works of John Dewey (1925-1953)*, ed. Boydston JA. Volume 4, Collected Works. Carbondale: Southern Illinois University Press, 2008.

27. Garden R. Disability and narrative: New directions for medicine and the medical humanities. *Med Humanit* 2010 36(2):70–4.
28. Williams WC. *Paterson*. Revised edition, Christopher McGowan. New York: New Directions Books, 1992.
29. Fins JJ. Vowing to care. *J Pain Symptom Manage* 2002 23(1):54–7.

19 MAGGIE IS IN TOWN

1. Fleming AA. A family's hope undiminished. *The Providence Journal.* November 14, 2006.
2. Michals D. We know she's in there. *Smith Alumnae Quarterly.* Winter 2010–11.
3. Baird S. 2006 Student address: Stacey Baird [Internet]. Commencement Archive, Smith College. North Hampton, MA. [Accessed 16 November 2012.] Available from: http://www.smith.edu/events/commencement_student2006.php.
4. This fax was received before the IRB approved study of family narratives. Prior verbal permission was obtained to use the quote without attribution.
5. Reiner R, director. *A few good men.* Columbia Pictures. December 11, 1992.
6. Fins JJ, Plum F. Neurological diagnosis is more than a state of mind: Diagnostic clarity and impaired consciousness. *Arch Neurol* 2004 61(9):1354–5.
7. Bauby JD. *The diving bell and the butterfly.* New York: Alfred A Knopf, 1997.
8. Rodriguez Moreno D, Schiff ND, Giacino J, Kalmar K, Hirsch J. A network approach to assessing cognition in disorders of consciousness. *Neurology* 2010 75(21):1871–8.
9. Worthen N. "Courage." Unpublished poem.
10. Elliot TS. *Burnt Norton.* Four quartets. Mariner Books, 1968.
11. Wieseltier L. *Kaddish.* New York: Vintage, 2000.
12. Fins JJ, Hammond C, Tarsney PS, Panero A, Martinez J, Kirschner KL. Surrogate decision making in the case of a pregnant woman newly disabled with brain injury. *PM&R* 2013 5(1):57–65.

20 WHEN CONSCIOUSNESS BECOMES PROSTHETIC

1. Callahan D, Nuland SB. The quagmire: How American medicine is destroying itself [Internet]. *New Republic.* May 19, 2011. [Accessed July 16, 2013.] Available from: http://www.newrepublic.com/article/economy/magazine/88631/american-medicine-health-care-costs#.
2. Schiff ND, Posner JB. Another "awakenings." *Ann Neurol* 2007 62(1):5–7.
3. Schiff ND. Recovery of consciousness after brain injury: A mesocircuit hypothesis. *Trends Neurosci* 2010 33(1):1–9.
4. Shah SA, Schiff ND. Central thalamic deep brain stimulation for cognitive neuromodulation – a review of proposed mechanisms and investigational studies. *Eur J Neurosci* 2010 32(7):1135–44.
5. Brown EN, Lydic R, Schiff ND. General anesthesia, sleep, and coma. *N Engl J Med* 2010 363:2638–50.

6. Cohen SI, Duong TT. Increased arousal in a patient with anoxic brain injury after administration of Zolpidem. *Am J Phys Med Rehabil* 2008 87(3):229–31.

7. Shames JL, Ring H. Transient reversal of anoxic brain injury-related minimally conscious state after zolpidem administration: A case report. *Arch Phys Med Rehabil* 2008 89(2):386–8.

8. Whyte J, Myers R. Incidence of clinically significant responses to zolpidem among patients with disorders of consciousness: A preliminary placebo controlled trial. *Am J Phys Med Rehabil* 2009 88(5):410–18.

9. Singh R, McDonald C, Dawson K, Lewis S, Pringle AM, Smith S, Pentland B. Zolpidem in a minimally conscious state. *Brain Inj* 2008 22(1):103–6.

10. Awakenings: Return to life [Internet]. *60 Minutes*. CBS News. November 25, 2007. [Updated August 28, 2008; accessed August 6, 2011.] Available from: http://www.cbsnews.com/stories/2007/11/21/60minutes/main3530299 .shtml?source=RSSattr=60Minutes_3530299.

11. Fridman EA, Beattie BJ, Broft A, Laureys S, Schiff ND. Regional cerebral metabolic patterns demonstrate the role of anterior forebrain mesocircuit dysfunction in the severely injured brain. *Proc Natl Acad Sci USA.* 2014 111(17):6473–8.

12. Monti MM, Vanhaudenhuyse A, Coleman MR, Boly M, Pickard JD, Tshibanda L, Owen AM, Laureys S. Willful modulation of brain activity in disorders of consciousness. *N Engl J Med* 2010 362(7):579–89.

13. Giacino JT, Kalmar K, Whyte J. The JFK Coma Recovery Scale-Revised: Measurement characteristics and diagnostic utility. *Arch Phys Med. Rehabil* 2004 85(12):2020–9.

14. Monti MM, Vanhaudenhuyse A, Coleman MR, Boly M, Pickard JD, Tshibanda L, Owen AM, Laureys S. Willful modulation of brain activity in disorders of consciousness. *N Engl J Med* 2010 362(7):585.

15. Mandela N. *Mandela an illustrated biography*. New York: Little Brown and Company, 1996.

16. Fins JJ. Neuroethics and the lure of technology. Epilogue. In *Handbook of neuroethics*, ed. Illes J, Sahakian BJ. New York: Oxford University Press, 2011. Pp. 895–908.

17. Bardin JC, Fins JJ, Katz DI, Hersh J, Heier LA, Tabelow K, Dyke JP, Ballon DJ, Schiff ND, Voss HU. Dissociations between behavioral and functional magnetic resonance imaging-based evaluations of cognitive function after brain injury. *Brain* 2011 134(Pt. 3):769–82.

18. Bardin J, Schiff ND, Voss HU. Pattern classification of volitional functional magnetic resonance imaging responses in patients with severe brain injury. *Arch Neurol* 2012 69(2):176–81.

19. Fins JJ. "Wait, wait – don't tell me"... tuning in the injured brain. *Arch Neurol* 2012 69(2):158–60.

20. Racine E, Waldman S, Rosenberg, Illes J. Contemporary neuroscience in the media. *Soc Sci Med* 2010 71(4):725–33.

21. Fins JJ. Affirming the right to care, preserving the right to die: Disorders of consciousness and neuroethics after Schiavo. *Palliat Support Care* 2006 4(2):169–78.

22. Carey B. New signs of awareness in some brain-injured patients. *The New York Times*. February 8, 2005: Sect. A:1.
23. Fins JJ, Schiff ND. In the blink of the mind's eye. *Hastings Cent Rep* 2010 40(3):21–3.
24. Conservatorship of the Person of Robert Wendland. Rose Wendland, as Conservator, etc., Petitioner and Appellant, v. Florence Wendland et al. Objectors and Respondent; Robert Wendland, Appellant. No. S087265. Supreme Court of California.
25. Ibid., p. 42.
26. Ibid., pp. 7–8.
27. Ibid., p. 43.

21   THE RIGHTS OF MIND

1. Strauss DJ, Ashwal S, Day SM, et al. Life expectancy of children in vegetative and minimally conscious states. *Pediatr Neurol* 2000 23(4):312–19.
2. Fins JJ, Master MG, Gerber LM, Giacino JT. The minimally conscious state: A diagnosis in search of an epidemiology. *Arch Neurol* 2007 64(10):1400–5.
3. Fins JJ, Schiff ND, Foley KM. Late recovery from the minimally conscious state: ethical and policy implications. *Neurology* 2007 68(4):304–7.
4. Letter from Peter R. Orszag, Director Congressional Budget Office, to Senator Edward M. Kennedy, Chair Committee of Health, education, Labor and Pensions. In V. Cost Estimate, Senate Report 110-140-Reauthorization of the Traumatic Brain Injury Act. July 23, 2007.
5. Nakase-Richardson R, Whyte J, Giacino JT, Pavawalla S, Barnett SD, Yablon SA, Sherer M, Kalmar K, Hammond FM, Greenwald B, Horn LJ, Seel R, McCarthy M, Tran J, Walker WC. *Longitudinal outcome of patients with disordered consciousness in the NIDRR TBI Model Systems Programs. J Neurotrauma* January 1, 2012 29(1):59–65. doi: 10.1089/neu.2011.1829. Epub August 4, 2011.
6. Final report of the ad hoc committee on a comprehensive and integral international convention on the protection and promotion of the rights and dignity of persons with disabilities. United Nations. General Assembly, Sixty First Session, Item 67(b). December 6, 2006.
7. I am grateful to Professor Laurence B. McCullough of Baylor College of Medicine for suggesting the relevance of McKeon's work to my argument.
8. McKeon R. The philosophic bases and material circumstances of the rights of man. *Ethics* 1948 58(3), Pt.1:180–7.
9. Ibid., p. 186.
10. Sen A. Well-being, agency and freedom: The Dewey lectures 1984. *J Philos* 1985 82(4):169–221.
11. Sen A. *Commodities and capabilities*. New York: Oxford University Press, 1999.
12. Venkatapuram S. *Health justice: An argument from the capabilities approach.* Cambridge: Polity Press, 2011.

13. Fins JJ. A review of Health Justice by Sridhar Venkatapuram. Cambridge: Polity Press, 2011. *JAMA* 2012 307(19):2106.
14. Sen A. Disability and justice. 2004 World Bank International Disability Conference. Washington, DC.
15. Amartya Sen. Second Day Keynote at 2004 World Bank International Disability Conference [Internet]. December 1, 2004. [Accessed July 16, 2013.] Available from: http://info.worldbank.org/etools/bspan/PresentationView .asp?PID=1355&EID=667.
16. Venkatapuram S. *Health justice: An argument from the capabilities approach.* Cambridge: Polity Press, 2011. P. 192.
17. Switzer JV. *Disabled rights: American disabilityp and the fight for equality.* Washington, DC: Georgetown University Press, 2003. P. 15.
18. Pedro Almodovar, director. *Talk to her.* Sony Classics. November 22, 2002.
19. Fins JJ, Plum F. Neurological diagnosis is more than a state of mind: Diagnostic clarity and impaired consciousness. *Arch Neurol* 2004 61(9):1354–5.
20. Fins JJ. Being conscious of their burden: Severe brain injury and the *Two Cultures* challenge. Proceedings from "Disorders of Consciousness." 87th Annual Conference of the Association for Research in Nervous and Mental Disease. *Ann NY Acad Sci* 2009 1157:131–47.
21. Fins JJ. The portrayal of coma in contemporary motion pictures. *Neurology* 2007 68:79–80.
22. Arroyo J. Interview with Pedro Almodovar [Internet]. *Guardian.* July 31, 2002. [Accessed July 16, 2013.] Available from: www.guardian.co.uk/film/ 2002/jul/31/ features.pedroalmodovar.
23. Freud S. *The interpretation of dreams.* Strachey J, translator. New York: Avon, 1980.
24. The many-sided life of Sir Charles Snow. *Life Magazine.* April 7, 1961:134–6.
25. Zafonte RD, Watanabe T, Mann NR. Amantadine: A potential treatment for the minimally conscious state. *Brain Inj* 1998 12(7):617–21.
26. Whyte J, Katz D, Long D, DiPasquale MC, Polansky M, Kalmar K, Giacino J, Childs N, Mercer W, Novak P, Maurer P, Eifert B. Predictors of outcome in prolonged posttraumatic disorders of consciousness and assessment of medication effects: A multicenter study. *Arch Phys Med Rehabil* 2005 86(3):453–62.
27. Schnakers C, Hustinx R, Vandewalle G, Majerus S, Moonen G, Boly M, Vanhaudenhuyse A, Laureys S. Measuring the effect of amantadine in chronic anoxic minimally conscious state. *J Neurol Neurosurg Psychiatry* February 2008 79(2):225–7. doi: 10.1136/jnnp.2007.124099.
28. Cohen SI, Duong TT. Increased arousal in a patient with anoxic brain injury after administration of zolpidem. *Am J Phys Med Rehabil* March 2008 87(3):229–31.
29. Shames JL, Ring H. Transient reversal of anoxic brain injury-related minimally conscious state after zolpidem administration: A case report. *Arch Phys Med Rehabil* February 2008 89(2):386–8.
30. Whyte J, Myers R. Incidence of clinically significant responses to zolpidem among patients with disorders of consciousness: A preliminary placebo controlled trial. *Am J Phys Med Rehabil* May 2009 88(5):410–18.

31. Singh R, McDonald C, Dawson K, Lewis S, Pringle AM, Smith S, Pentland B. Zolpidem in a minimally conscious state. *Brain Inj* January 2008 22(1):103–6.
32. Americans With Disabilities Act of 1990, Pub. L. 101–336.26, 104 Stat (July 1990).
33. Information and technical assistance on the Americans with Disabilities Act [Internet]. ADA.gov. [Accessed June 19, 2013.] Available from: http://www.ada .gov/2010_regs.htm.
34. OLMSTEAD v. L.C. (98–536) 527 U.S. 581 (1999) 138 f.3d.
35. Switzer JV. *Disabled rights: American disability policy and the fight for equality.* Washington, DC: Georgetown University Press, 2003. P. 31.
36. Meeting of author with the Honorable Chai R. Feldblum, Commissioner, the Equal Opportunity Employment Commsion. EEOC Headquarters, Washington, DC. May 8, 2013.
37. Switzer JV. *Disabled rights: American disability policy and the fight for equality.* Washington, DC: Georgetown University Press, 2003. P. 37.
38. Cook TM. The Americans with Disabilities Act: The move to integration. *Temple Law Review* 1991 64:393–470. P. 404
39. 42 U.S.C. § 12101 (b)(1) cited in U.S. Department of Justice, Civil Rights Division. 2011 Statement of the Department of Justice on the Enforcement of the Integration Mandate of Title II of the Americans with Disabilities Act and Olmstead v. L.C.
40. Feldblum CR. Antidiscrimination requirements of the ADA. In *Implementing the Americans with Disabilities Act, rights and responsibilities of all Americans,* ed. Gostin LO, Beyer HA. Baltimore: Paul H. Brookes Publishing Company, 1993. Pp. 35–54.
41. OLMSTEAD v. L.C. (98–536) 527 U.S. 581 (1999) 138 f.3d.
42. General Prohibitions against Discrimination, 28 C.F.R. Sect. 35.130(d) (1999).
43. Fins JJ and Pohl BR. Neuro-palliative care and disorders of consciousness. In *Oxford Textbook of Palliative Medicine,* ed. Hanks G, Cherny NI, Christakis NA, Fallon M, Kassa S, Portenoy RK. 5th edition. Oxford: Oxford University Press. In Press.
44. Fins JJ, Schiff ND. Conflicts of interest in deep brain stimulation research and the ethics of transparency. *J Clin Ethics* 2010 21(2):125–32.
45. Fins JJ, Dorfman GS, Pancrazio JJ. Challenges to deep brain stimulation: A pragmatic response to ethical, fiscal and regulatory concerns. *Ann NY Acad Sci* 2012 1265:80–90. doi: 10.1111/j.1749-6632.2012.06598.x.
46. Fins JJ. Deep brain stimulation: Calculating the true costs of surgical innovation. *Virtual Mentor* 2010 12(2):114–18.
47. Switzer JV. *Disabled rights: American disability policy and the fight for equality.* Washington, DC: Georgetown University Press, 2003. P. 40.
48. I am grateful to Chai Feldblum for this insight.
49. Hirshman L. *Victory: The triumphant gay revolution.* New York: Harper Collins Publishers, 2012.
50. Benjamin R. Banner days: "victory," by Linda Hirshman [Internet]. *New York Times.* June 21, 2012. [Accessed July 16, 2013.] Available from: http://www .nytimes.com/2012/06/24/books/review/victory-by-linda-hirshman.html.

51. Shapiro JP. *No pity, people with disabilities forging a new civil rights.* New York: Three Rivers Press, 1994. P. 128.
52. Switzer JV. *Disabled rights: American disability policy and the fight for equality.* Washington, DC: Georgetown University Press, 2003. P. 91.
53. Ibid., pp. 8–9.
54. Shapiro JP. *No pity, people with disabilities forging a new civil rights.* New York: Three Rivers Press, 1994. P. 117.
55. Ibid., p. 322.
56. Ibid., p. 324.
57. Coleman D. Assisted suicide laws create discriminatory double standard for who gets suicide prevention and who gets suicide assistance: Not dead yet responds to autonomy, inc. *Disabil Health J* 2010 3(1):39–50.
58. Dart JW. The ADA: A promise to be kept. In *Implementing the Americans with Disabilities Act: Rights and responsibilities of all Americans*, ed. Gostin LO, Beyer HA. Baltimore: Paul Brookes, 1993. P. xxi.
59. *Brown v. Board of Education of Topeka*, 347 U.S. 483 (1954).
60. Voss HU, Ulug AM, Dyke JP, Watts R, Kobylarz EJ, McCandliss BD, Heier LA, Beatty BJ, Hamacher KA, Vallabhajosula S, Goldsmith SJ, Ballon D, Giacino JT, Schiff ND. Possible axonal regrowth in late recovery from the minimally conscious state. *J Clin Invest* 2006 116(7):2005–11.
61. Mukherjee P, McKinstry RC. Diffusion tensor imaging and tarctography of human brain development. *Neuroimaging Clin N Am* 2006 16(1):19–43.
62. Blizzard CA, Chuckowree JA, King AE, Hosie KA, McCormaack GH, Chapman JA, Vickers JC, Dickson TC. Focal damage to the adult rat neocortex induces wound healing accompanied by axonal sprouting and dendritic structural plasticity. *Cereb Cortex* 2011 21(2):281–91.
63. Bob Woodruff. Personal communication with: Joseph Fins. July 10, 2007. New York.
64. Meili TE. *I am the Central Park jogger.* New York: Scribners, 2003.
65. Osborn CL. *Over my head.* Kansas City: Andrews McNeal Publishing, 1998.
66. Individuals with Disabilities Education Act, Pub. L. No. 101–476, 104 Stat. 1142.
67. Fleischer DZ, Zames F. Education: integration in the least restrictive environment. In *The disability rights movement: From charity to confrontation*, ed. Fleischer DZ, Zames F. Philadelphia: Temple University Press, 2011. Pp. 184–5.
68. Switzer JV. *Disabled rights: American disability policy and the fight for equality.* Washington, DC: Georgetown University Press, 2003. P. 107.

22 A CALL FOR ADVOCACY

1. Caro RA. *The years of Lyndon Johnson: Means of ascent.* New York: Vintage, 1990. P. xxii.
2. Harris JK, Godfrey HP, Partridge FM, Knight RG. Caregiver depression following traumatic brain injury (TBI): A consequence of adverse effects on family members? *Brain Inj* March 2001 15(3):223–38.

3. Relyea-Chew A, Hollingworth W, Chan L, Comstock BA, Overstreet KA, Jarvik JG. Personal bankruptcy after traumatic brain or spinal cord injury: The role of medical debt. *Arch Phys Med Rehabil* 2009 90(3):413–19.
4. Hollingworth W, Relyea-Chew A, Comstock BA, Overstreet JK, Jarvik JG. The risk of bankruptcy before and after brain or spinal cord injury: A glimpse of the iceberg's tip. *Med Care* 2007 45(8):702–11.
5. Woolhandler S, Himmelstein DU. Double catastrophe: Injury-related bankruptcies. *Med Care* 2007 454(8):699–701.
6. Fins JJ, Hersh J. Solitary advocates: The severely brain injured and their surrogates. In Transforming health care from below: Patients as policy actors, ed. Hoffman B, Tomes N, Schlessinger M, Grob R. New Brunswick, NJ: Rutgers University Press, 2011. Pp. 21–42.
7. Steinberg J. Recovering from injury, returning to TV, speaking for the wounded [Internet]. *The New York Times*. October 25, 2007. [Accessed August 2, 2011.] Available from: http://www.nytimes.com/2007/10/25/arts/television/25wood.html?ref=bobwoodruff
8. Steinhauer J, Zeleny J. For Giffords, House shows it can unite. *The New York Times*. August 2, 2011. Sect. A:1.
9. Woodruff L, Woodruff B. *In an instant: A family's journey of love and healing.* New York: Random House, 2007.
10. Fins JJ. Review of in an instant: A family's journey of love and healing. *JAMA* 2007 297(23):2642–3.

In Memoriam

Melva Baucom, December 3, 2008
Jean Brody
Angelo Donato, July 19, 2009
Kathy Hansen, April 19, 2012
John Harmon Jr., July 30, 2010
Josh Moore, April 29, 2009
Greg Pearson, September 7, 2011

Index

Printed in the United States
By Bookmasters